INFANT AND CHILDHOOD DEPRESSION

WILEY SERIES IN CHILD AND ADOLESCENT MENTAL HEALTH

Joseph D. Noshpitz, Editor

INFANT AND CHILDHOOD DEPRESSION

DEVELOPMENTAL FACTORS

PAUL V. TRAD

Laboratory of Developmental Processes
Payne Whitney Psychiatric Clinic

A Wiley-Interscience Publication

JOHN WILEY & SONS

New York / Chichester / Brisbane / Toronto / Singapore

Library of Congress Cataloging in Publication Data:
Trad, Paul V.
    Infant and childhood depression.

    (Wiley series in child and adolescent mental
health)
    "A Wiley-Interscience publication."
    Includes bibliographies.
    1. Depression in infants. 2. Depression in
children. 3. Infants—Development. 4. Child
development. 5. Depression, Mental—Etiology.
I. Title. II. Series. [DNLM: 1. Depression—
etiology. 2. Depression—in infancy & childhood.
WM 171 T763i]

RJ506.D4T72 1987   618.92'8527   86-28146
ISBN 0-471-85230-9

Printed in the United States of America

10 9 8 7 6 5 4 3 2 1

This book is dedicated to my four elder brothers and their families, who taught me how to share companionship; to my parents, Blanche and Jorge Trad, whose affection and faith in my abilities were always constant; and to my godson and namesake, Juan Pablo, whose development I have watched avidly over the years, and who has experienced the care and concern of a loving family. Someday, when he is old enough to understand the theories contained in this volume, I hope he will realize his good fortune. Finally, the following pages are dedicated to all infants and children who have or will experience feelings of loss in their lives.

Series Preface

This series is intended to serve a number of functions. It includes works on child development; it presents material on child advocacy; it publishes contributions to child psychiatry; and it gives expression to cogent views on child rearing and child management. The mental health of parents and their interaction with their children is a major theme of the series, and emphasis is placed on the child as individual, as family member, and as a part of the larger social surround.

Child development is regarded as the basic science of child mental health, and within that framework research works are included in this series. The many ethical and legal dimensions of the way society relates to its children is the central theme of the child advocacy publications, as well as a primarily demographic approach that highlights the role and status of children within society. The child psychiatry publications span studies that concern the diagnosis, description, therapeutics, rehabilitation, and prevention of the emotional disorders of childhood. And the views of thoughtful and creative contributors to the handling of children under many different circumstances (retardation, acute and chronic illness, hospitalization, handicap, disturbed social conditions, etc.) find expression within the framework of child rearing and child management.

Family studies with a central child mental health perspective are included in the series, and explorations into the nature of parenthood and the parenting process are emphasized. This includes books about divorce, the single parent, the absent parent, parents with physical and emotional illnesses, and other conditions that significantly affect the parent-child relationship.

Finally, the series examines the impact of larger social forces, such as war, famine, migration, and economic failure, on the adaptation of children and families. In the largest sense, the series is devoted to books that illuminate the special needs, status, and history of children and their families within all perspectives that bear on their collective mental health.

JOSEPH D. NOSHPITZ

Children's Hospital Medical Center, and
The George Washington University
Washington, D.C.

Preface

For me, the human infant represents an ineluctable paradox, a being of both exquisite fragility and infinite resilience. This book represents an effort to explain this most primal mystery and to reveal how the repercussions of early experience—dating from the first hours of life onward—can leave an indelible imprint on the child and adult yet to be.

Since I live amidst skyscrapers in a densely populated section of New York City, I seldom have the opportunity to observe children playing in the park. Sometimes, though, I visit Central Park on the weekend. There, in the midst of the wide open expanse of greenery, in a playground replete with jungle gyms, swings, slides, and sandboxes, I feel I am in a laboratory where a myriad of experiments are being conducted. Mothers (and occasionally fathers) and their infants engage in playful routines, each dyad rapt in its own unique universe of interaction. Other infants, generally older, play in the sandbox with brightly colored pails and shovels, digging or sifting the grains of sand, building or demolishing their castles. Sometimes one child will seem different from the rest. Such a child characteristically sits alone, his gestures in the sandbox are apathetic and lacking in purpose. His face is downcast, its expression somber. Is such a child experiencing depression, I wonder, and if so, what concatenation of events and what convergence of factors caused psychopathology to emerge in one so young?

Sometimes I imagine there are four such children, each with saddened visage, sitting in the sandbox. Mary, nearly 5 months old, is the daughter of a mother who suffered a bout of postpartum depression on the birth of her child. Billy, whose spasmodic gesturing reveals the telltale signs of cerebral palsy, suffered from anoxia at birth. A third child, Johnny, is the victim of abuse. Despite his being barely 1 year old, he has experienced more by way of physical beating than most people experience in a lifetime. Finally, Alice is a 2 year old who recently had open heart surgery to correct a congenital defect. Although she did not comprehend the motives of doctors and nurses in their white uniforms, her memory of being forcibly "put to sleep" lingers in her mind. Each of these four children has had a very different experience and yet, for each one an internal process has been triggered which manifests outwardly in a saddened face and sober mood. The primary goal of *Infant and Childhood Depression* is to articulate precisely the process whereby such infants and children come to display such saddened faces and to experience the affect of depression.

In essence, the scene in this fanciful playground of my imagination is not very different from the waiting rooms of many pediatricians and child psychiatrists. Indeed, many pediatricians and pediatric nurses are becoming increasingly more attuned to peculiar or uncharacteristic behaviors that may belie an underlying depression in their young patients. Nurse clinicians and social workers also have become increasingly adept at sensing when the infant and child is manifesting the kind of behavior that properly can be labeled psychopathologic. Moreover, the recent wealth of clinical and experimental data indicating that psychopathology does emerge among very young age groups has propelled these health care professionals to refer such infants and children to child psychiatrists and psychologists. It is hoped that the documentation provided in the following chapters will further encourage the growing network of referral to child psychiatric services for diagnosis and treatment, as well as for preventative purposes.

Those who are skeptical about the possibility that infants and young children can suffer from full-fledged psychopathology, and specifically from depression, need only focus on the feelings of loss they experienced when they were young. For, most theories on the origins of depression begin with the premise that an early encounter with object loss casts a shadow on the process of maturation, resulting in an episode of depression or depressive-like symptomatology. This symptomatology can recur in an unchecked fashion if measures are not taken to ameliorate the initial exposure to loss. Nor does loss affect only infants and children acutely; those who remain unpersuaded of the phenomenon of infant psychopathology need only remember the acute sense of loss, as well as the overriding confusion and despair accompanying shattered expectations when the space shuttle Challenger exploded in an incandescent fireball in midair in 1986.

Although the destruction of the space shuttle occurred in a sudden, condensed flash of light lasting only a few seconds, while the patient's loss of the love object is often diffused over the early years of infancy and childhood, the two events bear comparison. In both situations, we are challenged to give coherence to what—from the patient's point of view—is an incomprehensible and cruel twist of fate, and to painstakingly resurrect feelings of security and strength to replace the lost object. It is from these often incomprehensible and cruel twists of fate—the misfortune of being born with a handicap, the cruelty of child abuse, the irrationality of illness during infancy and childhood, and the discordance of being cared for by a parent suffering from depression—that psychopathology emerges and the therapist's task of directing the infant or child back to the pathway of healthy development begins. It is my fervent hope that this book will offer guidance in embarking on this journey.

My expressions of thanks and gratitude for those who encouraged my labors during the creation of this book are numerous. Among my professional colleagues for whom special warm acknowledgment is warranted are Daniel Stern, M.D., Donald McKnew, M.D., Paulina F. Kernberg, M.D., Cynthia Pfeffer, M.D., and Edward Tauber, M.D. of the William Alanson White Institute, and Gerald L. Klerman and the other members of the Selection Committee for Post Residency Fellowships at Cornell University Medical Center.

I also wish to convey cordial thanks to Beth Sandell, Brian Steller, and Vernon Bruete for their assistance in compiling a voluminous amount of research. For their invaluable editorial suggestions and commentary, special thanks to Morton Milder, Flora Lazar, and to Wendy Luftig, whose considered critical analysis was always of the highest quality, and for their consummate skill in assembling what often seemed to be an unwieldly mass of material and for reminding me of the shining light waiting at the end of all difficult journeys. I remain in debt to each of these gifted individuals for their patience, encouragement, and perpetual good spirits.

Thanks also to Richard H. White of Seattle, Washington, who exemplifies, for me, the rare qualities of courage and strength.

PAUL V. TRAD, M.D.

New York, New York
January 1987

Contents

CHAPTER ONE

A Developmental Perspective for Analyzing Infant and Childhood Depression

DEFINITION OF DEVELOPMENTAL PSYCHOPATHOLOGY

Since this book proposes to explore infant depression, a relatively uncharted terrain in the area of psychopathology, it is appropriate to offer an innovative perspective for defining, diagnosing, and treating this psychiatric disorder.

Before embarking on a discussion of infant depression, however, it is necessary to provide a glossary of words and phrases that recur throughout the text and that will be seminal for understanding the theories proposed. The articulation of all theory must rely on language—often an imprecise and elusive tool. Thus the following definitions are offered in an attempt to refine and clarify, as far as possible, the key building blocks subsequently used for devising a theory of infant depression.

Infant is a term which captures the full-bodiedness of a self-contained organism replete with myriad intricate capacities. For the purposes of this text, however, infant is first delimited in chronological terms: those children younger than 30 months are considered infants. This artificial demarcation arises from research indicating that the self expands at approximately this time. By *self* is meant the consolidation of sophisticated representational abilities. Infants possess a sense of self when they are capable of representing different perspectives of the same event and are capable of maintaining alternative schemas, or multiple scenarios, without confusion. The self, in essence, presents the infant with a paradox: he or she is now capable of representing alternatives and also of reflecting back on how his or her own behavior evokes phenomena in the external world, as well as within the self. By approximately 30 months then, the infant is capable of being his or her own omniscient narrator and of simultaneously perceiving of the self and others as separate actors in any given behavioral sequence. The infant has evolved from a state in which he or she perceived himself or herself as totally experienced/empathic and egocentrically united with the world, to a phase in which his or her autonomy is acknowledged. At this point, the infant has entered the world of childhood.

Regulation and its converse, *dysregulation,* are two of the overriding concepts alluded to in the following chapters. Regulation encompasses affective, cognitive, and/or neuroendocrine processes that are involved in generating a behavioral response. Such a *behavioral response* is a manifestation that is either overt or measurable and that contains affective, cognitive, and/or neuroendocrine components. Moreover, from the point of view of their outcome, behavioral responses may be characterized as being adaptive or maladaptive. When a behavioral response is *adaptive*, it permits the infant to balance his or her own repertoire of responses to environmental demands. Adaptive response may be described by such adjectives as flexible, fluid, plastic, and resilient. In contrast, *maladaptive* behavioral response prevents or thwarts the infant from balancing his or her own resources with those of the environment. Such response is typified by a rigid, stifled, inflexible, and pervasive quality.

When the infant manifests adaptive behavior, he or she selectively maintains a past response or chooses another response. That is, the infant displays a flexibility which permits him or her to recognize new stimuli, and as a consequence, either to maintain a prior response that is appropriate for the new stimuli or to generate a new response that is adaptive for the new stimuli. If, however, the behavioral response is maladaptive, the infant will maintain his or her former response in a self-perpetuating fashion. Thus the infant who exhibits maladaptive response will continue to relate to stimuli whether old or new in a manner ill-suited to the stimuli. Furthermore, maladaptive response can prevent the infant from recognizing and relating to new stimuli.

Lang, Levin, Miller, and Kozak (1983), from their studies of the psychophysiology of emotion in adults posit that affects are better understood if they are viewed as "activity" and "reactivity" phenomena, rather than as responses to inferred internal experiences. Adopting this view, the display of any particular affective state—anger, disgust, sadness, joy—may be interpreted as a disposition to either approach or avoid a given stimuli. That is, individuals who are regulating affective response may either attend to or reject a stimuli and display this preference via the manifestation of a discrete affect appropriate for the situation. In contrast, individuals who are dysregulated will also act or react affectively to environmental stimuli, but their response will be incompatible with the situation.

Substantiating the active orientation of affective response described by Lang et al., numerous researchers investigating affective development in infants have reported on the broad repertoire of response, and indeed, the versatility of infant affective display. Thus, infants of only several months old appear equipped to display a spectrum of emotions, including interest, joy surprise, sadness, anger, disgust, contempt, fear, shyness, and guilt (Izard & Schwartz, 1986).

In contrast to both the diversity of affective response in the infant and the flexibility with which it is displayed, cognitive capacities in neonates appear to be far less developed at birth, suggesting that affective displays manifest earlier than cognitive abilities. In discussing cognitive capacity, Greenspan (1979) refers to Piaget's notion that the infant engages in a series of well orchestrated "circular reactions" (Piaget & Inhelder, 1966). These prototypical responses are actually a form of goal corrected behavior, through which the infant incrementally refines his response in accord with previous action. Such goal corrected behavior is a form of self-regulation, and is semi-reversible. Semi-reversible means that the acts motivated by cognition cannot be completely reversed by other acts, but rather feedback impels further action which corrects earlier behavior retroactively.

This comparison between early affective and cognitive response suggests that during the first months of life the infant may rely more heavily on affective capacities. Indeed, since cognitive capacities are only semireversible, the infant may at least initially draw on his or her affective responses to interact with the environment precisely because affective display grants a fuller sense of control over external stimuli. If this is the case, then it becomes apparent that any assault or impingement on affective display might have serious consequences for the infant. As will be discussed in depth in subsequent chapters, any curtailment of the infant's disposition to actively orient to the environment through affective display—whether by caregiver rejection, lack of stimuli, exposure to noncontingency—might seriously damage future interaction. And if affective regulation is intruded on, the infant may respond by disorganizing affective behavior in an attempt to preserve the most available domain over which he or she can exert control. Disorganization of affective states at such an early age may then set the pattern for dysregulation which will permeate future development in both cognitive and affective areas.

Finally, at various points in the text, the term *internal mechanism* is used. Internal mechanism here does not refer to a concretized entity; rather, the phrase is indicative of the composite full spectrum of affective, cognitive, and neuroendocrine capacities emanating from the infant regarding interactions with the environment (Trad, 1986).

Another concept relied on in the text is *development*. In general, development should be conceived of as the temporal relationship that the behavioral responses described here maintain within themselves and with the environment. Moreover, development connotes nuances of evolution in the sense that new behavioral responses unfold over time.

Specific patterns or consolidations of behavioral responses within development are referred to in the text as *parameters*. These responses can be either continuous or discontinuous processes that result when biological, genetic, and environmental components interface. Crystallization and therefore measurement of these behavioral responses occur when they coalesce in discernible and predictable patterns. Within this text, the parameters selected for discussion include temperament, attachment, object permanence and constancy, and self-representation.

Given this glossary, it is possible to propose an initial hypothesis for the etiology of infant depression. Of course this hypothesis will be further elaborated in subsequent chapters. For now, however, depression may be defined as one of the processes generating a behavioral response. In this sense, it is a form of regulation. Moreover, depression may be adaptive or maladaptive. Depression is adaptive when, from his or her entire affective repertoire, depression is selectively and flexibly chosen by the infant for interacting with the environment. Here the affect displayed (e.g., sad face) can be described as a depressive-like phenomenon. That is, the infant displays his or her capacity to manifest a discrete response that may be characterized as "depressed affect." This does not mean that the infant is in fact depressed; rather it means that he or she possesses the ability to represent and hence experience depression. If the depression is adaptive, it also means that the infant is regulating the incidence of this depressive-like phenomenon.

As Klerman (1980) observed, depression manifested as a mood can represent an aspect of normal human experience. Perhaps the classic example of depressive mood exhibited within the context of adaptive human behavior is mourning. During periods of grief triggered by loss of a love object, a pervasive, depressive response, distinguished by features of intensity and duration, is generally evident. Although similar in symptomatology to a bona fide mood disorder, this reaction is not characterized as pathologic, since the precipitating factor is readily discernible, the response is in proportion to the loss, and the grief eventually resolves itself within a circumscribed period of time. Thus both affective depression and mood depression can be exhibited as normal nonpathologic phenomena. What differentiates these so-called depressions from psychopathology is that they signify regulated responses of the individual to external catalysts.

In contrast, if the depression is maladaptive, the implication is that the behavioral response of the infant is not manifested flexibly; it is virtually predetermined and self-perpetuating. That is, the depressive response has not been selectively chosen and is not coordinated or in balance with the environment. In this instance, depression is manifested either transiently as an intermittent affect or as an enduring mood that will transfer across tasks and situations. These forms of depression may be viewed as defects in the process of generating adaptive behavioral responses and are thus forms of dysregulation.

Developmental psychopathology, a diagnostic mode of analysis that first gained acceptance during the 1970s, represents a complex attempt to coordinate a variety of disciplines—including general developmental psychology, genetics, clinical psychiatry, behavioral psychology, and the medical model—under one rubric. Commentaries on developmental psychopathology have referred to the approach as a synthesis or a mosaic embracing the vast amount of data on infant research generated during the past few decades (Cicchetti, 1984). Thus the first notable feature of the developmental framework is that it is receptive to research gathered from a broad spectrum of diverse sources. In a word, the developmental model permits eclectic analysis: Phenomena derived from one particular discipline may be effectively integrated into the developmental model along with data extrapolated from an ostensibly unrelated discipline.

The developmental approach embodies this flexibility as a research tool primarily because it posits that fruitful psychiatric analysis can be achieved only when individual capacities and experiences are conceived of as occurring along a chronological continuum, a temporal axis, which spans birth through adulthood. This is not to suggest that behaviors will be continuous, undeviating, or stable over time. Rather, the totality of genetic factors with which the infant is endowed, as well as the myriad of environmental factors that sculpt experience, need to be viewed as elements contributing to the composite portrait of individual personality. Moreover, the developmental perspective permits us to analyze how various genetic factors intertwine with environmental factors at any given point in development, motivating the individual to devise effective coping strategies or in contrast, creating frustrating "snags" in development that may provoke subsequent psychopathology. Rutter (1986), in explaining the developmental process, noted that the approach accentuates mechanisms whereby interaction during one phase of development may modify responses at a later point of maturation by either sensitizing the individual to new stimuli or thwarting and stifling individual response.

The developmental psychopathology approach concentrates not merely on discernible abnormalities of development or on discrete episodes of psychopathologic responses. As Rutter (1986) has written, the developmental model does not seize upon abnormality or normality per se but instead seeks to draw parallels between normal affect and behavior and clinical aberration. In this sense, the approach enables the researcher to view infant behavioral response in terms of an integrated interactive mechanism that may be subject to periodicities of optimal functioning as well as episodes of dysregulated response.

Ultimately, however, the overriding value of the developmental psychopathology approach is that it both traces lines of predictability in the course of adaptive development and helps pinpoint aberrations of development. As a consequence, the model may yield insights into the evolving nature of psychiatric disturbances and may reveal mechanisms of interaction that have gone awry during the process of development. The model, then, may suggest heretofore overlooked clues about the etiology of depression and depressive like phenomena. Indeed, one of the major contentions of this book is that by applying the developmental model to the study of infants, one can trace back the origins of depression to phenomena occurring within the first months of life, and in some instances, the first days of life. The roots of depression may be found very early in life, but superficially, the connection between these depressive antecedents and later disorder may not appear obvious outside the developmental framework. In attempting to distinguish lines of predictive validity, developmental psychopathologists probe beyond the boundaries of specific empirical behaviors to the broader challenges facing individuals at different periods of development. Hence it is postulated that the coping strategies with which the infant resolves a particular developmental challenge will create an enduring residual imprint or pattern that will likely recur at a later stage of development. The precursors of disorder—the initial brief instances of disorientation that result in affective distress, cognitive impairment, and motivational paralysis—are as significant as the ultimate sequelae of full-fledged psychiatric disorder. If the coping strategy is effective, the infant will progress to a more advanced phase of development with a new mastery skill integrated within his or her behavioral repertoire. By contrast, if strategies for conquering the developmental challenge are thwarted, the infant will be frustrated and will likely experience distress (manifested through affective displays), which, in turn, will leave an enduring imprint. Although the distress may recede or be overshadowed by the skills acquired at a subsequent phase of growth, the damage to the affective and cognitive capacities may resurface or be triggered later when the infant is again subjected to a stress that he or she cannot resolve. Developmental psychopathology does not pose a model of linear development. Rather, it suggests that behavior will continually transform with both progressions and regressions along the developmental axis.

Finally, developmental psychopathology attributes preeminence to neither the "nature" nor the "nurture" aspect of development. The approach views the infant as an organism of infinite capacity, possessed of an intricately complex genetic endowment that interacts with unlimited stimuli in the environment. Although developmental psychopathology acknowledges the impact of specific variables that are primarily influenced by genetics or substantially derived from the environment, it is always the *interaction*, the moment of interface between these variables, positioned within the chronological frame of development, that seizes the attention of the researcher. For the developmental psychopathologist, this interplay of dynamic forces constitutes the matrix from which psychopathology will finally emerge.

DEVELOPMENTAL PARAMETERS

Armed with this working definition of the developmental psychopathology model, the next task is a pragmatic one: the determination of the artifacts of behavioral response, the evidentiary clues, on which the researcher should rely. In a sense the greatest virtue of the developmental model as a working model for understanding psychopathology—that the model is flexible enough to integrate data from a wide variety of sources—may also be one of its greatest limitations. Although it accommodates a plethora of data, it offers only the most general guidance for researchers seeking to extrapolate the key variables for devising lines of predictive validity. Until now, developmental psychology has devoted attention to pinpointing key developmental trends or continuities and discontinuities that arise during the typical course of infant development. Thus, as Rutter and Garmezy (1983) emphasize, age trends discerned through direct behavioral observation or detailed interviewing with caregivers have often been used in the developmental analysis.

A more effective method of using the developmental model, however, is to accentuate certain pivotal variables that play a seminal role in influencing infant interaction. Among the developmental parameters that have been isolated for discussion are "temperament," "attachment," "neuroendocrine changes," and "self-concept." Temperament refers to the predisposing personality, the individual behavioral style, each infant is endowed with constitutionally. As such temperament is predominantly a genetic or natural variable. As the developmental model so keenly reveals, however, infant temperament will be modulated by environmental stimuli and stressors and thus must also be construed within the context of interaction. Neuroendocrine changes represent a closely related variable (Derryberry & Rothbart, 1984) that may be categorized as genetic, because the neonate is equipped with an exquisitely responsive and sensitive mechanism geared to regulating internal hormonal states. Nevertheless, this mechanism does not regulate in isolation from the environment and, in fact, may be specifically designed as a vehicle for modulating the effects of environmental stress. Attachment behavior, which can be assessed via the Strange Situation Procedure (Ainsworth & Wittig, 1969) at one year of age, represents yet a further developmental parameter—one that is more clearly determined by environmental rather than genetic factors. Attachment response is largely a product of a series of interactive episodes between caregiver and infant. Yet here too it is not the environment alone that creates the form of the attachment bond forged within the dyadic exchange. The effects of both infant and maternal temperament will converge to shape and modify the nuances of this relationship.

Finally, the pivotal parameter for our analysis is the development of the self-concept. The self, as a consolidated, integrated aspect of the infant's internal mechanism, is too intricate a phenomenon to be attributed to either nature or nurture variables. Within the domain of the self, the innumerable effects of all the developmental parameters coalesce. The self, in essence, represents the cumulative encapsulated representation of the effects of all past experience and interaction. Thus, according to the model of developmental psychology, if the infant has been damaged or impaired, either subtly or blatantly, prior to the emergence of a full-fledged self-concept, such alterations will be embedded within the final realization of the self-concept.

REGULATORY CAPACITY AS A PHENOMENON OF DEVELOPMENT

Beyond its position on how infant behavior is molded by success or failure in attaining key developmental parameters, the developmental approach also provides the researcher with a perspective for uncovering the *process* of development. That is, infant capacities may be interpreted as constantly responding to fulfill the demands imposed by environmental stimuli and by intrapsychic responses to these and other stimuli. In this sense, development itself becomes an outgrowth of regulation, a form of perpetual regulation, during which the infant is continually challenged to respond to environmental stimuli, to react to responses generated internally, and to coordinate responses between these two realms.

We may argue that if development proceeds along expected pathways, and if each challenge is met by a counterpoised response of appropriate proportion, the infant will gradually assemble the skills necessary to adapt in a manner that promotes mastery and feelings of competence. Such an infant is exhibiting the capacity for highly effective *regulation* of the self. This type of regulation will entail integration of temperamental factors and neuroendocrine and attachment responses in a well-orchestrated format. Regulation is the process by which, for example, the infant decreases his level of activity and adjusts his or her hormonal output in a situation in which the maternal figure is emitting signals of soothing, calming behavior. Such a well-regulated infant, however, will respond equally appropriately to an instance of stress—for example, when the caregiver is momentarily absent—by elevating levels of hormonal emission and by exhibiting outward behavioral manifestions of distress. On the return of the caregiver, the infant will fairly rapidly and uneventfully return to his or her previous level of tranquility.

Thus a well-regulated infant will engage the full capacities of his or her internal mechanism to produce rapid, appropriate, and proportionate responses to the environment. Transitions between affective states will be accomplished smoothly and easily, and distress responses, to the extent that they transfer across tasks or situations, will not linger. Phrases used to describe this well-regulated response might include flexible, plastic, yielding, limber, appropriately sensitive, and most significantly, resilient.

By the same token, the developmental framework also provides new insights into the phenomenon of *dysregulation.* Just as regulation is characterized by a response that is highly fitting and balanced in terms of the situational context, dysregulation—its conceptual opposite—is manifested behaviorally by a characteristically exaggerated or muted response, inappropriate for the immediate stimuli. A catalog of adjectives that can be applied to the phenomenon of dysregulatory response might include stiff, stifled, inflexible, rigid, automatic, ingrained, brittle, and obdurate. Fluidity of response, which is the parameter of effective regulation, is conspicuously absent in instances of dysregulation.

In many respects, besides its emphasis on adaptation, the concept of regulation-dysregulation fits neatly into the developmental framework. First, dysregulation may surface when an infant or a child is grappling with any developmental challenge. For instance, an infant endowed with an irritable, petulant temperament may have a caregiver who is impatient with this type of response. Rather than seeking to modulate or soothe the infant, the caregiver will exacerbate the infant's impatience. Such an infant may grow increasingly frustrated, and his or her response will be poorly suited to adapt to the demands of the environment. Further, the infant will not devise alternative strategies for flexibly and resiliently learning to subdue irritability and incorporate it appropriately into his or her internal repertoire. A self-perpetuating cycle of dysregulation will ensue. This dysregulation may recede and appear to go into eclipse, as the infant develops more sophisticated skills, such as motor and verbal capacities, which promote adaptation to the environment. But the initial instance of dysregulation will leave a residual, encapsulated pattern that may surface at a later phase of development.

The concept of dysregulation also permits us to discern continuities in development. Although dysregulation may not be consistently present, the evidence of dysregulation—through inappropriate behavioral displays, avoidant or resistant attachment behaviors, or disinhibited neuroendocrine response—suggests that integration and coping at some earlier stage of development may not have been successfully achieved. Finally, one manner of conceptualizing infant depression may be as a form of dysregulation that can pervade the infant's entire behavioral repertoire at any point or resurface intermittently throughout development.

ADVANTAGES OF THE DEVELOPMENTAL MODEL OVER TRADITIONAL MODES OF DIAGNOSING DEPRESSION

The controversy about whether or not depression exists as a full-fledged entity in infants and young children arises, to a large extent, because researchers cannot agree on a precise definition of the disorder. Indeed it is difficult to arrive at a definition when part of the patient population (i.e., infants) has not yet acquired the verbal skills necessary to convey subjective affective states. Symptoms, in many cases, can only be inferred from outward behavioral manifestations, from measurements of hormonal output, or from prolonged observation of interaction. As a result, the researcher often must infer the nature of the inner reality the infant or child is experiencing.

The currently accepted approach to diagnosing depression in children relies on the adult-based criteria set forth in the *Diagnostic and Statistical Manual of Mental Disorders,* Third Edition (DSM - III; American Psychiatric Association, 1980). Perusal of the DSM-III criteria reveals that the symptomatology enumerated for major depressive episodes in children includes a dysphoric mood, characterized by a depressed or sad affect, hopelessness, and/or irritability. In addition, at least three of the following four symptoms must be present in children under six years: (1) failure to make expected weight gain, (2) insomnia or hypersomnia, (3) hypoactivity, and (4) signs of apathy. Although this symptomatology is accurate in diagnosing depression in children, given the data gleaned from the developmental model, the enumerated listing appears scant and incomplete. For example, the listing offers no suggestion of the role that temperamental factors may play in diagnosing depression or of the manner in which the attachment relationship may contribute to the fostering of an incipient depression. Indeed, perhaps the major shortcoming of the DSM - III criteria is that they identify depression at the chronological point when it has blossomed into a full-fledged syndrome. The developmental framework, in contrast, not only permits the researcher to investigate instances of depressive-like phenomena *not* enumerated by DSM-III (e.g., repeated affective distress following exposure to noncontingency), but it also enables the researcher to identify depressive-like phenomena, which may signify precursors of depression at any early stage. In this sense, the developmental model plays an instrumental role in the treatment and prevention of psychiatric disorder, as well as in the satisfactory articulation of the origins of infant and childhood depression.

The premise of the DSM-III approach is that childhood depression is merely an analog or an earlier version of adult depression. Thus measures of adult depression act as a lens through which to view the feelings and behaviors of infants. Not surprisingly, the DSM-III criteria have had only sporadic success in diagnosing childhood depression and often the articulated criteria appear underinclusive for encompassing the full range of depressive phenomena manifested by young children. As Carlson and Garber (1986) have noted, although there may be continuity between adult and childhood depression, the same disorder may present in childhood with a variegated clinical portrait as a consequence of the fact that the child is at a different developmental phase than the adult, and that development itself alters so rapidly in children that symptomatology may elude the researcher. They conclude, then, that the criteria used to diagnose childhood depression may need to be modified in order to reflect developmental alterations, commenting that while use of current adult criteria for diagnosing depression in children may offer a worthwhile initial strategy, these criteria should be used only as preliminary guidelines for empirical investigation.

Poznanski, Mokdros, Grossman, and Freeman (1985) investigated the efficacy of diagnostic criteria in childhood depression. They found that the symptomatology outlined by both the adult Research Diagnostic Criteria (Spitzer, Endicott, & Robbins, 1978) and DSM-III, while accurate in diagnosing depression in the majority of cases, failed in some vital diagnostic areas. For example, the criteria did not account for the integration of discrepant information from different sources, such as the child and parent. Moreover, it was found that nonverbal ratings—which may not be accurately or completely detected by these criteria—were strongly associated with a diagnosis of depression. This latter finding is significant because it is within the areas of nonverbal information that the developmental model is able to yield the most insights and provide the most data concerning the infant's cognitive and affective capacities.

The wealth of data obtained from the developmental approach is best illustrated in the following case study, documenting a longitudinal investigation spanning four generations. The case, reported by Engel, Reichsman, Harway, and Hess (1985), involved an infant named Monica who was diagnosed with "failure to thrive" syndrome and depression at the age of 11 months. The infant was born with a congenital atresia of the esophagus and received nourishment by a gastric fistula until 2 years of age, when surgical repair ultimately permitted the child to eat normally by mouth.

During the first year of life, Monica became cranky and irritable, and this period was followed by a withdrawn mood during which Monica spent most of her time lying on her back. Her apathetic response further reduced opportunities for stimulation and human interaction. Between 15 and 24 months, Monica developed a severe depressive-withdrawal reaction. Significantly, however, this response only occurred when the infant was confronted alone by a stranger. When the stranger departed and a familiar person returned, the reaction remitted.

Elaborating on the reaction, Engel and Reichsman (1956) observed that the infant's facial expression, posture, and activity all evoked a "mood of dejection" and sadness reminiscent of depression. Monica would tense her eyebrows and furrow her forehead, while the corners of her mouth turned downward. In addition to these physical manifestations of depressive-like phenomena, Monica's behavioral withdrawal was also apparent when she turned away from strangers and closed her eyes. Her immobility and hypotonia was interpreted as a withdrawal pattern, as well as an affective disturbance by the researchers.

Engel (1962) has commented that the depression-withdrawal symptomatology observed in Monica is a form of undifferentiated affect, indicating a loss of stimulation. It may be argued that these reactions were the result of the way in which Monica responded to the confrontation of a variety of stressors—including illness, separation from her caregiver, maternal depression, and neglect.

With respect to illness, Monica was born in 1952 and was diagnosed as having congenital atresia of the esophagus. A cervical esophageal fistula was established, along with a gastric fistula, in order that Monica could receive food. Separation from the caregiver was reflected in Monica's numerous hospitalizations during the first two years of her life. Overall, Monica stayed in the hospital for a total of 9 months. Moreover, during these hospital stays, the infant's medical condition mandated a degree of enforced passivity, coupled with a lack of meaningful human contact and stimulation.

Monica also experienced the phenomenon of maternal separation while at home, because her mother worked long hours in a factory. The infant's maternal grandmother performed the tube feeding when Monica's mother was working. As Monica approached 5 months, her mother became depressed, and the infant responded by withdrawing. The researchers noted that Monica's mother had not fully bonded with the infant. Additionally, with the onset of maternal depression, Monica's withdrawal further exacerbated interaction between the mother and infant. It was also discovered that Monica's mother often neglected her infant. Both a social worker and visiting nurse found the infant soaked in the drainage from her esophageal and gastric fistulas several times.

Longitudinal follow-up of the case approximately 25 years later, revealed that Monica remembered nothing about the fistula-feeding period other than what she was later told. Monica was married in 1971, and had four infants of her own, all of whom were bottle-fed. Curiously, all four infants were handled in the same manner by Monica. Rather than holding her infants en face, all were fed on the lap or alone with the bottle propped. This bottle propping behavior began as early as 2 weeks. On only three occasions did Monica support the infant fully on her lap. Support was generally abandoned within a few minutes, when Monica complained of the weight of the infant. Once the infant was able to hold the bottle by itself, Monica rarely held it during feeding. Despite the fact that Monica could not remember her own infant feeding period, her own manner of handling her infants during feeding bore a marked resemblance to the way she herself was handled while being fistula-fed.

Engel (1962) questioned how such a biological function as nursing achieved mental representation. Not only did Monica replicate the nursing experience she had as an infant with her own babies, but Engel et al. (1985) reported that films of Monica between the ages of 4 and 13 revealed that when playing with dolls she rarely held the doll en face, but instead, held the doll on her lap without support. Such data indicated a developmental continuity between Monica's fistula-feeding experience and her feeding practices with her own infants when she became a mother.

Equally noteworthy, Engel et al. (1985) reported on the behavior of Monica's children, all females, in their doll playing. It was found that earliest doll-feeding behavior closely imitated Monica's style. By age 5, Monica's daughters began to hold their dolls in their arms during feeding. Eventually, the en face position was preferred to Monica's lap support position. Commenting on this longitudinal pattern of feeding behavior that involved Monica's mother and grandmother, Monica herself and Monica's daughters, the researchers wrote that such behaviors as nursing can have enduring consequences for subsequent maternal behavior. This study, then, highlights the overriding importance of investigating caregiver history and observing interaction between infant and caregiver. The caregiver, in other words, plays a vital role in shaping the behavioral patterns of the infant that may be perpetuated in the infant's future development. Moreover, this study indicated that developmental phenomena often have their origins in previous behavioral experiences, suggesting that continuities in development exist.

NATURE VERSUS NURTURE VARIABLES WITHIN THE DEVELOPMENTAL MODEL

Since affective disorders are actualized by accumulated patterns of maladaptive development, resolution of these disorders depends on the deciphering of predisposing qualities and potentiating factors that trigger symptomatic patterns throughout the life span. Among the risk factors that the developmental model dwells on most extensively for diagnosing depression are those arising from infant environmental transactions. The model suggests that risk factors that shape these transactions may be characterized as either "genetic" or "environmental," and that these two categories of factors may interact in potentially subtle ways. Indeed, as Kendler and Eaves (1986) argue, discerning the etiology of psychiatric disorder necessitates an understanding of pertinent genetic risk factors, pertinent environmental risk factors, and the mechanism of interaction between these two sets of variables. They have further divided the domain of the environment into two states, the "protective environment" and "the predisposing environment." Contact with the protective environment (e.g., maternal nurturance) reduces the likelihood of psychiatric disturbance. Conversely, contact with the predisposing environment (e.g., maternal abuse) enhances the probability of illness.

Three basic approaches have been taken to understanding the balance between the impacts of genetic endowment and the environment. Family studies are useful for discerning the effect of shared—including both "shared" genes and "shared" environment—and nonshared influences on behavior among members of the same family. Adoption studies are valuable because they rely on subjects whose environments, but not genes, are linked and thus provide a direct method of assessing the effect of environmental influences shared by family members. Twin studies provide researchers with compelling insights into how nonshared influences, environmental, modify behavior (Rowe & Plomin, 1981).

Segregating the effects of genetic influences and environmental influences on behavior is of invaluable assistance for the developmentalist, whose goal is to ascertain the etiology of psychiatric illness. Essentially, as

Kendler and Eaves (1986) have noted, there are three basic configurations for the interplay of genetics and environment. First, nature and nurture factors may combine to produce an *additive* outcome determined by both genotype and environment. Second, genetics may modulate *sensitivity* to the environment. Third, genetic factors may modulate *exposure* to the environment. These models presuppose that genotype and environmental exposure contribute to the susceptibility to or the likelihood of illness.

The first model proposed by Kendler and Eaves (1986), which suggests that genetics and environment have an *additive* effect, postulates that liability to illness is an outcome of the combination of genetic and environmental contributions. Thus the effect of exposure to a given environment on illness liability will have to be gauged in terms of genotype, and the probability of an individual's exposure to a given environment functions independently of the individual's genetics. The model of genetic control of *sensitivity* to the environment hypothesizes that genes do not directly alter the probability of illness. Instead they control the degree to which the individual is sensitive to the risk-increasing or risk-reducing aspects of the environment. In other words, the environment controls gene expression or the environment modifies the manner in which genes influence risk of illness. Finally, the model of genetic control of *exposure* to the environment suggests that genetics influence liability to illness by altering the probability of exposure to a predisposing environment.

The researchers also suggest two additional models: in the first, genetics controls liability to illness, as well as sensitivity to the environment. Here genetics influences *both* susceptibility of the individual to the environment and the individual's sensitivity to the environment. In the second model, genetics controls susceptibility to illness and the probability of exposure to environment. In this case, genes influence both liability to illness and probability of exposure to a predisposing environment.

For the developmentalist, these models serve as useful tools for apportioning weight to either genetic or environmental factors when evaluating infant behavior within the developmental framework. By isolating risk factors attributable to the environment or to genetics, the developmentalist will be more adept at assessing the locus and the degree of the individual's susceptibility to psychopathology.

Depressive Correlates of Nature and Nurture Variables

The significance of segregating the influence of genetic factors from environmental factors in assessing psychopathology is underscored when we examine some studies that have highlighted the role of these factors in the etiology of depression. The complex nature of depression, as determined by multiple factors, was highlighted in an adoption study by Cadoret, O'Gorman, Heywood, and Troughton (1985), who studied 48 individuals with a diagnosis of major depression from a sample of 443 adoptees. These adoptees had been separated at birth from their biologic parents and placed with nonrelatives. Although the Cadoret et al. study involved adult depressives, its methodology may prove useful for developmentalists who seek to discern the effect of genetics and environment on infant populations at risk. The researchers found that depression was positively—although not significantly—correlated with a biologic background of affective disorder. In addition, however, both primary and secondary depression were positively and significantly correlated with several environmental factors. In analyzing the risk factors predisposing to depression in these cases, the researchers argued that environment should be viewed within a developmental framework in which the impact of environmental events depends on when they occurred.

The value of segregating and weighing environmental versus genetic forces is not merely academic. If the genetic and environmental factors can be segregated, prophylactic intervention can follow identification of a "population at risk" (Garmezy, 1985). Also, environmentally determined predispositions may be highly significant in a sizable proportion of depressed patients and, as advocated by Cadoret et al. (1985), could serve as a focus for research into methods for preventing depression.

The results of Cadoret et al.'s (1985) work are in keeping with a tentative truce that has finally been reached between the nature and nurture camps. They have long argued about the significance to be accorded each of these classes of factors. Both nature and nurture proponents are willing to concede that neither heredity nor environment considered in isolation can account for the complex totality of changes embraced by infant development. Indeed the one point on which both groups appear to concur is that development, as such, depends on input from both nature and nurture factors.

The crucial concept here is development and the manner in which the infant adapts to the challenges of *both* nature and nurture. As noted earlier, the developmental framework permits researchers to consider specific measurable characteristics and endogenous substances such as the temperamental trait of irritability or the level of the infant's blood cortisol, as well as to focus on maturation as an unfolding process witnessed through evidence of memory recall.

Increasingly investigators are calling for an alliance between nature and nurture schools of thought, lest research become compartmentalized and inflexible (McCall, 1977). The techniques used are partly responsible for the perpetuation of this debate. Developmental psychologists have embraced unquestioningly the experimental model, whereby cause and effect relationships are derived from an environment within which variables have been artificially manipulated. This adherence to a cause–effect model creates an incentive to attribute outcomes to *either* a nature or a nurture component. Rather than continuing with this approach, McCall urges that developmental psychopathologists attend more to the actual process of development as it unfolds within a naturalistic setting. During observation of infants and children in actual life circumstances, long-term patterns of development will emerge.

McCall's (1977) rationale for advocating this approach relies on developmental psychopathology's emphasis on changes that occur over extended periods of time and need for a continuum of observation at different ages. Moreover, the developmental approach mandates that maturation be viewed as a fluid process, in which capacities emerge and grow in a cumulative fashion, rather than as a rigid, static process. As a result, developmentalists must constantly inquire as to which behaviors emerge over age, which developmental events constitute the antecedents of these behaviors, and how developmental changes in one behavior are related to developmental changes in other behaviors.

McCall (1977) also alerts researchers to the concepts of individual differences and developmental function. These concepts may serve as a more precise manner of framing the issues raised by heredity versus environment advocates. When McCall speaks of individual differences, he is referring to the rating of an individual subject on a given attribute, in contrast to the rating of other individuals on that same attribute. As thus conceived, individual differences seem to be primarily attributable to hereditary factors. In contrast, developmental function refers to the degree to which behaviors can replace, supplement, or evolve out of one another during chronological development. Thus developmental function may be more attributable to environmental pressures.

After extensive review of developmental studies, McCall (1981) applied these concepts to an analytic model. He hypothesized that during the first 18 months of life developmental function is largely maturational and hence predictable, whereas individual differences are unstable and not highly correlated with either genetic or environmental factors. Infants who deviate from this normal course generally return to typical patterns of developmental function once the environmental factor causing the deviation is removed. In contrast, most individual differences exhibited during the first 18 months will neither be chronologically stable nor correlate with genetic or environmental factors. At approximately 2 years of age, however, individual differences will emerge more forcefully, will be consolidated, and will demonstrate increasing stability across time. Developmental function, by contrast, will become less continuous.

The Confluence Model

One theoretical analysis that may shed further light on the developmental approach to the nature versus nurture controversy is the confluence model

(Berbaum & Moreland, 1980). This model focuses on the dynamics of interaction that exist between an individual family's configuration and a child's intellectual functioning. The confluence model is appropriate for studying the impact of the variables of external environment and biological endowment because it isolates two factors that, in traditional analysis, have been viewed as being primarily representative of *either* genetics or environment. That is, intellectual functioning, as measured via IQ scores, has been interpreted as being dependent largely on the child's genetic endowment, while family configuration has been conceived of as a variable subject to environmental fluctuation. While it is not the purpose of this chapter to trace the origins of intellectual functioning, a discussion of the confluence model's approach may shed some light on how nature and nurture variables can be integrated successfully. Thus the study of affective development may borrow this conceptual approach from the study of cognitive development.

Confluence theory is first and foremost developmental in that it emphasizes change within individuals over time (McCall, 1985). Second, as McCall notes, the major independent variables highlighted in the theory are *intra*familial, (rather than *inter*familial)—a domain which may be pivotal to understanding overall cognitive development. The theory also pays heed to how parental and sibling environment affect individual intellectual performance. Most significantly, for the purposes of this discussion, the confluence theory postulates that intellectual functioning—a domain previously thought to be genetically determined and hence virtually impervious to either direct or indirect environmental influence—may in fact be altered or at least modified by manipulation of environmental phenomena.

In one review of data from longitudinal studies that focused on intraindividual variation in IQ over time, McCall (1983) commented that such intra-individual variation may be attributed in significant part to "nonshared, within-family environmental variation." Indeed such intrafamilial factors may account for 15 to 25 percent of all variability in IQ and for 30 to 50 percent of environmental variability in IQ.

McCall (1983) notes further that intrafamilial factors exerting impact on cognitive development may be of two distinct types. First is a category of environmental factors impinging on one child as opposed to another in the family. Such factors are dubbed by the researcher as "continuous nonshared within family environmental factors" (p. 409). As an example, a first-born male might be subject to parental encouragement in the area of athletics or intellectual activities that another child in the family might not experience. Another category of nonshared environmental factors includes situations or events that are of shorter duration and occur at a particular chronological period of development. Moving to a new neighborhood or parental divorce are instances of this latter type of environmental influence. Such latter factors are discontinuous, exerting more of an acute influence on cognitive development. To give credence to the notion that individual variation in IQ may be strongly influenced by environmental factors, McCall cites an earlier study (McCall, Appelbaum, & Hogarty, 1973) which reveals substantial intra-individual variation in IQ when correlated with age. Specifically, IQ was found to fluctuate by a range of 28.5 points between the ages of 2.5 and 17 years.

According to McCall, while changes in IQ scores over age may be attributed to several causes, such as gene–based developmental trends or the emergence of greater genetic control, the most plausible hypothesis remains that of discontinuous intrafamilial environmental influences. In discounting the effect of genetics on variability over time in intellectual performance, McCall notes that if, in fact, gene-based developmental trends were responsible for IQ variability, then siblings would display similar trends. But evidence indicates (McCall, 1970, 1972) that no such pattern exists. Moreover, if genetic control, which increases with age, accounts for increased test scores, one might expect greater similarity in later childhood than in earlier years when some siblings are younger. However, when patterns of IQ change among siblings were charted for preschoolers (aged 3 to 6 years) and for school-aged children (aged 6 to 13 years), siblings were not found to be more similar to one another than unrelated children during either age segment (McCall, 1972). Intrafamilial environmental factors, in contrast, have been related to individual variations in measurable intellectual functioning. It has been demonstrated, for example, that parental efforts to accelerate a child's development or severity of punishment do correlate with IQ changes (McCall et al., 1973a).

The main thesis of McCall's argument, and indeed of the confluence model in general, is not that intrafamilial environmental factors alone determine the level of IQ functioning, but rather that the impact of such variables may be more dramatic than previously supposed. The confluence model proposes that certain characteristics previously viewed as largely a function of unalterable biological endowment may be more susceptible to alteration and to the effect of interventive strategies than has been articulated in the past. In a recent study conducted by Berbaum and Moreland (1985), the confluence model was used to estimate intellectual development for a family sample of 321 children from 101 adoptive families. The confluence model, used to predict mental age, accounted for up to 50 percent of individual variance in this variable. Although the predictive power of the model was reduced when the relationship between chronological and mental age was taken into account, the predictive power of the model was not eliminated. The model generated a good fit for data derived from both biological and adopted chldren. The researchers noted that as a paradigm for explaining cognitive development on the basis of environmental rather than genetic factors, the confluence model may be used to explain partially the intellectual development of an individual child within a family. Thus the confluence model offers researchers a tool for modifying intellectual functioning to some extent through environmental manipulation.

Critics of the confluence model (Price, Walsh, & Vilberg, 1984) have argued, with some justification, that the empirical support for the model is largely invalid, because mental age is generally correlated in these studies with chronological age. McCall (1985) concedes that the model may not be highly efficient from the standpoint of prediction, since only modest increments in accuracy are associated with family configuration variables once chronological age is included in the formula. That is, gene-based developmental trends, which manifest themselves through the variable of chronological change, do appear to exert a significant effect on individual cognitive functioning. Nevertheless, McCall (1985) stresses that the value of the confluence model lies not in the fact that it offers a complete explanation for individual variability in cognitive capacity, but rather that it poses a new set of variables which have been demonstrated to exert some alterable effects on intellectual functioning. As such the confluence model does provide some suggestions for the formulation of interventive strategies.

Connel and Furman (1984) present another conceptual framework for development. Beginning with the premise that certain continuities and discontinuities in development occur within any one individual, they observe that changes in individual characteristics should be viewed in terms of transition. Individual characteristics may be biological, cognitive, affective, or interpersonal. The researchers posit that individual changes, rather than being attributed to either a genetic or environmental component, should be interpreted in terms of a transitional event, a transitional period, and a transitional mechanism. By transitional event, the researchers mean a catalyst that provokes change. The transitional period refers to the duration of time during which the transition lasts. The transitional mechanism refers to the reorganizational processes that maintain the change in the organism's pattern of functioning. Significantly, transitional events may be *exogenous* or *endogenous*. Exogenous events occur in the external or environmental milieu and might include such factors as entering school or the death of a significant other. Endogenous factors focus instead on internal alterations in physiology or psychology.

The transitional analysis has proven fruitful in devising strategies for studying infant and child development. Since entrance into the school environment is a known exogenous transitional event, researchers have theorized that developmental changes will be more dramatically displayed in the individual characteristics of children entering the first grade than of a group of children moving from second to third grade. An example of the use of transitional analysis in which the precipitating event leading to the developmental change is primarily endogenous might be an infant born with a physical handicap. In such a case, the precise impact of the event on development may be difficult to determine in an individual case. But longitudinal comparison studies between handicapped and nonhandicapped infants may provide data on the manner in which such an endogenous factor serves as a catalyst for altering the expected course of development.

These studies, focusing on the confluence model of intellectual functioning and the transitional analysis as applied to development, suggest that exogenous factors can impinge on the infant or young child in many ways. The studies offer hints for devising strategies that alter the environmental milieu of the child and thus modify development. From these studies, we can discern that cognitive functioning, which embodies a strong genetic component, is capable nevertheless of being altered to a heretofore unsuspected degree.

Research in the area of affective functioning presents developmentalists with a somewhat different dilemma. Various studies have confirmed that genetic transmission plays a significant role in the manifestation of affective disorders. In a study exploring the precise nature of genetic transmission, Baron, Klotz, Mendlewicz, and Rainer (1981) devised a threshold model of inheritance. This model postulates that the first-degree relatives of patients with bipolar and unipolar affective disorders may have an underlying attribute linked to the etiology of the disorder. This attribute is referred to as a vulnerability or liability. Assuming such a vulnerability, the researchers developed a liability curve hypothesized to have a normal distribution. The point on the curve beyond which all persons were expected to manifest disorder was termed the threshold. Relatives of affectively disordered patients were postulated to have a higher mean liability to depression than individuals in the general population. Using this threshold analysis, the researchers reported a significant morbidity risk for affective disorder among first-degree relatives. A genetic mechanism operated as a primary catalyst for affective disorders.

However, the ultimate role of this genetic determinant is not clear. Armed with the knowledge that infants and children of parents with affective disorders (most notably depression) are at high risk of developing a similar disorder, should the developmentalist assume that such infants will inevitably fall prey to mental illness? The Baron et al. study (1981) is valuable in that it phrases the issue in terms of "risk" and "thresholds of vulnerability," rather than in terms of inevitability. Developmentalists need to be alert to the factor of risk in infants of parents with these disorders. In addition, specific interventive strategies, geared to suppress, circumvent, or underplay the genetic vulnerability of such infants and children, need to be devised.

A variety of studies have confirmed the relatively high incidence of genetic transmission of affective disorders. Thus Mahmood, Reveley, and Murray (1983) note that a review of the literature indicates that the morbidity risk of first-degree relatives of affective disorder patients is in the range of 10 to 15 percent—a significantly higher rate of risk than in the general population. Mendlewicz and Rainer (1977) focused on the genetic transmission of manic-depressive illness. By comparing adoptive parents with biologic parents, they reported a greater degree of psychopathology, particularly of affective illness, in parents genetically related to manic-depressive patients than in parents who adopted and raised depressed individuals.

In a study on a similar theme, Klein, Depue, and Slater (1985) investigated 37 offspring (adolescents and young adults aged 15 to 21) of parents with bipolar affective disorder and 22 offspring of parents with nonaffective psychiatric disorder. A control group was also included. Results included the fact that a significantly greater number of offspring of bipolar (43%) than of control (18%) parents met criteria for a psychiatric disorder. This difference was primarily due to substantially higher rates of affective disorders among the offspring of bipolar subjects (38%) than of control subjects (5%).

As a final footnote to this discussion of the respective roles played by genetics and environment in shaping infant and child development, several studies focusing on infant populations have revealed that nurture and nature variables intertwine and affect one another as factors creating behavioral change. Plomin and Rowe (1979) applied a twin analysis to infant social behavior, comparing responses to mother and to a stranger. A group of 21 identical twin pairs and 25 same-sex fraternal twin pairs (average age 22.2 months) were studied. The researchers studied behavior in seven situations including stranger approach, play and cuddling with mother or stranger, and separation from mother.

The researchers reported that hereditary traits appeared to affect more individual differences in social response to strangers than differences in response to mothers. These data indicate that the environmental influence on behavior may occur primarily within families, rather than among families. In a related study, Matheny and Dolan (1975) observed twins in a longitudinal investigation at 9, 12, 18, 24, and 30 months of age in two settings—unstructured free play and relatively structured test taking. Behaviors relating to adaptability to the two settings were rated and the scores analyzed for evidence of continuity. It was found that identical twins were more similar than same–sex fraternal twins in both settings, but correlations were consistently stronger in the playroom setting. The researchers concluded that situation variables contribute to the low stabilities frequently reported for personality dimensions, but that the ultimate degree of behavioral change is genetically programmed. Phrased another way, the results indicated that environmental factors are filtered through the individual's intrinsic hereditary endowment before behavior emerges.

Taken as a composite, these studies suggest that the debate over genetics versus environment may oversimplify interpretation of infant behavioral manifestations. Ultimately, some personality characteristics—cognitive and affective functioning, temperament—have strong genetic components. But such characteristics may be susceptible to modification by factors that interact with genetic variables to create particular behaviors that may be more multifaceted than previously supposed. The task of the developmentalist is not to delineate precise genetic or environmental etiologies. Rather, infant and child care specialists must use the framework offered by the developmental continuum to devise strategies geared toward accommodating both hereditary and environmental factors.

Bond (1982) captured the simultaneous fluidity and stability offered by the developmental model when she noted that development must be perceived as "multilinear, multidirectional, heterogeneous, and plastic." In addition, the developmental model accommodates data derived from transactions. Such transactions occurring between infant and caregiver constitute a large portion of the evidence currently available in the area of infant maturation. Moreover, the developmental approach examines both typical patterns of behavior, as well as manifestations that deviate from the norm. For this latter reason, a developmental approach is particularly appropriate for devising a therapeutic model of treatment.

Given the chameleon-like qualities of the developmental model, it would appear to be an ideal method for studying the infant. Yet there is another, more pragmatic reason for advocating such an approach. Parents often seek out professional advice when their child is going through a puzzling stage of development (Daws, 1985). The situation is often more acute in the case of infants; insecure new parents, untutored and unaccustomed to their new role as caregivers, may harbor fears that they are incapable of properly caring for their infant. A consultation with a pediatrician or child psychiatrist for such parents may provide the caregiver with needed reassurance and can enhance the mother's skills at meeting the infant's needs (Daws, 1985). In cases of medically high-risk infants—such as handicapped infants—early intervention on the part of a therapist can facilitate adaptation to infant interaction. The developmental model, which permits nonintrusive remediation at virtually any level of development, is especially suited to these situations (Sigman, 1982). Thus the developmental model is appropriate for studying infants not only because it uniquely integrates data from a wide variety of sources, but also because therapists are so often confronted with examples of caregiver-infant interaction for observation, diagnosis, and treatment.

A DEVELOPMENTAL PERSPECTIVE FOR INFANT DEPRESSION

The central premise of this book is that the multidimensional approach offered by the developmental model is mandatory for understanding how depression can evolve in infants and young children. Research on depressive states in early life strongly indicates that symptomatology should be analyzed from the developmental perspective. Children who are capable of verbalizing coherently often express such affective states as guilt, self-blame, dejection, negative self-image, and apathy, according to Rutter and Garmezy (1983). But verifying such symptomatology in infants is, needless to say, a greater challenge because the researcher must rely on behavioral manifestations almost exclusively (Trad, 1986).

In a landmark study, Spitz and Wolf (1946) identified such depressive symptomatology as weeping, withdrawal, apathy, weight loss, and sleep disturbance in institutionalized infants during the second half of the first year. Moreover, between the ages of 6 months and 4 years separation from or loss of the major caregiver causes children to go through a recognizable series of stages including protest, despair, and detachment (Bowlby, 1969). Prior to 6 months, however, no studies have discerned infant depressive reactions to loss of the type Bowlby identified.

Despite the dearth of specific evidence concerning the sequence of responses that follows loss of the caregiver in the first months of life, several researchers have demonstrated that presentation of extreme discrepancies or of disrupted contingencies can trigger a facsimile of learned helplessness, described by Seligman and Maier (1967), that can evolve into the kind of despair and detachment that Bowlby (1969) has described. Although full-fledged depressive symptomatology may not be manifest for prolonged periods of time prior to 6 months of age, the developmental process, whereby the infant integrates patterns of response, may become part of the regulatory process well before 6 months of age.

The following chapters will focus on the multidimensional factors that contribute to depression in early life. The developmental framework will be used as an orienting perspective, within which the variables of temperament, attachment, and self-concept evolution will be assessed. Particular emphasis will be placed on how deviations of behavioral manifestation or dysregulations may emerge either at a particular developmental phase or from the interaction and coordination of variables at any phase of development. Such dysregulations will be interpreted as potential signals that the infant is prone to developing full-fledged depressive symptomatology if the dysregulation is not remedied. This book posits that depression in early life is a function of the dynamic interplay of these variables within the process of regulation.

To bolster this theory of the etiology of infant depression, specific "at risk" populations have been isolated in order that the mechanisms whereby depression becomes entrenched may be fully articulated. Infant depression may, at times, appear to be an elusive phenomenon—difficult to define, diagnose, and treat. It is the goal of this book to demonstrate that, by assiduously applying the developmental approach to analysis of hallmarks and to the integral process of regulatory capacities, researchers can achieve breakthroughs in this area of infant psychopathology.

CHAPTER TWO

The Concept of Childhood Depression

The past 40 years have seen remarkable change in attitude and approach to the question of infant and childhood depression. Recent research suggests that depression in childhood is a real and widespread phenomenon and that risk factors for depression (lack of parental and social support) are growing in our society (Lin, 1986). Both childhood and depression are concepts that are continually evolving, and the specific meanings associated with each of them have changed and compounded over time. The most basic question that confronts researchers today is whether depression is a single entity in both childhood and adulthood. There are two facets to this question. First, does depression in childhood present the same manifestations as adult depression, and second, are the dynamics of depression the same in both childhood and adulthood?

To define the manifestations of depressive disorders throughout childhood, it is essential to devise a descriptive system that allows for the investigation of disorders across developmental epochs. The various cognitive, physical, and self-regulatory stages of infancy and childhood present a clinical picture that has different features contributing to a composite diagnosis. During both infancy and childhood, depressive manifestations may change as they move from being transitory developmental phenomena to more clinically significant phenomena.

The term "depression" has been applied to a wide range of conditions; precise definition is difficult. Consequently, when discussing depressive disorders, it is imperative to differentiate among depression as an affective state, as a dysphoric mood, and as a syndrome. As an *affect*, depression is the external representation of the subjective experience of emotion. Depressive affect may be one of the symptoms of a depressive disorder or a symptom of a host of other disorders. Equally, it might represent a normal outcome of the consolidation of a developmental milestone—what one might call a developmental equivalent of depression. An example of such a depressive affect might be the developmentally expected depressive affect described by Mahler (Mahler, Pine, & Berman, 1975) during the rapprochement phase of separation–individuation. As a *mood*, depression is understood to refer to a sustained-feeling tone, the predominant conscious, subjective emotion, which colors one's perception of the world. Finally, as a *syndrome*, depression is identified as a cluster of symptoms causing varying degrees of incapacity, having a commonly occurring clinical picture, a natural history, a number of biobehavioral correlates, and a predictable response to treatment. According to DSM-III, the symptom cluster for major depressive disorder includes changes in sleep patterns and/or appetite, and anhedonia (lack of pleasure).

With respect to infant depression, we asked whether the diagnostic criteria of DSM-III can sufficiently describe the wide expression of depression in childhood. The study of childhood depression may be able to borrow from some of the methodologies, such as biological markers, developed for the study of depression as a syndrome in adults. Some methodologies currently being used to assess the phenomenology of depression in children will be reviewed in this chapter. However, we need specific methodologies tailored for the study of depressive phenomena as affects in children—for example, coding systems to study affects revealed by the facial display of emotions.

The neuroendocrine model is a promising paradigm that may help in revealing the dynamics of adult and childhood depression. This model may provide insight into the genesis of depression, especially when a developmental approach is undertaken, as for example, when biological markers are studied in conjunction with a difficult temperament. Self-regulation guides the process of self-development, and maladaptive self-concepts can develop from defective self-regulation. (See Chapter Four—Regulation and the Development of the Self.) This chapter examines how a defective self-concept may contribute to a predisposition for depressive psychopathology.

In recent years, depression in children has been studied through its endogenous correlates. What is more likely involved, however, is the activation of some latent predisposition by exogenous environmental factors, a process akin to that described in the learned helplessness paradigm (Abramson, Seligman, & Teasdale, 1978). In this model, depression is a product of adverse effects of the environment impinging on a vulnerable self or, in children, a developing self with its emerging regulatory capacities. Children who are unable to regulate affective changes effectively, risk developing depression in the face of repeated assaults on their sense of self. Neuroendocrine dysregulation may provide evidence of which environmental cues guide neurochemical development and which environmental deficits put the child at risk (Trad, 1986).

FOUR APPROACHES TO CHILDHOOD DEPRESSION

A critical review of the literature reveals four approaches to childhood depression. Each theoretical model, in an attempt either to prove or disprove the existence of childhood depression as a distinct clinical entity, raises questions of definition, approach, and methodology. These questions are examined by each subsequent school of thought.

Developmental Symptomatology Argument

Although the writings of the classic psychoanalytic researchers on depression (Abraham, 1912; Freud, 1917; Rado, 1928) reveal differences in approach and theory, all regard certain early childhood experiences as necessary for the subsequent development of depression. However, with the exception of Renè Spitz (Spitz, 1945; Spitz & Wolf, 1946), none of these investigators correlated these experiences to childhood depression per se.

Depressive symptoms in adults were viewed retrospectively as manifestations of trauma in a developmental stage, but little attention was paid to symptoms in childhood. Instead these researchers took the approach that depression, as a syndrome analogous to that in adults, does not occur in childhood (Rie, 1966; Rochlin, 1959).

This argument was bolstered as late as the 1960s by findings from a study conducted by Lapouse (1966). Using 482 randomly selected children, ranging in age from 6 to 12 years, he found that various forms of behavior commonly classified as depressive symptoms were markedly widespread. Lapouse questioned, however, whether the high prevalence of symptomatic behavior might not be more indicative of normal developmental phenomena than of a psychiatric disorder. The strength of Lapouse's viewpoint served to delay recognition of childhood depression as a distinct clinical entity until the late 1960s.

The "Depressive Equivalents" Argument

In the 1960s, a theoretical model was developed that posited equivalents to depression in childhood but noted that the overt manifestations of this syndrome were not the same as in adults (Cytryn & McKnew, 1974; Glaser, 1968; Renshaw, 1974; Toolan, 1962a). In this model, the diagnosis of depression was assigned to children with a variety of behavioral problems, even if there were no clear mood changes or dysphoria. These behaviors, which included aggression, hyperactivity, enuresis, sleeping and eating disturbances, and somatic complaints, were thought to be signals of an underlying, yet unseen, depressive disorder and were called "masked depressions" or "depressive equivalents."

The validity of the depressive equivalents argument has been questioned. First, symptoms that are transient, which were disqualified for purposes of diagnosis by these researchers, may nevertheless be clinically significant. Second, the various classificatory schemata used often contradicted one another and probably confused investigators attempting to define depression in children. Even when these criteria were defined, they were not reliable for use in validation studies (Cytryn & McKnew, 1974). Hence if masked depression and depressive equivalents were to be considered before formulating a diagnosis, childhood depression would be ubiquitous. These problems together have led to a general disavowal of this model. Nevertheless, it is valuable in that it calls attention to some of the atypicalities, particularly in the form of antisocial behavior, that occur in the presentation of some childhood depressions. Indeed the aggressiveness of the 2-year-old children of manic-depressives studied by Zahn-Waxler, Cummings, McKnew, Davenport, and Radke-Yarrow (1984) and the high degree of overlap between depression and conduct disorders discerned by Puig-Antich (1984) among prepubescent boys, suggest that symptoms such as aggression may be correlates of certain types of depression. This is not to say, however, that aggression is synonymous with depression.

The Single-Factor Approach

The single-factor approach accepted the concept of depression in childhood as a clinical entity analogous to depression in adults (Albert & Beck, 1975; Arajarvi & Huttunen, 1972; Ling, Oftedal, & Weinberg, 1970; McConville, Boag, & Purohit, 1973; Poznanski & Zrull, 1970). Epidemiological research focused on attempts to isolate a single factor that would provide a necessary and sufficient explanation for childhood depression. However, these studies gave an uneven portrayal of the syndrome, in terms of both diagnosis and prevalence. The most important reason for the inconsistent results was the use of subjective, nonstandardized criteria for the diagnosis of depression. This use reflected a lack of agreement concerning the definition of depression and, in some cases, a disinclination to formulate a definition. The approach is being supplanted, especially in psychiatric research, by multifactorial models of causation.

The Adult Model Approach

Most recently, a fourth school of thought has emerged. The adult-model approach posits, as does its predecessor, the single-factor approach, that childhood depression is analogous to adult depression, but holds that it can best be studied, like adult depression, through a multifactorial orientation. The investigative strategy of this school of thought is to start with a known disorder, that is, the understanding of depression in adulthood, and find the similarities and dissimilarities with childhood depression. The hypothesis is that if it is possible to delineate and measure depressive syndromes in adults, it should also be possible to do the same with children, using the same diagnostic criteria. Depression is seen as continuous from infancy to adulthood, that is, as a disorder in which the symptomatology, treatment, and correlates are continuous, yet affected by development.

In 1973, one of the pioneers of this approach, W. A. Weinberg, modified the Feighner Adult Diagnostic Criteria (Feighner, Robins, Guze, Woodruff, Winokur, & Munoz, 1972) for use in children. (These criteria later became the basis of DSM-III criteria for depression.) Using these criteria, Weinberg diagnosed depression in 42 of 72 children, 6 to 12 years of age, who were referred to a diagnostic center. He thus demonstrated that a single set of criteria for depression could, with some modification, be applied to both children and adults.

The acceptance of the adult model for childhood depression evolved as the result of a series of studies that, over time, led to the elimination of certain concepts held by the previous schools of thought. For example, after reviewing the records of 547 psychiatric patients, aged 1 to 17 years, Pearce (1977) divided them into two groups according to the presence (25% of the sample) or absence (75% of the sample) of dysphoric mood. Through further analysis, he found the symptoms that clustered with dysphoric mood, but not dysphoric mood alone, differentiated between depressed and nondepressed children. This further cemented the concept of a depressive syndrome, identifiable by a constellation of correlates rather than by any single factor.

Investigators for the development of DSM-III recognized these achievements and developed one set of criteria to be used for both adults and children. DSM-III is one of the instruments currently being used to diagnose depression during childhood. In addition to offering a standard set of diagnostic criteria, DSM-III also provides the clinician with multiaxial criteria. These additional diagnostic tools can be used to recognize the symptoms of depression in childhood that differ from adult symptoms due to developmental changes. Exposing these differences will allow the clinician to see how, at each developmental stage, the child's abilities and limitations impose their characteristic stamp on affect, mood, and symptom complexes.

One such difference may involve the duration of symptomatology needed for a diagnosis of depressive syndrome. The National Institute of Mental Health Subcommittee on Clinical Criteria for the Diagnosis of Depression in Children (1977) recognized that since depressive symptoms in children may be transitory, a minimum symptom duration of 4 weeks for the diagnosis of childhood depression is required. The DSM-III requires a symptom duration of only 2 weeks for both adults and children before the diagnosis of major affective disorder can be applied.

The notion of a nosological continuum of depressive disorders is supported by evidence of a shared positive response to pharmacological treatment of depression. For example, both adults and children showed a positive therapeutic response to appropriate blood levels of imipramine, a psychopharmacologic agent that acts to increase plasma concentrations of norepinephrine and dopamine by blocking their reuptake (Puig-Antich, 1979).

Another apparent link between childhood and adult depression involves seasonal affective disorder (SAD). This disorder, which usually occurs during the winter months, has recently begun to be documented in children (Rosenthal et al., 1986) and has been described in a way that resembles SAD in adults (Rosenthal et al., 1984). Although the precise etiology of the disorder is uncertain at this time, it appears that the condition is triggered by a type of neuroendocrine dysregulation. The disorder involves symptoms of irritability, fatigue, depressed affect, and sleep changes. Since the frequency of seasonal affective disorder is relatively unknown, parents and teachers may misinterpret the child's moods and respond to him or her in an inappropriate manner, thus exacerbating the situation. Parents may simply come to see their children as being "moody" during the winter months. Rosenthal et al. (1986) made their observations after investigating a group of seven children with a mean age of 12.3 years and a mean duration of the illness of 5.1 years. All subjects received and responded to environmental light therapy and responded in a manner similar to adults. The recession of symptoms once light therapy is administered suggests that in some instances childhood depression may be triggered primarily by endogenous factors.

The similarities between adult and childhood forms of depression are probably significant. However, the differences may be equally significant, as DSM-III recognizes, albeit in a limited way. DSM-III does not deny the existence of developmental change over the course of infancy and childhood, or that such change affects the course of psychological disorders. Moreover, the establishment of a single set of criteria for diagnosing depression in both children and adults has helped to clear away some of the confusion as to the nature of depressive disorders, and prepared the way for developing a clearer picture of how such disorders function throughout life.

Indeed, DSM-III has proven superior to other diagnostic criteria that have been applied to children. Cytryn, McKnew, and Bunney (1980) compared the reliability of DSM-III criteria and criteria developed based on the "depressive equivalents" argument by reviewing the charts of 37 children whom they originally diagnosed as having acute ($N = 12$), chronic ($N = 11$), or masked depressive ($N = 14$) reactions. Using DSM-III criteria, the authors independently rediagnosed each case. The results were in total agreement with the DSM-III diagnoses in 89 percent of the children, and of the four cases in which there was disagreement, three were in the masked category and one was in the chronic. Accordingly Cytryn and his associates (1980) revised their thinking and reported that masked depression has not been as accurate as DSM-III in diagnosing affective disorders.

Comparisons of DSM-III with other diagnostic criteria have also supported the reliability of adult-based criteria for children. In one study attempting to clarify the concept of masked depression, Carlson and Cantwell (1980) found it possible to diagnose these children using criteria developed from the adult model. The study involved 102 children, ages 7 to 17 years old. The researchers also found that a systematic interview identified more children with depression than standard evaluation procedures, which, in fact, had overlooked depression in 60 percent of the cases. In a later study, Carlson and Cantwell (1982) compared the DSM-III depression criteria with Weinberg depression criteria (WDC; Weinberg et al., 1973). They found diagnostic agreement in 78.4 percent of the depressed children using WDC and DSM-III. WDC was seen as less accurate than DSM-III. More recently, Lobovits and Handal (1985) compared DSM-III criteria for major affective disorder with the results of two other depression scales, the Personality Inventory for Children (PIC-D; Froman,

1971) and the Children's Depression Inventory (CDI; Kovacs, 1978). Their purpose was to establish a reliable estimate for the prevalence of depression among latency-aged children using DSM-III criteria. The subjects, 50 children aged 8 to 12 years and referred to an outpatient clinic, were interviewed by two clinicians; parents were interviewed separately. The children filled out the CDI, while the parents filled out the PIC-D. The clinicians assessed the children according to DSM-III criteria for depressive disorders. Results showed a 90 percent agreement between the two clinicians who judged the interviews to determine a diagnosis. Thus DSM-III criteria were judged to show an acceptable level of diagnostic agreement in assessing depression in children of this age. The DSM-III criteria showed 32 percent prevalence for depression in this sample, based on assessments of the child interviews, and an estimate of 22 percent based on the parent interview. The authors stated:

> *The results of this study indicate that DSM-III criteria for major depressive episode offer a useful starting point in untangling the confusion surrounding the diagnosis and prevalence rate of childhood depression. (p. 52)*

Thus several studies show that DSM-III provides alternatives for those cases that were originally diagnosed as masked depression, for example, conduct disorders, overanxious disorders, and attention deficit disorders. This result is further supported by evidence of a similar response to treatment as detected by Puig-Antich (1982), who found that in a population of boys with both major depression and conduct disorder, both conditions responded to treatment with imipramine. While behavior problems do appear in depressed children, they may overlap with depression or may predict the onset of depression and they tend to be less severe than those diagnosed with genuine behavior disorders, which are often chronic and of greater magnitude.

Although perhaps the most solid foundation of the three schools of thought on the characteristics of depression in childhood, the DSM-III criteria for depression have many limitations. The most significant is their failure to account in a comprehensive way for the likely age-sensitivity of the disorder. Developmental considerations relating to both the onset and course of the disorder in childhood are currently major topics of research.

Admittedly DSM-III includes a section for the associated features (prodromal symptoms, onset, and course) that may be unique to children and may vary with age. Using these guidelines, which take developmental and symptomatic factors into account, helps to differentiate between transient and more enduring states. DSM-III also recognizes that, with the varying capacities of children, there is information that can and should be obtained from a variety of sources, including the child, parents, and school personnel, since patients often do not accurately observe their affective state and do not always present the clinician with classical histories (Carlson, 1979).

In some instances, prodromal manifestations may occur acutely in predisposed individuals—those whose natures are influenced by their age and personality structure or who are genetically predisposed to depression and exhibit an incomplete form of the illness, such as atypical depression, atypical dysthymia, or adjustment disorders with changes in mood.

Despite increasing recognition that age affects the development and expression of depression in childhood, it is still unclear, even at the grossest level, what form the effects of age assume. In their sample of 80 school-aged (8 to 13 years) depressed children, Kovacs and Paulauskas (1984) reported that the less mature children suffered the most chronic depressions and, during major depressive episodes, they required much more time to recover than the more mature children. However, a study of depression in female children by Garber (1984) yielded just the opposite results. In this trial with 137 girls between the ages of 7 and 13, Garber found an increase in the frequency of both depressive syndromes and symptoms with increasing age. These results are consistent with most other studies (Pearce, 1978; Rutter, 1986), which show a noticeable rise in the incidence of depression in early adolescence. Garber notes that within the developmental context, there are a number of possible explanations for these findings. They include, but are not limited to, hormonal changes associated with puberty, genetic factors, frequency of environmental stressors, and the possible presence of the cognitive set associated with learned helplessness.

The complicated nature of the impact of age on depression and whether this results in different disorders, with different clinical pictures, different clinical courses at different points in development and different prognoses has been clarified to some extent in two major studies by Kovacs et al. (1984a,b). These researchers assessed the various diagnoses [major depressive disorder (MDD), dysthymic disorder (DD), and adjustment disorder with depressed mood (ADDM)] that can overlap with other psychopathology. In two prospective studies involving the same cohort of 65 subjects, 8 to 13 years of age, these diagnoses were studied with respect to age of onset, length of episode, and incidence of coexisting disorders.

Many similarities emerged between the clinical picture and prognosis of childhood depression as described by these researchers and adult depression described by others. A high incidence of co-occurring psychiatric disorders is common in both depressed children and in depressed adults. Nearly all of the DD group had concurrently diagnosed conditions and over three quarters of the MDD group had another psychiatric diagnosis.

Multiple affective disorders are common in most forms of both childhood and adult depression. Over half (57%) of the children with DD had concurrent MDD and 38 percent of those with MDD also met criteria for dysthymia. In adults, the rate of MDD superimposed on chronic depression is also significant, although somewhat lower, ranging from 26 to 30 percent (Kovacs, 1984a,b). In a family study by Weissman et al. (1986), slightly less than 30 percent of adult probands with major depression had depressive personality.

The high degree of overlap between affective disorders and anxiety disorders in childhood provides another striking parallel with adult depression. For example, roughly one third of those with DD and MDD had simultaneous anxiety disorders (36% of DD cases and 33% of MDD cases). Among adults, well over half (58%) of adults in a case-control family study of depression also had sufficient anxiety symptoms to meet DSM-III criteria for agoraphobia, panic disorder, or general anxiety disorder. Conversely, Breier, Charney, and Heninger (1984) found that of 60 adult subjects with either agoraphobia or panic, 68 percent had had a past or current episode of major depression. This figure is almost identical to that detected by Bernstein and Garfinkel (1986), who found that 69 percent of chronic school refusers, an overwhelming majority (62 percent) of whom met criteria for anxiety disorders, also met criteria for some type of affective disorder.

With respect to the prognosis for different affective disorders, the similarities between childhood and adult depression are less clear cut. Each of the disorders studied by Kovacs et al. (1984a) had a different prognosis and clinical course. Utilizing a prospective, longitudinal controlled format, Kovacs et al. (1984a) found that the mean duration of DD was the longest (3 years), with MDD typically lasting 32 weeks and ADDM persisting 25 weeks. A maximal recovery rate of 92 percent for MDD was reached at 1.5 years from onset. Depressed adults, however, appear less resilient. Only half of the adults studied by Keller, Shapiro, Lavori, and Wolfe (1982) recovered from major depression within a year of the episode's onset. By contrast, when Kovacs et al. (1984a) compared the rate of remission of depressive disorders among children of different ages, they found that the rate of remission in MDD, while not affected by the child's sex, was negatively correlated with age. That is, children who were older when a major depression occurred for the first time appeared to recover more rapidly. Similarly, they found that in children with DD, the younger the child at onset, the longer it took for the child to recover. Therefore, in both disorders, the age of onset had a negative correlation to time for recovery. For ADDM, however, age of onset did not relate to time of recovery.

In another trial involving the 133 subjects of the New York Longitudinal Study (NYLS), Chess and Thomas (1984) found, despite the limited sample size, little to support a correlation between age of onset and severity of disease. They identified six children with affective disorders in childhood or adolescence and followed them prospectively for decades. Two were diagnosed as having recurrent MD. Three had DD and one was classified as having ADDM. Semistructured interviews with parents were conducted when the children were 2 to 4 months of age and thereafter at prescribed intervals until the children were 6 to 8 years of age. After 16 years, separate interviews were conducted with the subjects and their parents.

The two cases of MD first showed symptoms at 8 and 12 years, respectively, but both were still diagnosed as MD at their most recent followup interview in early adulthood. Of those with DD, depressive symptoms were first noted at 5, 17, and 16 years of age, respectively. The children whose symptomatology began at 5 and 17 years continued to function poorly, while the child with onset at 16 was diagnosed as having had depressive neurosis and recovered at age 20.

Along these same lines, another study tested the hypothesis that bipolar manic-depressive illness (BMDI) with onset in childhood or adolescence might have a worse prognosis than adult-onset BMDI because early onset may reflect a more severe form of the disease. From a review of 99 cases of adolescent-onset BMDI, Carlson, Davenport, and Jamison (1977) cited 28 BMDI patients having a mean age of onset of 15.8 years that were compared with 20 whose mean onset was 50.6 years. The authors concluded that early onset does not necessarily represent a worse form of the disease. However, Kovacs et al. (1984a,b) and Puig-Antich et al. (1985) found evidence in their studies that early onset of MDD may be associated with higher lifetime morbidity.

Interestingly, results were largely unchanged in cases of multiple diagnoses. The recovery rate of juveniles with MDD superimposed on DD ($N = 16$) was not found to be significantly different from the rate at which juveniles with MDD without DD ($N = 26$) recovered. Likewise, DD subjects with superimposed MDD ($N = 16$) and those without ($N = 12$) were not seen to differ with respect to the accumulative probability of recovery from DD. This marks an important prognostic distinction from the adult form of the syndrome where recovery from MDD superimposed on DD is more likely than from cases where MDD is not superimposed. Keller, Shapiro, Lavori, and Wolfe (1982), for example, found that MDD superimposed on chronic depression remitted faster than cases of MDD alone. (This relationship did not hold, of course, when measuring the remission of both the acute and chronic conditions.) Subjects with DD with superimposed MDD ($N = 16$) or with anxiety disorder ($N = 11$) did not differ from the way subjects with DD recovered when no other disorder was superimposed.

These findings imply that childhood depression is a very heterogeneous disorder. Its basic operation is largely similar to adult depression, but it is, in some respects, also influenced by developmental changes and therefore dissimilar. Kovacs et al. (1984a,b) concluded that the fact that earlier age of onset predicts a more protracted recovery for both MDD and DD invalidates the common belief that depressive episodes in younger children are brief and transient. However, all the data in the literature do not agree regarding this point, and data such as those of Freeman, Poznanski, Grossman,

Buschbaum, and Banegas (1985) and Carlson (1983), which run counter to this argument, continue to appear with a frequency that cannot be ignored. This conflict has led to the investigation of biological markers in children to see if and how they compare with those found in adults. Clearly the adult model of childhood depression would gain further credence if adults and children were found to share the same markers.

PHYSIOLOGICAL MARKERS FOR DEPRESSION

Several researchers (Lowe & Cohen, 1980; Puig-Antich, 1986) have attempted to isolate biological correlates to depression. These "markers" differentiate and identify depressed patients, or people at risk for depression. Puig-Antich (1986) defines biological markers as "characteristics that have been shown to be specifically associated with the disorder in question, during an episode, during the symptom-free intervals, or both" (p. 342).

With this definition in mind, biological markers can be differentiated as "state markers," which are associated only with the active period of the disorder, or "trait markers," which are associated with the patient throughout his lifetime. State markers show abnormalities with the onset of the disorder and subside during symptom-free periods. True trait markers are measures that are persistently abnormal even in fully recovered patients, and usually predate the first appearance of the disorder. Future editions of the *Diagnostic and Statistical Manual of Mental Disorders* should incorporate trait markers, to aid in diagnosis between pathological episodes.

The prominent biological markers for affective disorders in adults include a group of endocrine metabolite and sleep EEG abnormalities relating to central nervous system functions. Biogenic amines such as dopamine, norepinephrine, and serotonin serve hormonal functions in the regulation of neurotransmitter operations. These amines and their metabolites appear in abnormal quantities in depressed adult patients (Carroll, 1983; Schildkraut, 1965). Markers can show changes in circadian rhythm of secretion, amount of secretion, and basal levels. Whether these same alterations in neuroendocrine response and sleep patterns appear in depressed children, thus indicating a further resemblance between the childhood disorder and the adult model, remains to be documented.

Metabolite Studies

McKnew and Cytryn (1979) conducted one of the first investigations into biological markers of depression in children. They analyzed the urinary excretion of 30 methoxy 4-hydroxy-phenyl-glycol (MHPG), norepinephrine, and vanilly mandelic acid (VMA) in 9 children suffering from a chronic depressive reaction and in 18 normal control subjects. The depressed children excreted significantly less MHPG than the control subjects, but there were no major differences in norepinephrine or VMA excretion. This contrasts with the findings for clinically depressed adults, whose MHPG secretion is usually found to be abnormal—higher than average in some groups and lower than normal in others. In one subgroup of bipolar manic-depressives, MHPG levels increased during the manic phase and decreased during the depressed phase of the disorder (Lowe & Cohen, 1980).

Cortisol Secretion

Plasma cortisol, a hormone secreted by the adrenal cortex, has been shown to be hypersecreted in adults with affective disorders. A concrete example of the elusive nature of age-specific features in depression is revealed in Cantwell's (1983a) review of childhood depression. Cantwell noted that approximately 50 percent of melancholic adults with major depressive disorder show hypersecretion of cortisol during the acute phase of their illness. However, when children and adults with major depressive disorder of the melancholic type are compared, only about half as many children as adults hypersecrete cortisol. Cantwell points out that the reason for this finding may be the presence of an age effect, and the presence of subtypes among children with regard to their tendency to secrete cortisol. This was demonstrated by measurement of the plasma cortisol levels of four prepubertal children who met requirements for endogenous depression (Puig-Antich et al., 1979). In two of the four subjects, cortisol hypersecretion was documented during the depressive episode, and the levels were reduced on clinical recovery. Furthermore, Puig-Antich, Novacenko, Goetz, Corser, Davies, and Ryan (1984) studied the cortisol and prolactin responses to insulin-induced hypoglycemia through the use of the insulin tolerance test (ITT). Both during the depressive episode and on full recovery these levels remained unchanged in both the depressed children and in those children with neurotic disorders. However, cortisol levels were seen to be higher in the endogenous depressive subgroup. With regard to these observations, Puig-Antich (1986) suggests that the contrast between plasma cortisol levels in depressives and nondepressives becomes more significant with age, and is not a significant marker in prepubertal patients.

Dexamethasone Suppression Test

The Dexamethasone Suppression Test (DST) has provided one useful, although not uniformly reliable, means of measuring the cortisol levels associated with depression. When dexamethasone is administered to patients with affective disorders, suppression of cortisol levels fails, due to the dysregulated secretion of this steroid. Depressed patients "escape" from the effects of dexamethasone earlier than nondepressed subjects for whom the presence of dexamethesone normally suppresses cortisol production for 24 hours. According to Puig-Antich (1986), this pattern of cortisol hypersecretion occurs only during a depressive episode and returns to normal on recovery, thus making it a state rather than trait marker.

Typically dexamethasone is administered orally by tablet at 11 PM. On the following day, blood samples are extracted and tested at 4 and 11 PM, or several times throughout the day. If an elevated level of plasma cortisol is measured in any of the samples, an abnormal, or positive, test result is said to occur (Carroll, 1983). While this test has proven to have clinical value in adults, it may be of even greater specificity in children, particularly preadolescents, who do not typically develop certain conditions, such as alcoholism, anorexia nervosa, bulimia, and opiate addiction, which also cause cortisol nonsuppression and therefore make the DST unreliable in certain adults (Dackis et al., 1983; Edelstein et al., 1983; Hudson et al., 1982; Swartz & Dunner, 1982).

Carroll et al. (1981, 1982 in Lingjaerde, 1983) have found that nonsuppression of cortisol in adults occurs in approximately 67 percent of patients with endogenous depression and in 4 percent of patients with nonendogenous depression and other psychiatric disorders. These results show a sensitivity (percentage of people correctly identified by the test as having the disorder) of 67 percent and a specificity (percentage of people correctly identified as not having the disorder) of 96 percent for this test (Lingjaerde, 1983).

The DST has not been used as extensively with children as with adults. Based on the available evidence, it is somewhat difficult to evaluate whether the test provides a comparable level (i.e., between adults and children) of discrimination between depressed and nondepressed individuals (and between different subtypes of depression) and ultimately whether neuroendocrine markers validate the adult model approach. It is known that, at least among adults, the DST shows some age sensitivity, with abnormal findings increasing, although not linearly, with age (Feinberg & Carroll, 1984). Whether there is a comparable developmental trend in children is not yet known. Most studies have examined the DST's discriminatory power on a very global level for children, and have overlooked developmental considerations. Freeman et al. (1985) recently reported cross-sectional and longitudinal assessments of six children between 6 and 12 years of age who were diagnosed as both psychotic and depressed. A diagnosis of depression was based on administration of semistructured parent and child interviews and the Schedule for Affective Disorders and Schizophrenia for School Aged Children (K-SADS; Chambers, Puig-Antich, & Tabrizi, 1978). Dexamethasone suppression tests were given to five of the six children. Of these, four showed positive results.

The ability of the DST to discriminate among different subtypes of depression has also been shown to be somewhat comparable for children and adults. These results further support the notion of childhood depression (or perhaps, more accurately, childhood depressions) as analogous to adult depression. Dexamethasone suppression tests administered to a group of 30 children, aged 5 to 12 years, were able to differentiate between those children with major depressive disorder, dysthymia, and two control groups, those "definitely not depressed" and those with dysphoric mood (Petty et al., 1985). Among adults, the test can discriminate between endogenous and nonendogenous depression (Feinberg & Carroll, 1984).

While the DST differentiates better for unipolar than bipolar endogenous depression (the latter condition still being rare in childhood), its sensitivity and specificity are sufficiently high to warrant its continued use and refinement. This seems true for use in preadolescents, who lack many confounding conditions that may also lead to cortisol hypersecretion (Trad, 1986).

TRH-TSH Test

An abnormal DST result is considered to indicate a disinhibition of the limbic hypothalamo-pituitary-adrenal (HPA) axis (Carroll, 1983). Another test, the TRH-TSH (thyrotropin releasing hormone-thyroid stimulating hormone), also provides a measure of limbic regulation, in this case along the pituitary-thyroid axis (Lingjaerde, 1983). This test measures serum thyrotropin response after a test dose of thyrotropin-releasing hormone (TRH). Baseline measures of serum TSH are taken prior to an intravenous injection of TRH. More samples are then taken over the next two hours (Loosen & Prange, 1982, in Lingjaerde, 1983). Normally a marked increase in TSH occurs, peaking 30 minutes after injection.

A blunted TSH response has been measured in many patients (approximately 25%) with primary endogenous depression. However, as in the DST, blunted responses have also been noted in patients with alcoholism and anorexia nervosa—again, a consideration that may make these tests of greater value or specificity in preadolescents (Loosen & Prange, 1982, in Lingjaerde, 1983).

Neither the DST nor the TRH-TSH differentiates between unipolar and bipolar endogenous depression, but a blunted TSH response, unlike nonsuppression in the DST, sometimes carries over into remission. This suggests that while abnormal DST is largely state dependent, blunted TSH response may be more trait dependent. In terms of the mechanism of action, a deficiency of norepinephrine has been implicated in the abnormal responses to the TRH-TSH and DST alike (Lingjaerde, 1983).

Growth Hormone

Atypical secretions of growth hormone (GH), another biological marker, have been detected in depressed children. Puig-Antich et al. (1984a) compared 10 children with the melancholic subtype of major depressive disorder to 10 children with major depression, nonmelancholic subtype, and 7 nondepressed children with other emotional disorders. There were significantly different levels of plasma GH concentrations between groups at 30, 45, and 60 minutes after insulin injection. All differences were seen to be related to the fact that those with the melancholic subtype of major depression produced elevated amounts of GH.

During the depressive episode, the secretion of GH was increased during sleep and was decreased in response to insulin-induced hypoglycemia (ITT; Puig-Antich, Tabrizi, Davies, Goetz, Chambers, Halpern, & Sachar, 1981; Puig-Antich et al., 1984). The level of nonresponse to insulin is apparently similar for children and adults as revealed in the studies of Puig-Antich et al. (1984) and Lewis et al. (1983). Puig-Antich et al. (1984) compared the GH response to ITT in 46 drug-free prepubertal children from 6 to 12 years of age. Thirteen children met unmodified Research Diagnostic Criteria (RDC; Spitzer, Endicott, & Robbins, 1978) for definite endogenous MDD subtype, 17 children met RDC for nonendogenous MDD, and 16 met DSM-III criteria for nondepressed neurotic disorders (separation anxiety, phobia, obsessive compulsive, or overanxious) without a history of minor or major depression or persistent depressed mood. Three baseline samples before and 8 consecutive samples after insulin injection (every 15 minutes) were obtained. Findings showed that low GH response to ITT identified 13 or 14 (43%) (depending on the cutoff level of GH hyposecretion used) of 30 prepubertal children with MDD. In Lewis et al., 40 percent of those children with pure major depressive disorder (as distinguished from bipolar disorder or depressive spectrum disease) exhibited nonresponse to insulin.

Different responses to ITT among different subtypes of depressives—a marker that has been demonstrated for certain subtypes of adult depression (Lewis et al., 1983)—have also been noted. A peak GH plasma concentration of 3.5 nanograms per millimeter or less during the first 60-minute post-insulin injections showed maximal discrimination in the Puig-Antich et al. (1984a) study. The use of this single criterion positively identified 62 percent of 13 children with endogenous MDD, 35 percent of 17 with nonendogenous MDD, and 13 percent of 16 neurotic subjects. Thus GH response to ITT seems to be approximately two-thirds sensitive for endogenous depression, and positively identifies about one third of those with depressive disorder, with an 87 to 94 percent specificity for nondepressed children with emotional disorders. These findings indicate that GH blunting during ITT is a biological marker specific to endogenous MDD in prepubertal children.

Whether GH levels are state or trait markers is still unclear. In Puig-Antich et al. (1984), although depressive prepubertal groups secreted significantly higher amounts of GH during sleep than did nondepressed neurotic or normal children, increases in GH concentrations in the depressive groups have not been positively linked to depressive episodes. The study included 71 prepubertal children (22 with endogenous MDD, 20 with nonendogenous MDD, 21 with nondepressed neurotic disorders, and 8 normal). Findings from this study leave open the question as to whether the increase in GH was a residual of a previous episode or a true trait marker.

Puig-Antich et al. (1984) have attempted to shed some light on the pattern of response as related to depressive episodes. They reported that both findings persisted in prepubertal major depressive patients after at least 4 months of sustained clinical recovery and at least 1 drug-free month. In this study they examined GH response to ITT in 18 drug-free prepubertal children who had at least 4 months of sustained recovery from an episode of MDD (11 subjects had definite endogenous subtype). These responses were compared to those found in a control group of 16 prepubertal children with nondepressed neurotic disorders. Findings from this study indicated that the prepubertal subjects with a past episode of endogenous MDD continued to have significant hyposecretion of GH when compared with the control group. Blunted GH response to ITT might be a marker of a past episode or a true trait marker for endogenous MDD.

Prospective studies of prepubertal offspring at risk for the development of depressive illness, as well as continuous follow-up of these patients over time, are needed to further elucidate this possibility. In any event, the degree of blunting of GH to ITT seems to be most pronounced in the endogenous subtype, which suggests an abnormal endocrine function in prepubertal children with a past episode of MDD. This abnormality may change in the course of development. In a recent examination of ongoing studies of GH concentration in adolescent depressives, Puig-Antich (1986) states that while prepubertal major depressives hypersecrete GH during sleep, adolescent and adult major depressives tend to hyposecrete GH during sleep. This suggests that the effect of major depression on GH secretion is reversed during puberty.

Sleep EEG Studies

Several researchers report findings that adult major depressives show decreased first rapid eye movement period (REMp) latency, decreased slow-wave sleep time, increased REMp density, decreased sleep efficiency, and abnormal temporal distribution of REMp (Kerkhofs et al., 1985). None of these markers was found to be consistently associated with depressive episodes in prepubertal children (Puig-Antich et al., 1984a). Puig-Antich attributes this lack of direct correlation to the influence of age on sleep EEGs. However, Puig-Antich and associates (1982) did find sleep EEGs to be trait markers in recovered prepubertal depressives. These researchers found 28 fully recovered, drug-free, prepubertal patients with major depressive disorders to have highly significant shortening of the first (REMp) latencies, and a higher number of REMps compared to themselves when depressed, and to nondepressed normal and neurotic children. The authors suggested that these findings might be markers of a past episode or a trait in prepubertal major depressives before a depressive episode is developed. These findings are consistent with findings of most adult patients compared during periods of depression and remission.

Summary

Children share many of the biological markers that are useful for the diagnosis of depression in adults, but the direction and specificity of biological abnormalities may differ in different age groups. Abnormalities in MHPG and cortisol secretion are found among both children and adults, but the efficacy of the cortisol response to the DST and the ITT for children remains unclear. The TRH-TSH test, however, may prove more useful in children than adults, due to the lack of complicating syndromes. Hypersecretion of GH is likely to prove a valid trait marker for depressive disorders in children, although the response is reversed in adolescent and adult depressives, who tend to hyposecrete GH during sleep. Due to developmental effects, sleep EEG studies of depressed children have shown only few direct correlations with those of adult depressives.

PSYCHOSOCIAL STRESSORS AND DEPRESSION IN CHILDHOOD

Diagnosis according to DSM-III requires assessment on five different axes:

   I. Clinical syndromes
  II. Personality disorders
 III. Physical disorders and conditions
  IV. Psychosocial stressors
   V. Level of adaptive functioning

Axes I and II have already been addressed in discussion of the growth of the syndromal approach to childhood depression. But the developmental experience of the child can be more effectively incorporated into diagnosis and treatment by using axes IV and V in addition to the primary diagnosis.

This synthesis allows the clinician to differentiate the way in which developmental adaptation takes place in the face of a psychosocial challenge. It also helps to qualify the expected (i.e., congruent) or unexpected (i.e., incongruent) socioemotional responses during specific developmental epochs within the life of the child. By utilizing all the elements of the diagnostic armamentarium we will be able to delineate more clearly the more adaptive from the pathological manifestations in the child.

Psychosocial stressors for children center mainly on the behavior of significant adults. Such stressors have slightly different implications for children than they have for adults. This notion was examined in several studies. Poznanski and Zrull (1970) found that the families of depressed children are marked by a high rate of mental discord and parental depression, and that the parents themselves are often rejecting, hostile, and suffering from various personality problems.

Similarly, Brumback, Dietz-Schmidt, and Weinberg (1977) found a history of affective disorder, especially with the mother, in 89 percent of the families of those depressed children studied. Puig-Antich et al. (1979) found serious family discord or mistreatment of children in 11 out of 13 cases of depressed children and a family history of psychiatric disorder in 61 percent of the relatives of their index children. An equally compelling figure was reported by Freeman et al. (1985). Among six children diagnosed as both psychotic and depressed, there was only one child whose parents did not have either affective or alcohol and/or substance abuse disorders.

The predominant response to caregiver depression was passive or active depression, and the response to caregiver disability was outwardly directed aggression or passivity and withdrawal, according to the observations of Philips (1979). A disruptive, hostile, and generally negative environment is associated with depression in both the parent and child, and is also associated with children who might become or remain depressed as adults.

A LEARNED HELPLESSNESS MODEL FOR CHILDHOOD DEPRESSION

Difficulties in diagnosing depression in infants and children may be related to the serious shortage of studies describing the nature of the changes in self-understanding during development (Brim, 1976). This shortage in turn may be related to the fact that research on the development of self-concept has been largely limited to assessing self-esteem in children (Damon & Hart, 1982). Such an approach stems from the fact that self-esteem can be measured more accurately than the more general concept of self-understanding. Studies attempting to correlate self-esteem to interpersonal relations, achievement, and other factors have not yielded compelling results (Wylie, 1979).

This section proposes an alternative developmental pathway for understanding childhood depression—learned helplessness. The learned helplessness model suggests that depression can be induced from environmental factors, that the repeated experience of negative affect can result in depression identical to endogenous depression. Learned helplessness involves an acquired perception of lack of control over events in an individual's environment. This has been shown to be a function of the individual's sense of self—that is, his or her ability to reflect accurately on the impact of his or her interactions with the environment—as well as of his or her general concepts of causality. Various researchers have suggested that full-fledged depression or depressive-like phenomena cannot exist before the development of a sense of self. Indeed, Seligman (1975) and Abramson, Seligman, and Teasdale (1978) have noted that learned helplessness depression cannot occur without the element of negative self-esteem which presupposes some basic sense of self.

Both the development of the self and the development of concepts of causality have proven sensitive to developmental status and converge in a mutually, although not necessarily symmetrically, reinforcing system (Trad, 1986). The overall concept of causality affects many aspects of the self and, to a lesser but not insignificant extent, the self affects notions about causality. Since these factors are critical to an understanding of how learned helplessness arises, we will explore each separately before turning to a discussion of their convergence in depression.

Development of Self

Lewis and Brooks-Gunn (1979) postulated a developmental sequence in which affective and cognitive development coalesce, by the age of 24 months, to produce a self that is capable of self-representation. Within the schema of these researchers, self-development may be delineated along a four-stage model. From birth to 3 months, infant response is geared to biological control and is primarily reflexive. Between 4 and 8 months, social activity emerges and, with it, a biological control over behavior becomes evident. Lewis and Brooks-Gunn observed that by the first year of life the infant has emerged as a truly social organism. During the crucial juncture between 12 and 24 months, the repertoire of emotional expression enlarges dramatically, as does the capacity for cognitive skill. Responses suggestive of empathy, self-representation, and symbolic representation become apparent through the infant's behaviors.

Piaget (1952, 1954) also discussed self-development, both implicitly and explicitly, in his writings on cognitive development. He defined four demarcation periods pertaining to cognitive maturation: sensory-motor, preoperational, concrete operational, and formal operational. External behavioral manifestations at the end of the sensory-motor period (2 years of age) indicate the acquisition of object permanence.

Bertenthal and Fischer (1978) were able to recognize a pattern underlying the development of self-recognition and object permanence. By 24 months, infants were able to identify themselves by reciting their own names in response to the query "Who's that?" when facing themselves in a mirror.

Emde (1984) concurred with these observations that the self coalesces by the end of the second year of life. He noted that dimensions of this concept include a sense of continuity over time and space, a differential identification of the self-image, and verbal self-expression through use of pronouns. Emde also suggested that during the second to third year, children's sense of continuity and stability becomes more entrenched in their internal self-schema, with such qualities being reflected in capacities of self-awareness, self-consciousness, symbolic play, advanced cognitive abilities (including development of a sense of causality), socialization of affect, and organization of inner states. Combined, these qualities or ingredients become part of the dynamic process of self-development and are components of the self.

Emde's theories are consistent with the work of Mahler, Pine, and Bergman (1975), who described the growth of the self as a process of individuation from the environment. Mahler distinguishes three stages in the journey from birth to complete individuation: autism, symbiosis, and separation-individuation. During the autistic stage, the infant does not differentiate between itself and the environment. During the symbiotic stage, the infant has gained an awareness of the environment, but is not differentiated from the caregiver. In the final stage, the infant comes to possess a sufficient sense of separateness from the mother to have a stable mental representation of her as a separate person. During this stage, usually between the ages of 16 and 24 months, the child will go through a period of increased risk for depression, when the internal representation of the mother is still fragile. At this time, called the "rapprochement" subphase of the separation-individuation period, the child may be subject to new feelings of separateness and aloneness. When the representation of self and mother as separate, continuous entities solidifies, this risk diminishes.

Between the ages of 3 to 5 years, the child's sense of self is most dramatically expressed through activity, and in fact, children of this age conceive of themselves in terms of an action, rather than a body-image concept (Keller et al., 1978). Broughton (1978) noted that during the early years of childhood, this physical concept of self dominates. However, at approximately the age of 6 years, children express comprehension that inner psychological reality differs from physical reality. By the age of 8 years, the distinction between internal and external reality becomes more sharply defined, as the child begins to understand that the self can be the object of its own reflection and of independent behavior. A full-fledged sense of self emerges with adolescence, during which, as Selman (1980) wrote, self-reflection permits the individual to comprehend that he or she can exert some degree of control over behavior.

Implicit within all of the developmental stages outlined above is a variety of mechanisms that propel the emergence of the self-concept. One is empathic signals from the environment. Kagan (1981, 1982, 1984) notes that the orchestration of empathic signals emitted by the caregiver and directed toward the infant represents a behavioral prerequisite for the infant's ability to distinguish later between external and internal realities. Kagan has reported that when infants receive sufficient positive affective cues and responses from their caregivers, their response is displayed through smiles of mastery. Such smiles, which peak between 19 and 25 months, suggest that infants are endowed with an innate mechanism designed to set goals and to attain mastery over such goals.

Central to Kagan's (1981,1982,1984) observations is the notion that the relationship between caregiver and infant is vital for the development of the infant's incipient sense of self. It should be noted at this point that Kagan's notions about the relationship between infant and caregiver are predicated on the idea that a coherent, sustained attachment bond is essential for the normal development of the self. Moreover, it has been shown that the attachment bond is constructed through early infant-caregiver interactions (Ainsworth, 1973). In turn, these social interactions (mirroring, affect attunement, empathy) are affected by each partner's temperamental rhythms. Thus both temperament and attachment are vital to the infant's early maturation and subsequent development of a sense of self.

Self-esteem, the individual's personal assessment of worthiness, may thus have its roots in early interactions between infant and caregiver (Harter, 1983). Returning to Kagan's notion of smiles of mastery, it may be argued that such smiles, external manifestations of a sense of accomplishment, may represent the earliest evidence of a positive sense of self-esteem.

A developmental framework which enables researchers to view the spectrum of maturation from infancy through adolescence and beyond provides a distinct sequence of normative development. The self develops as a concept by approximately the second year of life and signifies a coalescence of such factors as infant and caregiver temperaments and infant and caregiver attachment bonds. Additionally, mechanisms of response pertaining to the self begin to emerge during this period and assume prominence during the early years of childhood. Such mechanisms include self-regulatory and control capacities, and self-esteem and self-attributional dimensions.

Regulation Versus Dysregulation in Children at Risk for Affective Disorder. Since affect regulation is a critical mechanism necessary for the development of the self, we may infer that if an infant or child exhibits dysregulation with regard to affective states, this faulty mechanism of response will be incorporated into his or her developing sense of self. Thus it becomes significant to include the full ramifications of affective regulation and modulation in any discussion of self-development.

Kopp (1982) has pinpointed the ability to regulate one's behavior as an integral component of the development of the self. In her schema, the growth of object- and self-representation is paralleled by an increased ability to control the self and the environment. This regulatory capacity derives from the growth of cognitive skills and affective responses, which are, in turn, primarily reflective of the role played by caregivers. The rhythms of exchange between infant and caregiver expand the infant's repertoire of responses, which become the building blocks for the developing self. Kopp identifies five stages in the development of self-regulation, beginning with the infant's control of waking and arousal states and culminating in regulation of behavior based on an awareness of self and others as individuals.

The role of regulation in the development of the self and in the sustaining of a mature self has been commented on by other researchers as well. Bandura (1978) noted that adult behavior involves a continuous reciprocal interaction between behavioral, cognitive, and environmental influences, which reveals the self-regulatory processes engaged in by individuals. Harter (1983) has also written extensively on the development of the self and self-regulation. For example, she notes that the development of the self has traditionally been conceptualized as emerging from interaction. Once again, the underlying notion is that interaction—implicitly with the caregiver during the primal dyadic relationship—is crucial to the emergence of a normative sense of self. Harter also observes that self-control is an essential element of a healthy sense of self. Self-control, as reviewed by Harter (Harter, 1983, pp. 339-366), includes the organism's possession of an internal organization capable of avoiding or minimizing anxiety and of enhancing gratification. Self-control appears, therefore, to be similar to self-regulation.

Regardless of which factors are thought to precipitate affective displays, however, it seems clear that infants and children of parents with affective disorders characteristically regulate differently from children whose parents are emotionally healthy. With regard to regulation, three key studies investigated young children of parents suffering from affective disorders and found that such children exhibited distinctive difficulty in regulating affective states (Gaensbauer et al., 1984c; Radke-Yarrow, Cummings, Kuczynski, & Chapman, 1985; Zahn-Waxler et al., 1984).

In the Gaensbauer (1984c) study, the authors observed infants longitudinally from 12 to 18 months. Attachment and affiliative response was measured by laboratory investigations during which the infants were exposed to a series of stressors combining separation from the mother and from objects with which the infant was playing. It was found that during such stressor episodes children of affectively ill parents, in contrast to a control group of children, displayed aberrant and unexpected affective responses that were out of synchrony with the situation. For example, at 12 months of age, such children exhibited more fear than control infants in situations such as free play and reunion with the mother; situations in which one would normally expect the infants to experience less negative affect. Also these children exhibited less fear in situations where more would be expected (i.e., during brief maternal separation) at 15 months. The researchers postulated, as a result of this finding, that children of depressed parents may prolong the experience and expression of affect and may thus respond with slow recovery time from a disruptive emotion. The children's affective response is not only muted but also less flexible. Gaensbauer et al. (1984c) state:

> *Affectively, the proband infants appeared to be showing a generalized disturbance in their capacities to adaptively regulate their emotions involving a number of different affects and different contexts. (p. 228)*

Zahn-Waxler et al. (1984) examined a group of two-year-old children, some the offspring of bipolar parents, to assess social functioning in children of parents with affective disorders. They found that by 2 years of age, these "at risk" infants encountered difficulties in their interpersonal interactions and appeared easily overcome by obstacles. In a study of two and three-year-old children of mothers with affective disorders, Radke-Yarrow et al. (1985) found insecure attachments (avoidant, resistant, and A/C—mixtures of avoidant and resistant—categories) more common among children of depressed parents than control families.

Locus-of-Control Beliefs. Expressions of hopelessness and worthlessness as aspects of self-concept are common among adult depressives. These self-descriptions, which tap, in part, an individual's perceptions of who or what controls the outcome of events, may take special form in childhood. Such perceptions may be loosely referred to as locus-of-control beliefs. Seligman (1975) distinguished between two types of locus-of-control beliefs, internal and external. He observed that a person with an internal locus of control perceives that he or she can exert sufficient control over events to master the environment. Such an individual, in other words, is motivated to employ personal skill to overcome a problematic situation. An individual with external locus of control perceives outcomes as being the result of chance, luck, or forces beyond his or her control. How each of these locus-of-control beliefs may engender a depressive response is not a function of externality or internality alone, but instead a combined function of the locus-of-control and the nature—positive or negative—of the environmental event. The strongest predictive validity for depressive affect has been demonstrated with the combination of an internal locus of control and negative events (Seligman & Peterson, 1986).

ATTRIBUTIONAL STYLE.   Individual variations in locus-of-control beliefs are captured operationally in what has been called attributional style. What is significant, particularly from a developmental psychopathology perspective, is that a depressive attributional style, in certain environments, may be as much a function of normal as of pathological development in causal understanding.

Kun (1977), for example, examined the logical structures with which children and adults related the causes of success or failure. In children aged 5 to 6 years, Kun identified a "magnitude co-variation" schema, in which degree of success at a given task was perceived as being positively related to a change in the degree of a facilitative factor endogenous to the individual—either ability or effort—but did not incorporate exogenous inhibitory factors such as the idea of task difficulty. Kun's conception is closely related to an attributional schema developed by Nicholls (1978) and labeled the "halo" schema. According to Nicholls, young children at this age believe that a positive outcome is directly attributable to both effort and ability. In this conception, greater effort is associated with greater ability. Kun also identified a direct "compensation" schema, developing in children between the ages of 6 and 9. Children of this age are able to perceive that either ability or effort will affect the outcome of the task. Finally, among children over age 9 and predominating among adolescents, Kun identified a cognitive attributional style which she labeled "inverse compensation." Under this schema, subjects perceived that high ability can compensate for a lack of effort and high effort can compensate for a lack of ability.

Nicholls and Miller (1985) conducted further investigations into causal schema which enabled them to disclose that among young children under 6 years of age, the concepts of luck and skill are not differentiated. With age, these two concepts do in fact diverge, so that by adolescence, the split between an outcome attributable to luck factors and one attributable to skill factors is readily apparent.

Thus a child's developmental status may lead to certain inaccuracies in the child's perceptions of his or her role in a situation. Nondepressed children typically attribute positive outcomes to internal causes and negative outcomes to external factors, inconsistent as this may seem. Depressed children, on the other hand, do not make such a distinction; thus they risk self-esteem deficits (Seligman & Peterson, 1986). If children wrongly attribute authorship of an event, particularly one with an unpleasant outcome, to themselves, they may be vulnerable to negative affect. Most child psychiatrists are familiar with the situation of a child who has wished or fantasized that some adult die or become ill. When this adult coincidentally falls ill or dies within a relatively short period of time, the child is often overcome with guilt, genuinely believing that he or she caused the event. The pathogenic factor is the attribution of bad events to internal causes. The stability and the globality of the internal causes will predict the pervasiveness of the learned helplessness. We shall see other examples of this in the chapters on populations at risk in which children faced with certain adaptive demands at different stages in their development may display an inaccurate, yet to some extent developmentally expected, perception of their contribution to the event.

ILLUSIONS OF CONTROL AND ILLUSORY CONTINGENCY.   One specific developmental progression that may be most significant for understanding how certain children's evolving concepts of causality may predispose them to depression concerns phenomena known as illusions of control and illusory contingency. These are naturally occurring phenomena whereby young children have been shown to assume more responsibility for the outcome of events than is objectively warranted. Thus in environments that are consistently negative, the natural progression in children's causal understanding may induce them to accept responsibility that is unrealistic. Guilt and self-reproach may ensue (Trad, 1986).

Piaget (1930) was one of the first researchers to report on the phenomenon of illusions of control, when he observed that children younger than 6 or 7 years of age evince an illusion or fantasy that they can, in fact, exert control over objectively uncontrollable events. Langer (1975) further investigated the concept of illusions of control, defining the concept as the expectancy of personal success being inappropriately higher than the objective dimensions of a situation would warrant. Weisz (1980) points out that control over an outcome requires that (1) the outcome must be contingent on a person's behavior, and (2) the individual must be competent to produce the required outcome. The illusion of control is a misperception of both the nature of contingency and the level of personal competence. In infants, this phenomenon may result from insufficient differentiation between self and environment, when the infant fails to distinguish between its desires and external events. Illusory contingency is a mistaken perception regarding the nature of causality regarding an event or class of events. The individual mistakes an externally caused event for one within the realm of personal or another's control, or denies the level of control that is available to him or her.

Weisz (1980) explored the concept of illusory contingency within the context of a card game experiment involving kindergartners and fourth graders. Experimenters drew cards blindly and randomly from a shuffled deck of cards. Children were told that each time a yellow chip was drawn they would win. Children were then asked to predict winnings of other children who differed from them in age, intelligence, effort, and previous practice. Objectively, winning was a purely random event, but the younger children displayed more illusory contingencies by predicating the chance of winning on age, intelligence, or effort. Children under the age of 8 years appeared incapable of cognitively integrating the notion that success could be a random occurrence; instead, there appeared to be a need to attribute outcome to some controllable identifiable factor.

Learned Helplessness in Children

Now that this preliminary outline of development has been provided, it is appropriate to broach the issue of how impairment in the development of the self-concept or schematic phenomena associated with the self can result in childhood depression. According to the learned helplessness model, the organism perceives events to be uncontrollable and beyond mastery (Abramson, Seligman, & Teasdale, 1978). Feelings of uncontrollability lead to high levels of anxiety, which are in turn neutralized by depression, along with its concomitant feelings of helplessness. The depressive affect serves to allay the anxiety, but at the same time, reinforces feelings of helplessness and the sense that events are beyond mastery.

This model may apply to childhood depression as early as the first months of life. As discussed earlier, temperament and attachment factors are integrated to define the characteristics of the early infant-caregiver relationship. If the caregiver misperceives the infant's temperamental cues or is, for some reason, incapable of establishing a sufficiently harmonious relationship, the infant is likely to experience the negative affect associated with deprivation. Moreover, such an infant probably fails to receive adequate positive reinforcement, along with its concomitant positive affect. As noted earlier, negative affect correlates with negative self-attribution, while positive affect correlates with positive self-attribution.

If the self-concept of a child who has experienced a high degree of negative affect is considered contaminated from the start, by 2 years of age, when the sense of self coalesces into a coherent concept, such a child may already be vulnerable to depression. Subsequently, this child will inevitably develop the cognitive schemata of illusions of control, illusory contingencies, attributional schema, and impaired locus of control. Unlike children whose development is normative, the deprived child may experience these phenomenologic states as exacerbating his or her already vulnerable sense of self.

While illusions of control may provide a child who has experienced sufficient gratification from the caregiver with feelings of mastery, the deprived child undergoing the experience of illusions of control will emerge increasingly more debilitated. Such a child may come to perceive events as being completely beyond his or her control, and thus may be described as having an external locus of control, with increasing susceptibility to learned-helplessness depression. The child may possess an equally debilitating internal locus of control, but may perceive himself or herself as the cause of negative outcome. Such a child will engage in a high degree of negative self-attribution.

It is still not clear, however, which factors other than development will determine whether the child forms external locus-of-control beliefs or internal explanations for negative outcomes. The mechanisms of development embodied within the concept of self discussed earlier, including self-control and self-regulation, may also play a part in determining whether a child will become vulnerable to learned-helplessness depression. The caregiver who provides sufficient experiences of contingency and affect attunement for the infant may be additionally instilling in the child the capacity to self-regulate and modulate between variant affective states. In contrast, a caregiver who fails to engage in sufficient intersubjective interaction with the infant may be preventing the child from developing the necessary flexibility to modulate different affective states. By early childhood, such a child has, in effect, become handicapped in his or her abilities to control the environment. For such children, illusions of control and illusory contingencies, rather than serving the purpose of immunizing the child from experiencing failure, with its concomitant negative affect, serve to exacerbate the child's feeling of helplessness by convincing him or her that either he or she is responsible for the failure, or that failure is an inevitable occurrence beyond his or her control.

Substantiation for learned helplessness has come in many forms: studies of animals, studies of adults and, most recently, studies of children (Seligman & Peterson, 1986). One particularly important confirmation involves evidence of neuroendocrine correlates to learned-helplessness depression (Weiss, Glazer, Pohorecky, Bailey, & Schneider, 1979). In these studies, rats that were confronted with a series of inescapable shocks showed lowered levels of norepinephrine (NE) compared with control rats that received no shocks. Rats that were given shocks but were able to find a way to escape showed higher NE levels than controls. Weiss et al. theorized that the rats that experienced shock overproduced NE to the degree that the regulatory system eventually failed, leaving the rats unable to cope with further shocks. Learned helplessness in infants and children may follow a similar path of neuroendocrine dysregulation (Trad, 1986).

SUMMARY

In review, the concept of childhood depression can be observed as having evolved sequentially through four primary schools of thought. Each school of thought has created its own methodology to prove or disprove evidence for depression in childhood.

The first school of thought, the developmental symptomatology argument, denied the existence of childhood depression. The second school of thought, the "depressive equivalents" argument, established the idea that childhood depression did exist but with "depressive equivalents." The third school of thought, an epidemiological approach, accepted childhood depression as a separate and distinct clinical entity and rejected the idea of "depressive equivalents." This school adopted an epidemiological approach, looking for a single factor of causation. The fourth school accepted the idea of childhood depression, rejected the concept of equivalents, and suggested that childhood depression is analogous to depression as it is found in adults and that a multifactorial approach is needed for the diagnosis of both.

The continuity of depressive manifestations over time still needs to be verified through longitudinal studies of patients from infancy through adulthood. The presumption that long-term subclinical affective disorders that have their onsets during childhood continue into the early years to adulthood has yet to be verified. One theoretical model that would help test this hypothesis is the phenomenon of learned helplessness. The repeated experience of failure or low self-esteem in infancy and childhood may lead to feelings of helplessness and hopelessness. Such learned helplessness may easily continue into adulthood and contribute to a depressive state (Seligman & Peterson, 1986).

There is another, more fundamental puzzle for which any diagnostic school of thought must provide a solution. It is necessary to make the distinction between sadness and depression. Feelings of sadness derive from an internal or external loss, whereas depressive feelings encompass dejection, helplessness, and hopelessness that may or may not result from a real or perceived loss (Furman, 1984). It is an important task to distinguish between the affect, the dysphoric mood, and the syndrome of depression and to factor out the different causes for each.

To achieve a resolution to these and other problems, future research must be designed to take into account not only the developmental context, but the extreme heterogeneity of depression itself. Quantitative and qualitative comparisons are needed of the various subgroups with multiple diagnoses. An examination of similarities and differences may lead to the identification of child groups that present identically to adult depression and of other child groups whose members are completely different from adults in the way they express depression. Currently, DSM-III offers only the adult model for both childhood and adult depression.

One area that holds great promise for determining the appropriateness of DSM-III classification of depression is psychoendocrinology. Specifically, it may prove feasible to relate aspects of the dysregulation hypothesis of affective disorders to observed changes in temperament over time from infancy to childhood. This may well provide a more accurate picture of the developmental correlates of depression and of the nature of depression itself.

The idea of depression in children and adults has been well established. However, the concept of infant depression has not been so well defined. Perhaps a similar progression of ideas will be observed in the study of the development of a concept of infant depression. In the past, the existence of such a phenomenon has been denied based on the belief that infants are too young to experience depression. Through a historical study of the development of the concept of childhood depression, parallels can be drawn between childhood and infant depression, and various phenomena in infant depression can be delineated.

CHAPTER THREE

Identifying Infant Depression

This chapter examines the symptomatology of depression in infants, beginning with the identification of the "hospitalism" and "anaclitic depression" syndromes described by Spitz and Wolf (Spitz, 1945; Spitz & Wolf, 1946). The cases identified by Spitz and Wolf present examples of gross depressive symptomatology including extreme withdrawal, weight loss and failure to thrive, and lack of affect. Since that time, other signs of depressive phenomena have been documented in infants and correlated with various dynamic models of depression. It is not the purpose of this chapter to identify and evaluate each of these models. Indeed many theories still lie largely within the realm of speculation and are thus scarcely validated. This chapter focuses instead on developing an understanding of the most well-accepted description and theory of infant depression—that which has coalesced around observations of the impact of loss of a love object as occasioned by separation. In this chapter, several case histories of such deprivation and its associated psychopathology are examined.

Kashani, Husain, Shekim, Hodges, Cytryn, and McKnew (1981) report that "the current literature suggests that depression as a clinical entity is observable in children" (p. 150). Their review of the literature on childhood depression includes biochemical, genetic, learned helplessness, life stresses, cognitive distortion, behavioral reinforcement, and sociological models. Nevertheless, as Carlson and Garber (1986) point out,

> *The absence of a generally agreed-upon and objective set of guidelines for diagnosing depression in children has been a major obstacle to progress in the field, and has made generalizations across studies and communication among researchers difficult. (p. 399)*

These deficiencies have been even more prominent in the study of depression in infancy (Trad, 1986).

Depression is correlated with deficits in three areas: cognitive, affective, and self-conceptual. Tracing the etiology of underlying depression during infancy requires a theoretically and operationally valid terminology analogous, but not limited, to that which appears in the current edition of DSM-III (American Psychiatric Association, 1980).

One of the difficulties encountered in formulating such guidelines has been the interweaving of areas of continuity and discontinuity in affective development. There is, as we have seen, impressive evidence of both in the course of early development. Hyson and Izard (1985), for example, demonstrated continuity of emotional patterns during toddlerhood. These researchers measured proportions of interest expressions, anger, emotion blends, and frequency of emotion changes during two tests given 5 months apart. It was determined that such emotional continuities across time may be related to individual differences in the temperament dimension of emotionality (Buss & Plomin, 1975) or may be indicative of continuities in early socialization with the caregiver. Even within patterns of continuity, however, changes did occur. The researchers found that there was a rise in complex emotional expressions over time. For example, there was more frequent display of emotion blends (e.g., sadness-anger, interest-anger, interest-sadness) at 18 months than at 13 months.

Such changes are not surprising given the different levels of cognition and capacities for expressing emotion at different phases in an infant's or child's development. Therefore, as Cicchetti and Schneider-Rosen (1986) emphasize in advocating a developmental approach to depression, it is not possible to delineate a fixed set of characteristics yielding a diagnostic profile for depression that may be applied across different ages. Indeed, this has been one of the chief criticisms levied against the predominantly static quality of DSM-III criteria (Garber, 1984), as well as one of the major obstacles to overcoming the lack of epidemiological studies on depression among preschoolers (Earls, 1984).

In order to recognize pathology at various age levels, it is crucial to understand normal development in the affective, cognitive, and social domains. One issue central to this discussion concerns the precise chronology of when certain emotional capabilities first exist and are manifested in recognizable form. Any evaluation of affective development must consider both the number and kind of emotions expressed, as well as their intensity, range, and degree of differentiation. It must also assess the ability of the infant to modulate these emotions. Two major theories have been posed concerning the ontogenesis of emotions (Cicchetti & Schneider-Rosen, 1986). The first holds that the individual's full range of emotion is differentiated throughout infancy and childhood from two or three primary affects, which are in existence, albeit dormant, when the child is born. According to this perspective, cognition plays a central role in the differentiation process (Bridges, 1933; Sroufe, 1979).

The second theory maintains that biological and expressive components for a wide number of emotions—which, based on this theory, encompass neurophysiological, biochemical, social, and experiential components (Izard, 1977)—are already differentiated at birth. Hence the name differential emotions theory applies to the latter hypothesis. Emotional expressions and feelings are activated by changes in activities of underlying neurochemical substrates in a manner similar to that described in Derryberry and Rothbart's (1984) model of affect as a function of neurochemical regulation. As the infant develops, discrete emotional units are linked with cognition (Izard, 1977). Implicit in the differential emotions theory is the belief that although certain emotions may be experienced at earlier stages, specific cognitive advances have to be made before the emotions can be expressed (Cicchetti & Schneider-Rosen, 1986).

In Izard's theoretical construct, emotions are viewed as evolutionary in origin and as having an adaptive function. In the social sphere, the adaptive function is signaling. Emotions and their accompanying behavioral manifestations serve to cue the caregiver. With maturation, the adaptive function of emotions changes. For example, sad affects, as Izard and Schwartz (1986) point out, can serve as a stimulus for prosocial behavior and social bonding. The distress reaction to pain during the first six months of life tends to signal the mother. During toddlerhood, this reaction may be replaced by one of anger, which helps to focus energy for coping mechanisms.

An interpretation of depression from the viewpoint of differential emotions theory would suggest that the emotions thought to play a central role in the etiology of depression—anger, guilt, sadness, shame, fear—exist in infancy, but that the cognitive associations with these affects have not yet developed to a mature extent. Only when the infant can experience the affect in terms of an emotional reaction to an object, such as a psychologically or physically unavailable parent, can the emotion be viewed as having etiological significance for infant or childhood depression (Cicchetti & Schneider-Rosen, 1986).

Attempts to validate each of these views of an infant's emotional and cognitive capacities trace back to the time of Darwin, who sought to isolate the earliest signs of particular emotions. It was apparent to Darwin in 1877, when he observed the signs of affective development in his own children, that emotional differentiation begins very soon after birth. Darwin charted the development of emotions by noting signs of distress, indicated by frowning, on the eighth day and signs of violent passion, indicated by flushed complexion, in the fourth month. He observed fear to be one of the earliest emotions, beginning as early as a few weeks after birth. This reaction, as indicated by the infant appearing startled at any sudden sound, was always followed by crying. Pleasurable sensations, as exhibited by smiles with brightened eyes and slightly closed eyelids, were present by day 45–46. At 6 months, 11 days, Darwin described more complex emotions, such as sympathy. The infant showed a melancholy face, the corners of the mouth being well depressed, when his nurse pretended to cry. Based on these observations, Darwin asserted that significant individual differences existed in the emotional displays of infants.

Recent investigations tend to confirm Darwin's observation of a high degree of affective differentiation in the infant. In her study of the development of affect in infants, Provence (1978) described the infant in a healthy affective state as revealing a broad spectrum of vivid feelings that have manifold and subtle nuances, demonstrating an affective life that is rich and colorful. Provence felt there should be cause for concern if the range of affective expression was narrow, or if the emotions displayed were relatively sparse in number when compared with those of other infants of the same age. Phrased differently, a relatively affectless state in an infant might be evidence of maladaption.

A well-developed organization of discrete facial expressions denoting the presence of a variety of affects at an age when cognitive and social abilities are very immature may also substantiate the claims of the differential emotions theory. Evidence from observations of infants' facial expressions lends support to the hypothesis that discrete affective systems may be part of genetically programmed neurophysiological structures that are independent of perceptual or cognitive development in their qualitative differentiation.

Differentiated expressions of emotion have phenomenological significance at psychological as well as biological levels. From the first weeks and months of life, perception and cognition are essential components of affective experience. The differentiation of these responses permits flexibility in organizing the multiplicity of events that the infant encounters in the environment. Simultaneously, of course, the infant's adaptive capacity will benefit from the opportunity for stimulus generalization provided by the associated complexes.

Whether or not discrete affective systems are neurologically present at birth, they cannot be manifested without the opportunity for stimulus generalization. Theoretically, the infant lacks a sophisticated repertoire of internal coping responses and external coping resources that would otherwise help to alleviate distress. If the infant is deprived of the opportunity to develop and exercise these systems in the context of environmental stimuli, affective and cognitive development will be delayed. If the stimulus deprivation is severe enough, the infant's ability to respond affectively may be permanently impaired.

Freedman and Brown (1968) compared the effects of the sheltered and minimal life experience of a brother and sister raised in virtual isolation to the effects of the much richer, but highly abnormal, experiences of children who were reported to have been raised shortly after birth by wild animals, most notably wolves. While the experiences of these "feral" children were extremely distorted, the children were nonetheless provided with a substrate of experience from which they could draw. The consequences of the minimal experience were much more severe than those of the highly distorted experience. The brother and sister reared in isolation developed little more than the rudiments of psychic structure, manifesting echolalia and largely failing to demonstrate an awareness of separation from the environment. The feral children, however, evolved psychic structures showing clear elements of ego organization and drive, such as the ability to form strong libidinal attachments. Freedman and Brown theorize that adequate physical contact in the first months of life is essential for subsequent psychic structural development.

There appears to be a minimum input threshold below which the level of experience is insufficient to allow for adequate affective differentiation. However, there is still much work to be done in discovering how the specific experiences of the infant interact with cognitive and affective complexes to produce depressive constructs such as low self-esteem, guilt, or hopelessness. The problem is compounded by the fact that representations of these constructs are not readily detectable until approximately 18 months of age (Piaget, 1954).

Clearly several questions must be answered before the progression of depression in infancy can be delineated. For example, what specific prerequisites exist for the development of depression in infancy? Is there a threshold at which a symptomatic attribute might shift from being a transitory developmental phenomenon that is unreliable over time to one that is clinically reliable? How does the biological fragility of the infant affect subsequent developmental processes? How do the cognitive achievements of the infant facilitate the regulation and representation of the affective experience?

The approach to answering these questions would have to include the following elements:

Tracing the components of attachment behavior (e.g., proximity seeking and exploratory behavior);

Examining the individual (temperamental) differences in affect and in correlates to sad affect;

Determining the way in which these individual differences may influence the infant's affective experience and expression;

Determining analogous or dissimilar biological markers of depression in infancy, when compared to markers of childhood or adult depression.

An understanding of each of these dimensions would not only facilitate the diagnosis of depression in infancy, but they may also be antecedents of depressive syndromes in childhood and adulthood. Viewed prospectively, such dimensions may enable the researcher to identify a risk for depression throughout the life cycle. Once this goal has been achieved, the notion of "depressive equivalents," once popular in the treatment of childhood depression, may be replaced by the more accurate criteria of "developmental equivalents."

DEVELOPING A CONCEPT OF INFANT DEPRESSION: VALIDATING THE CONCEPTS OF HOSPITALISM AND ANACLITIC DEPRESSION

In the attempt to formulate a valid construct of infant depression, it is useful to examine the historical events that first led researchers and clinicians to identify a cluster of symptoms that would eventually be labeled as depression in infancy. The events culminating in the description of the syndrome of hospitalism (Spitz, 1945) and anaclitic depression (Spitz & Wolf, 1946) will help illustrate some of the basic premises that shape thought concerning infant depression to this day.

Hospitalism

Observations of infants in a variety of institutional settings—hospitals, nurseries, and foundling homes—provided the initial context from which a clinical portrait of seriously disordered infants emerged. In the early part of this century, it was recognized that infants confined to these institutions fared poorly, both physically and psychologically (Bakwin, 1942; Lowrey, 1940; Parrot, 1922; Spitz, 1945). Indeed, through the end of World War II, many infants failed to survive such periods of confinement. The term "hospitalism," coined by Spitz (1945), describes the syndrome encompasss-ing many of these effects. Spitz defined hospitalism as "a vitiated condition of the body due to the long confinement in a hospital or the morbid conditions of the atmosphere of a hospital" (p. 55). The term incorporates psychological components and has increasingly been used to describe the long-term effects of institutional care on infants placed in hospitals or nurseries at an early age.

Lowrey (1940) was one of the first to document systematically the far-reaching deleterious effects of institutionalization. In 1940, Lowrey studied 28 infants between the ages of 2 weeks and 11 months, beginning at the time of their admission to an institution where they were to remain for 2 to 3 years. Over 50 percent of the infants in this sample entered the study before they reached the age of 6 months, and all showed symptoms of inadequate personality development as revealed by an inability to give or receive affection or to relate to others. Over the entire course of the study these inadequacies manifested themselves in frequent aggressive temper tantrums, which were often extremely violent, enuresis, speech defects bordering on muteness, attention-demanding behavior, shyness or sensitivi-ty, eating difficulties, stubbornness, negativism, selfishness, thumb-sucking, and excessive crying.

Bakwin (1942) describes a number of similar characteristics of hospital-ized infants. They sleep, smile, and babble less spontaneously than infants are likely to do at home and appear unhappy, listless, and apathetic, lose weight, often have respiratory infections and run fevers, according to this researcher. Moreover, these infants are indifferent in their appetites and receive food without enthusiasm. When they return to their homes, however, defervescence occurs within a few days and is accompanied by an immediate, striking weight gain.

Spitz (1945) followed the contrasting longitudinal responses of 164 infants, of whom 69 were institutionalized in a nursery and 61 in a foundling home. These two subgroups were compared with 34 children of the same age who remained in their parents' homes. The infants placed in foundling homes were found to be at significantly higher risk for various kinds of infection and illness from the third month after admission. Toward the end of the first year, the developmental quotients of these children dropped from an average of 124 in the first month to an average of 72 in the last 4 months. (The developmental quotient is a measure for intellegence and quantifiable data for development.) The home-nurtured children in this study did not develop these changes. In addition to severe developmental retardation, the foundling home infants showed specific patterns of response to strangers, ranging from extreme friendliness combined with anxious avoidance of inanimate objects to a generalized anxiety expressed in lengthy "bloodcurdling screams." In contrast, the nursery infants who were fed, nursed, and cared for by their own mothers or surrogates did not respond in such a fashion.

There has been broad recognition of the prevalence of some of the symptoms of depression among infants in institutions since the early part of this century, and explanations for the phenomena have evolved over the last 75 years. An incomplete knowledge of nutrition during World War I was given as the reason why infants failed to thrive in hospital settings (Bakwin, 1942). As more information was gained concerning nutrition and sanitation, the death rate decreased among these infants. Still, however, they continued to do poorly in hospitals, presenting a definite clinical picture in which they did not gain weight normally despite the provision of diets sufficient for growth in a home setting.

The inadequacy of the argument concerning the impact of the quality of physical care on institutionalized infants' physical and mental development prompted researchers to search for other explanations for the seemingly devastating consequences of institutionalization. By the era of World War II, several researchers began to abandon explanations based on the quality of physical care and to turn to theories implicating lack of stimulation. This new emphasis was not without precedent. As early as 1915, Chapin, founder of the boarding-out system of care for neglected children in America, recognized that infants require individual care, affection, and psychological stimulation. Broad experience in children's hospitals and foundling homes also led Parrot (1922) to believe that lack of adequate stimulation was responsible for the failure of some children to survive in these institutional settings. Brennerman (1932) also recognized the importance of stimulation. When mothers were not available to nurture their infants, Brennerman ordered that every infant on his service be picked up, carried about, and otherwise amused several times each day.

Bakwin (1942), too, focused on the harmful effects of lack of stimulation. He presumed that psychological neglect dulled infants' responsiveness to emotional stimuli, noting that even after they had been in the hospital only briefly, responses could be elicited from these infants only after repeated attempts. He believed that during early human life, the mother and infant form a biological unit and that when it was necessary for the mother to be absent, a surrogate mother should be provided. It was thus not entirely unexpected for these infants to do poorly when the warmth and security derived from maternal contact were withdrawn.

Given the general drift away from purely physical explanations (i.e., those focusing on the quality of nutritional and sanitary conditions) toward those revolving around the adequacy of stimulation, it is not surprising that Spitz's (1945) attempt to isolate pathogenic factors responsible for the outcome of infantile development also dwelled on the isolation that many institutionalized infants experience. Spitz concluded that because of their isolation, infants were cut off from any meaningful stimulation. For example, the foundling-home infants were left in solitary confinement after they demonstrated the ability to stand up in their beds. Often they lay supine in their cots for many months. By the time they were able to turn from their backs to their sides, the indented configuration of the mattresses prevented them from turning in any direction at all. Moreover, as soon as they were weaned in the fourth month, contact with their nurses ceased and their development fell below normal. Referring to the fact that one nurse had been assigned to every eight infants, Spitz noted that "Foundling Home does not give the child a mother, nor even a substitute-mother, but only an eighth of a nurse" (p. 65).

The repercussions of isolation in infancy are summarized well by Lowrey (1940), who wrote that

> *The conclusion seems inescapable that infants reared in institutions undergo an isolation type of experience, with [a] resulting isolation type of personality, characterized by unsocial behavior, hostile aggression, lack of patterns for giving and receiving affection, inability to understand and accept limitations, [and] marked insecurity in adapting to [the] environment. (p. 585)*

Lowrey felt strongly that children should not be raised in institutional settings and that if they must be institutionalized, it should be for the shortest possible time, in an atmosphere providing adequate planned, personal contact by a minimum of one adult caregiver.

Anaclitic Depression

A syndrome related to hospitalism, anaclitic depression, has also helped sharpen investigators' focus on the causes and correlates of infant depression. In describing this syndrome, also based on observations of institutionalized infants, Spitz and Wolf (1946) moved beyond discussion of the importance of early coenesthetic stimulation and drew a more explicit connection to disruptions in the caregiver-infant bond. They used the term depression because both the clinical picture and the facial expressions of these infants were similar to those found in depressive adults. However, they employed the word anaclitic (leaning up against, or dependent) to distinguish the syndrome from adult depression: "I have called anaclitic depression 'anaclitic', because it is structurally different from depression as seen at a later age" (Spitz, 1954, p. 97). This concept is based on the theory that an infant chooses an anaclitic object (generally, the mother) according to his or her original dependence on the caregiver to provide food and protection. Thus the term anaclitic depression describes "partial emotional deprivation" in infants who were separated from their maternal object, particularly where the relationship between mother and infant had been satisfactory. The etiologic role of disruptions in the caregiver-infant bond in this form of depression distinguishes it from adult depression, which is predicated, according to psychoanalytic theory, on the existence of a punishing superego which the infant has yet to develop.

Spitz and Wolf (1946) observed 123 unselected infants (62 females, 61 males). Each infant remained in a nursery from the age of 14 days through the end of its first year, with a few staying until they reached 18 months. Forty-five infants developed the syndrome. The main premorbid experience shared by all infants who developed the syndrome was the loss of the caregiver for a nearly unbroken period of 3 to 5 months. Moreover, the better the caregiver-infant relationship before the separation, the more frequently and severely the syndrome appeared at separation.

Of the 45 infants in Spitz and Wolf's study who developed depression, 26 had "mild" and 19 had "severe" depression. After numerous episodes of displaying a happy mood and outgoing behavior, the infants with severe depression began showing sadness and weepiness, developing a rigid, frozen expression in the following months. This depressed affect was accompanied by withdrawal, loss of appetite, loss of interest in the outside world, dejection, retardation, and finally stupor. All infants showed greater susceptibility to intermittent colds or eczema and gradual decline in their developmental quotient (Spitz and Wolf, 1946).

Spitz and Wolf (1946) classified the signs and symptoms of anaclitic depression into three distinct groups. The first, which they labeled "static" signs and symptoms, refers to observable phenomena in the infants under study. Although pathognomonic, these phenomena were at times represented more subtly, by dejected physiognomonic expressions and postures, ranging from apprehensive to sad or depressed. In the early stages of the development of the illness, the child is capable of engaging the observer's attention, but he or she loses this ability as the illness progresses. Indeed, the infants initially clung to the observer but eventually grew sad and disappointed when the observer withdrew. Over time, the infant's apprehensiveness, expressed by crying and screaming, increased as the observer approached and there was no expression of disappointment at the observer's withdrawal. As the clinical course worsened, the infants exhibited complete withdrawal, dejection, and a disengagement from the environment. When the infant finally established contact, it was severely retarded and the infant's pathognomonic expression did not brighten by showing happiness or active play. Spitz and Wolf believed that the difference between normal stranger anxiety (which develops between the sixth and eighth month) and the behavior manifested in anaclitic depression was both quantitative and qualitative, taking place during the period of depression.

The second group of signs, which Spitz and Wolf (1946) referred to as "genetic," were discernible only through longitudinal investigation of the child's development. The researchers relied on evidence of sudden behavioral changes, considered in relation to the infant's overall progression through the major developmental periods of the first year (e.g., the eighth-month anxiety period). Sudden changes (e.g., from being pleasant, smiling, and friendly to being withdrawn) that they could not attribute to organic causes, but could link to a period of separation from the mother, provoked suspicion of anaclitic depression.

"Quantitative" signs of depression, the last of the three classes of symptoms outlined by Spitz and Wolf (1946), tap the progression of the disorder as indicated by consecutively administered developmental tests. Typically these signs reveal a declining developmental quotient as the disorder progressed.

According to Spitz and Wolf (1946), the youngest age at which the syndrome of anaclitic depression first became manifest was the beginning of the sixth month, although age of onset could also occur up to the eleventh month of age. Sex and developmental quotients were not found to play a significant role in the formation of the syndrome. The mothers of those infants that developed the syndrome had been removed from the child between the sixth and eighth month for a period of 3 months during which time the child either did not see his or her mother at all or saw her no more than once a week. Four to 6 weeks following the mother's departure, the syndrome of anaclitic depression was observed.

Since not all children whose mothers were removed developed the same syndrome, maternal separation was seen as a necessary but not sufficient cause for its development. Spitz and Wolf (1946) found that when the mother did not return or an adequate substitute caregiver was not provided, the infant's depression progressed rapidly. They observed that if the mother returned within 3 months, the infants would recover at least partially from the emotional damage. Upon the mother's return, the infants showed a dramatic behavioral change. Not only did they resume previous friendliness and approachability, but even more striking was the increase in their developmental quotient. Unfortunately, although Spitz and Wolf followed the cases in their study for one and a half years, they did not note whether the depression in infancy resulted in any longer-term sequelae.

This study demonstrated that when a good caregiver-infant relationship was disrupted, the clinical picture was frequently distressing with severe symptomatology. However, in the sample with poor caregiver-infant relationships, not a single severe depression occurred. Spitz and Wolf suggest that the depression is caused by the loss of a love object, and thus an unsatisfactory love object is more easily replaced than a satisfactory one.

Anaclitic depression and hospitalism therefore lie along a continuum of emotional deprivation. Spitz (1965) has portrayed hospitalism and anaclitic depression as two variants in severity of a single syndrome. Hospitalism, or "total emotional deprivation," is the more severe of the two, and anaclitic depression, or "partial emotional deprivation," the less severe. Severity, according to Spitz, is largely a function of the length of the maternal deprivation. When the period of maternal absence exceeded five months and the clinical picture changed radically, developing into a syndrome with a much poorer prognosis, Spitz (1945) referred to this phenomenon as hospitalism.

While there has developed a general consensus about the harmful impact—in terms both of depression and other psychopathology—of lack of stimulation and emotional availability in early life, theorizing has not stopped since the 1940s. The most recent theoretical refinement accepts the premises of Spitz and others concerning the etiological significance of infant isolation in psychiatric disorders of infancy and later life. However, it has narrowed the focus to a specific time period, often referred to as the "sensitive period," during which lack of stimulation is thought to have lasting repercussions. Klaus and Kennel (1976) have been among the most ardent supporters of the view that the bond established (or not established) between caregiver and infant in the earliest hours of life sets a pattern for all subsequent interactions and the expectations associated with such interactions. This idea has sparked a flurry of research activity, and it is not clear whether it can be validated empirically, however appealing it may be in light of currently popular practices in postnatal care. We shall turn to a discussion of some of these empirical data later.

Case Studies of Infant Depression

Since the time of Spitz (1945; Spitz and Wolf, 1946), a number of cases of infant depression have been reported in the literature. Some closely resemble the phenomena of anaclitic depression and hospitalism as described by Spitz. The common theme running through all these histories appears to be a separation or loss experienced by the infant. At first observed only in hospitalized infants and foundlings—cases where the infant suffered a total loss of the mother—depressive symptomatology has since been associated with other forms of loss or perceived loss. For the infant these losses can include short-term separation from the mother, separation from siblings or other attachment figures, abuse, neglect, or contact with a depressed parent. (These various "losses" are discussed in depth in Chapters Seven, Eight, and Nine, which are devoted to the different populations thought to be at risk for depression.)

Engel (1962) hypothesized that the depression-withdrawal reaction may even occur anticipatorily to protect against experiences of loss and helplessness and to indicate a need for the conservation of energy that the infant achieves by erecting heightened barriers to incoming stimuli. Engel quotes Bibring (1953), who says "Depression represents a basic reaction to situations of narcissistic frustration [the prevention of which] appears to be beyond the powers of the ego" (Engel, 1962, p. 95). Engel and Schmale (1973) later called this response the "conservation-withdrawal reaction" syndrome. It is primarily reactive, serving the infant's need to preserve his or her integrity when confronted with stress from its environment (Menahem, 1984).

Engel and Reichsman (1956) described two qualitatively different emotional reactions in a single female infant as she grew from 15 months to 24 months of age. Born with congenital atresia of the esophagus, this infant was hospitalized twice for weight loss at the age of 1 year and again at the age of 15 months. During the lengthy hospitalizations, the patient showed symptoms both of hospitalism, in the form of physical and mental retardation, and anaclitic depression, as depicted by facial expressions and overall improvement when the caregiver relationship was reestablished. It was after the infant's recovery from depression and the marasmatic state that the authors observed two well-delineated behavioral patterns, which they described as "depression-withdrawal reaction" and "depression-unpleasure reaction." The depression-withdrawal reaction occurred rapidly, but only when the infant was confronted by a stranger while alone. During this reaction, a prompt loss of muscle tone was seen. Occasionally the corners of the infant's mouth would turn down. The inner corners of her brows would also be elevated, producing a furrowed, frowning brow. This picture gradually developed into a closing of the eyes and proceeded to a state of sleep. (The empathic sensation on the part of the observer was one of sadness and helplessness.) Heart and respiratory rates were unchanged or slightly diminished.

The "depression-unpleasure" which was considered to include elements of depression-withdrawal and anxiety occurred if the stranger tried to communicate with the infant. She would assume a protective posture by pulling her tights up to her abdomen or by turning away. Her facial expression was anguished, with her face puckered, the brow deeply furrowed, and the mouth opened to a square shape (Engel & Reichsman, 1956).

The authors classified the patient's condition as "depression in infancy" and compared this clinical picture to that often seen in adults. They clearly defined the facial expressions in both reactions, comparing them very closely with Darwin's (1877) classic descriptions of grief, dejection, and despair. (The details of this case are discussed in Chapter One, A Developmental Perspective for Analyzing Infant and Childhood Depression. Significantly, the behavior of this infant, who experienced early depression, was replicated both in her doll playing patterns during childhood and in the feeding behavior she demonstrated toward her own infants, suggesting the continuity and endurance of early behavior patterns [Engel et al. 1985].) Along the same lines, Spitz and Wolf (1946) observed that in infants who developed anaclitic depression, crying would often give way to withdrawal, during which they would lie down with their faces averted, refusing to engage in their surroundings.

Menahem (1984) presents two other examples of this depressive withdrawal response. In Menahem's two cases, the infants were breast-fed by the mothers, but suffered weight loss. The infants failed to thrive, even though they were with the mother, while the mothers refused to admit that their feedings may have been insufficient. The babies initially protested their inadequate feedings, but eventually stopped. They manifested no dissatisfaction, although they did not gain weight. Menahem suggests that the infants were attempting to conserve their energies and adapt to the lowered level of care.

Cases in which an existing caregiver-infant bond ruptures and those in which that bond never develops may differ significantly (Casler, 1961). Ainsworth's (1962) conceptual approach to early pathogenic caregiver-child relations also recognizes the multiplicity of forms that deprivation of stimulation can assume. She used the term "deprivation" to denote insufficient caregiver-child interaction and the term "separation" for discontinuity in the relationship. Separation could thus occur with or without deprivation (Trad, 1986).

Emde, Polak, and Spitz (1965) described a case in which the caregiver-infant bond never developed. Nonetheless, the progress of this case is notable for its similarity to Spitz's original description of anaclitic depression. The infant, raised in a residential nursery from the age of 8 days, had no further involvement with his biological mother. Beginning at the age of 9 months, a depressive syndrome developed gradually, with a total estimated duration of 7.5 months. Onset was related to the transfer of this patient at the age of 6 months to another room in the nursery where there were fewer regular staff members. The clinical picture of the patient's depression fused with symptomatology of anxiety at the age of 8 months. Spitz and Wolf (1946) note that many of their cases of anaclitic depression were observed at around 8 months of age, the same time that the onset of stranger anxiety is generally observed.

Several aspects of the infant's behavior appeared to the researchers to suggest that he was suffering from depression. Premorbid levels of functioning were observed during the first month in the nursery, when the patient exhibited substantial "fussy crying," demanding more attention than other infants of the same age. At other times, the infant was described as being shy. The infant's smiling response to a human face began to diminish a few weeks before 6 months of age. One week after transfer to the nursery, his developmental quotient dropped. The smiling response again disappeared 3.5 weeks after the transfer. Consistent with Spitz and Wolf's (1946) findings, the infant's recovery from the depression was reflected by a reengagement with the environment. Two weeks before the depression resolved itself, the infant related well to volunteers who provided care. One notable and perhaps promising aspect of this case that represents a departure from Spitz's original description of the clinical course of anaclitic depression was that the enduring depressive episode resolved itself 7.5 months after onset—despite Spitz and Wolf's earlier contention that if depression was not resolved 3 months after onset, it appeared to be irreversible.

Separation appears to have played the determining role in a case reported by Meyendorf (1971) in which a 19-month-old female infant reacted with depression, retardation, and starvation 1 week after being separated from her parents and, subsequently, from her two siblings. Neurological symptoms of ataxia, ptosis, and incoordination of eye movements, similar to those seen by Spitz in his studies of hospitalism, were observed even after she was reunited with her parents, ostensibly because she had not yet been reunited with her siblings. Her condition began to improve 1 week after she was reunited with her siblings even though this occurred outside the environment of the home. This observation supports Spitz's claim that the object-loss is not necessarily the primary caregiver in every case. Once the siblings were reunited with the infant, her recovery from one "brief, single-depriving separation episode" seemed prompt and complete. When the threat of new separation became apparent 6 weeks later, however, she reacted with another brief depressive episode after a 1-hour trial placement in a nursery. Clearly the earlier separation heightened her vulnerablity to a depressive reaction since prior to her traumatic separation from her siblings, she had reacted normally to the same situation.

Taylor (1973) reported a case in which an infant became listless and lethargic, despite slight weight gains, after being weaned abruptly from breast-feeding at 9 weeks of age. Once maternal support was reestablished, however, the infant recovered in a short time. This case, like the Meyendorf report, confirms Spitz's findings regarding the rapidity with which the syndrome progresses from anaclitic depression to hospitalism and the promptness of the patient's recovery. Taylor's report also concurs with Meyendorf's studies in documenting a similar degree of vulnerability for a relapse in the face of any threat of further separation.

The earliest age at which a case of anaclitic depression has been reported is about 4 months (Gaensbauer, 1980, 1982). Jenny, a 3.5 month-old female infant, had been taken at 2 weeks of age to the emergency room where she was found to have a fractured arm. During a routine examination at 7.5 weeks of age, a bruise was found on her back. At 3 months, after another broken arm and a nondepressed skull fracture, it was decided to hospitalize her. Although appearing happy and highly sociable, Jenny presented the hypervigilant aftermath of trauma. On discharge 5 days later, she was transferred to a foster home, where she spent most of the first day crying. This reaction was related to loss of contact with her mother and abrupt weaning. As time passed, further evidence of neglect was shown by the foster mother, and Jenny developed feeding and sleeping problems (regurgitation and waking at night). Her withdrawal was progressive as the number of her positive responses decreased. Jenny still showed evidence of good maternal attachment, however, when visited by her mother.

Nevertheless, after 3 weeks, Jenny was observed to be more subdued following a visit by her biological mother, cried easily, and was less active and less interested in her toys. When she was evaluated at 3 months and 25 days of age, her behavior was lethargic, apathetic, and disinterested, which was consistent with a diagnosis of depression. She showed evidence of stranger anxiety, avoided eye contact, and tended to withdraw from her mother.

Observed in a laboratory playroom setting, Jenny's gaze aversion became more evident during the playful interaction with her mother and during a maternal reunion episode. Her mother tried to soothe her but overstimulated her in an effort to gain her attention. Gaensbauer (1980) and Schmale (1972) state that avoiding eye contact with the mother may be a depressive emotion measure aimed at avoiding distressing affects. This phenomenon can be recognized as an example of the motivational force affects can have.

The early age at which Jenny exhibited signs of depression compelled researchers to place greater reliance on facial expressions that accompany other behaviors suggestive of sadness. To test the validity of this approach Gaensbauer and Hiatt (1984) used the maximally discriminative facial movement scoring system (Izard, 1979). Gaensbauer and Hiatt's findings support Spitz's descriptions, but the former established that by the age of 4 months, rather than 6 months, facial expressions and behavioral manifestations of sadness may be observed in infants. Sad facial expressions, as evidenced by a "raising or triangulation of the inner corners of the eyebrows, and a drawing down of the corners of the mouth" (p. 209), occurred frequently in Gaensbauer and Hiatt's observations. Other emotions, such as happiness, interest, anger, disgust, surprise, and possibly fear, as well as sadness, have been shown in studies by Gaensbauer and other researchers to be at least rudimentarily formed by the time the infant reaches 3 to 4 months of age. Expressions of interest have been observed from birth, while documentation on infants seeking stimuli has been overwhelming in recent years (Izard, 1977). According to Gaensbauer and Hiatt, these discrete facial expressions, reflecting discrete affect systems, may be rooted in and controlled by specific neural pathways.

At an early age, however, many of the negative affects may still be more difficult to interpret than positive affects. Hiatt, Campos, and Emde (1979) determined that in infants aged 10 to 12 months, fearful expressions were less discrete than were expressions that denoted happiness and surprise. Facially, these expressions were fleeting, often lasting only 1 or 2 seconds. While the facial expressions identified seemed to be associated with an underlying emotional state, they were not deemed to be synonymous with it.

Indeed, Jenny's case illustrates the wide array of affects available to even a very young infant, as well as their evanescent—hence difficult to interpret—quality. Although she exhibited a predominantly subdued, and often inscrutable facial expression, other transient emotions, including sadness, fearfulness, anger, joy, and interest/curiosity were also noted. These facial expressions demonstrated consistent patterns of association with specific behaviors. Sadness occurred in conjunction with psychomotor retardation, fear in conjunction with bodily withdrawal and gaze aversion, and anger in conjunction with hitting and arm swinging. These discrete emotional expressions were observed to be highly transient and intermittent, even when Jenny's behavior suggested a more enduring motivational state.

Specific contexts similar to her early traumatic experiences appeared to elicit the fear, anger, and sadness observed in Jenny. The precipitating events for the depressive episode were consistent with the triple loss—separation from the mother to whom the patient showed a clear and positive recognition, abrupt weaning, and affective and stimuli deprivation—concept of depression previously described by Spitz and Wolf (1946). This study also demonstrated that a crucial factor in the infant's depression was a loss of the mothering function, rather than the actual loss of the mother, as Jenny's depression recurred with each new separation from a foster home. As most other studies of anaclitic depression have shown, Jenny's case was not sudden or transient. Rather, it emerged over time, and while it improved after adequate caregiving was reestablished, it persisted for several days.

Prospectively Studied Cases

Spitz and Wolf (1946) stated that it was impossible to determine at the age of 1 to 1.5 years whether early depression left any visible psychological imprint. The following two case reports, in which infants were followed for many years, address Spitz's (1945) original question about the nature of the pathogenic factors underlying hospitalism and anaclitic depression and also provide data on the impact of early depression. In the first, Davidson (1968) followed a female infant intensively from the age of 28 weeks. The patient had several demonstrated depressive episodes throughout the course of follow-up. People who had contact with the patient at age 5 described her as being underweight, nervous, unhappy, withdrawn, and avoidant under stress. By age 8, she was said to be too quiet and self-contained, and at age 12, sad, sullen, and bitter. When interviewed at the age of 15, the patient's responses tended to be psychosomatic and depressive.

Retrospectively, this patient showed three noteworthy characteristics at the age of 7 months: a tendency toward excessive sleep, uncoordinated muscular development, and a thin, undernourished appearance despite adequate food intake. Constant regurgitation prevented her from digesting food. She spent as many as 17 hours a day in the depression-withdrawal state but could be awakened and would smile when stimulated. She was an extremely undemanding baby. Her motor development was also retarded, and she expressed depression through lassitude, apathy, and feeding difficulties.

Harmon, Wagonfield, and Emde (1982) for 12 years followed a child who had been placed in a residential nursery at 8 days of age. They observed repeated depressive episodes, the first of which began at the age of 9 months and lasted 7.5 months before lifting. Three other depressive episodes occurred in infancy, at 2 years and 1 month, at 3.5 years, and at 4.5 years. The central theme of each was separation from the primary maternal figure and the sequence of protest, despair, and detachment [articulated by Robertson & Bowlby (1952)] was severe during these episodes. The patient had a transient school phobia on entering kindergarten. One year after psychiatric treatment began at 8 years and 3 months, an outbreak of eczema occurred in response to his therapist's vacation. The patient soon became depressed again in reaction to the loss of some of his orphanage mates. During termination of treatment at age 12, another outbreak of eczema was observed. At both 1.5 and 2.5 years after the third adoption, he was reported to have successfully adjusted to his new family.

In the cases reported by Davidson (1968) and Harmon, Wagonfield, and Emde (1982), a number of depressive precursors are noteworthy, including a high degree of interactional dysregulation as evidenced by an innate ability to seek and demand attention in a strikingly active and tenacious manner that later subsides into withdrawal. The more subtle disorders could be detected in pathognomonic expressions and postures. As in the above mentioned cases, the infant's discrete emotional expressions are highly rudimentary, transient, and intermittent, showing only short-term stability, even when the infant's behavior suggests a more enduring motivational state. Such affective functioning appears highly flexible, with affective states capable of rapid changes according to the variability of stimulus conditions. This flexibility enables the infant to monitor and organize his or her responses to constantly changing environmental conditions (Gaensbauer, 1982).

The clinical process of tracking variations in ideas and thoughts is inherently limited, often neglecting affects as they change from moment to moment. Affects occur in mixed and fused states. Therefore, rigid compartmentalization of affective, cognitive, and motivational human behavior violates the complex connectiveness of human experience (see Table 1). The property of flexible modulation between affective states is the quality that we refer to as spontaneity that characterizes the emotionally healthy child (Trad, 1986).

SEPARATION: A PROBABLE COMMON PATHWAY TO DEPRESSION IN INFANCY

The work of Spitz and Wolf (1946) and Harmon et al. (1982) and others, amply demonstrates the existence of hospitalism and anaclitic depression in infancy. Since separation from a caregiver is the central dynamic triggering these specific depressive states, it seems reasonable to hypothesize that perturbations in the attachment bond are central to the development of other forms of functional depression that may surface during infancy. Attachment theory, elaborated after Spitz (1945; Spitz and Wolf, 1946) and others' work on institutionalized infants, provides a good conceptual foundation for understanding these earlier findings and for explaining how they may relate to depression in infancy. A clear understanding of attachment bonding and an examination of infant reactions to separation may prepare the way for developing early diagnostic criteria of depression in infancy.

Attachment Behavior

The study of attachment behavior concerns those characteristics and actions that comprise the connection observed between mother and infant. Bowlby (1969) proposes that attachment behavior has been observed clearly during a baby's first year of life, but that in children older than 1 year, it is less well chronicled. During the second and third years of life, attachment behavior is not reduced in either intensity or frequency of display, but the contexts in which it occurs change as the child matures and develops broader and more refined perceptual abilities. Bowlby suggests that attachment behavior is exhibited with some strength and regularity until almost the end of the third year of life and that this expression continues to constitute a major part of behavior until the fourth year. At this point, the child's display of attachment behavior decreases in intensity and frequency, although it is still observable and persists throughout the early school years.

Bowlby (1969) describes six actions taken by the infant to strengthen attachment to the caregiver: crying, smiling, following, clinging, sucking,

Table 1. Clinical Studies of Infant Depression

	A. Spitz (1945)	B. Spitz and Wolf (1946)	C. Engel and Reichsman (1956)	D. Emde, Polak, and Spitz (1965)	E. Meyendorf (1971)	F. Ossofsky (1974)	G. Gaensbauer (1980, 82)	H. Harmon and Wagonfeld (1982)
DSM-III								
I. Major depressive disorder		Depression	Depression	Depression	Depression	Depression	Depression	Depression
Dysphoric disorder	Feeble smile Dull	Sad face Dejected	Sad face	Sad face Less smiling	Sad face		Sad face Loss of pleasure	
Eating disturbances		Eating disturbances Weight loss			Eating disturbances		Eating disturbances Food refusal	Food allergies
Sleep disturbances		Sleep disturbances Insomnia			Sleep disturbances		Sleep disturbances	
Psychomotor activity		Stupor	Loss of tone Immobility		Restlessness Retardation Fidgeting Ataxia	Hyperactivity Clumsiness	Retardation	
Loss of interest	Apathetic	Withdrawal	Withdrawal	Withdrawal	Withdrawal	Withdrawal Apathetic	Withdrawal Apathetic Lethargic Hypervigilence	
Loss of energy								
Attentional disturbances	Unresponsive	Unresponsive			Unresponsive	Short span		
II. Dysthymic disorder								
Irritability/anger				Irritable/angry Demanding Fussiness	Irritable Monotonous cry	Tantrums	Irritable	Difficult
Tearfulness/crying		Weepiness				Tantrums	Irritable	Tantrums
Affective								
Developmental retardation	D. retardation	D. retardation		D. retardation	D. retardation	D. retardation		
Avoidance	Avoidancy		Avoidancy	Avoidancy			Avoidancy	
Abnormal stranger reactions	A.s. reacions	A.s. reactions	A.s. reactions				A.s. reactions	
Shyness				Shyness				
Anxiety/apprehension		Apprehension		Anxious				
Physical						Allergies		
Decreased immune functions	D. i. functions							Multiple viral infections
Dejected posture				Dejected posture	Dejected posture			
Enuresis/Encopresis						Enuresis/Encopresis		
Other					Ptosis Change in voice	Allergies Colic		Atopic dermatitis Occult GI bleeding

and calling. Crying, smiling, and calling tend to draw the mother to the infant, while following and clinging draw the infant to the mother. The function of sucking is less easily assessed and Bowlby calls for a closer examination and interpretation of this activity. He notes that calling may begin at any time after 4 months of age and, in the infant, is manifested as short, sharp calls and, later, by use of names.

Proximity seeking behavior is only one facet of attachment theory. Bowlby (1969, 1982) suggests that several systems—each with its own activators, terminators, predictable outcomes, and functions—comprise the phenomenon of attachment. The connection between exploration and attachment is stressed as a particularly important aspect of development in a species possessing high potential for adaptation to a wide range of environments. The motivations for attachment and exploration interact dynamically with each other. When the attachment system is intensively activated, the infant tends to seek proximity to the mother. Conversely, when the attachment system is at low intensity, the infant will act on the impulse to explore and respond to the pull of novelty. Bowlby (1969) observed a marked difference in children's exploratory behavior in the presence of the mother, as distinguished from such behavior displayed in her absence. Alteration in behavior is compounded if the child is confronted with a strange person or place. When the mother is nearby, most children are more confident and ready to explore. In her absence, they are more timid and may become quite distressed.

Separation Behavior

Attachment theory (Bowlby, 1969) evolved from studies of children between 6 months and 3 years of age who had been separated for prolonged periods from their mothers. According to attachment theory, a crucial bond develops between caregiver and infant, and when this bond is severed through any kind of separation, the infant suffers a loss experienced in the same way that adults experience mourning. The response to separation is instinctive and may, in part, resemble the response of other species, such as monkeys. Observations with animals provide an opportunity to gain insight regarding the physiological and behavioral responses that occur during separation, without some of the complicating influences encountered in work with human infants. Bowlby (1960) has argued that, with the exception of differences in mobility, humans and lower primates share many behaviors during the second year.

Reite, Short, Seiler, and Pauley (1981) observed the behaviors of eight pigtailed macaque monkey infants. They concluded that a shared evolution between higher primates and humans, as witnessed in part by similarities in their response to disruption of the attachment bond, may make the monkey model of affiliative behavior useful for understanding the functions and processes of attachment. The eight monkey infants were followed over the course of a 10-day separation from their mothers in order to observe any changes in behavior and physiology. Behavioral variables were classified into one of five groups: activity, social contact, environmental contact, self-directed, and caregiver-infant. Physiological changes were measured through the use of a surgically implanted multichannel biotelemetry system. Implantation was performed at a mean age of 19 weeks (range 15-26 weeks). Records were kept of EKG, body temperature, eye movement (EOG), muscle activity (EMG), and three channels of EEG.

Study results revealed that although there were profound individual differences in response to separation, monkey infants experienced behavioral changes similar to those often found with human subjects, including slowing of movement, decreases in play, increases in oral behaviors, assumption of a characteristic slouched posture, and sad facial expressions. Among the physiologic alterations observed were decreases in heart rate and body temperature, sleep disturbances, and changes in EEG.

Reite et al. (1981) characterized some physiologic changes as "relatively long lasting" and concluded:

> The data demonstrate that the disruption of an attachment bond may be accompanied by pronounced physiological changes suggestive of a general impairment of autonomic homeostatic regulatory processes. The findings have important implications for our understanding of the pathophysiology of grief and the physiological concomitants of separation, loss, and depression in children. (p. 165)

Human responses to separation typically follow a three-phase pattern (Robertson & Bowlby, 1952). A stage called protest occurs first and is characterized by separation anxiety and by the child's wish to return to the mother. Grief and mourning, which Bowlby refers to as despair, dominate the second stage. The child in this stage fears that the mother will not return. In the third and final stage, called detachment, the child displays disinterest even in the mother's presence.

While these states may theoretically be described as separate entities, the child moves from one to the next and may spend from days to weeks in a transition period among phases or may alternate between two phases (Bowlby, 1969). Protest may begin either immediately after separation or after some delay and may last a few hours or extend to a week or more. Signs of protest include loud crying, shaking in bed, or thrashing. A protesting infant or child may also exhibit an eager response to any sight or sound that might indicate the return of an absent parent.

During the succeeding phase, despair, the infant or child continues to exhibit a preoccupation with the missing parent, but behavior also suggests an increasing hopelessness. Physical movement diminishes or ceases, and the infant becomes withdrawn and inactive. Often the infant ceases to make demands of the people in the environment. When the infant reaches the detachment phase, the observer may be misled into believing the child is recovering from the loss since, at this time, he or she begins to show more interest in the environment. However, it is difficult to reestablish the severed attachment at this stage.

For the child whose stay in a hospital or residential nursery is prolonged, the entire experience of loss is likely to be repeated several times as he or she becomes transiently attached to a series of nurses or caretakers who eventually leave. This series of disturbed attachments of short duration will gradually result in the child's withdrawal of commitment and cessation of all attachment behavior. Although some researchers have suggested the term withdrawal for this phase, Bowlby (1969) proposes that "detachment," as the natural counterpart to attachment, is a more accurate term. An infant who reaches this state eventually becomes unresponsive to any family members who may visit. He or she becomes increasingly self-centered and may show enthusiasm only for material goods.

Jenny's case, described earlier (Gaensbauer, 1980, 1982), provides a good illustration of this behavioral sequence. Her initial behavior, which consisted of distress, fussiness, and crying in response to separation from her mother and placement in foster care, can be seen as a protest. This protest has been described by Gaensbauer (1982) as part of the "fight-flight" response—a depressive withdrawal from stress to which the infant has failed to adapt. After reinstatement of adequate caregiving in this infant's second foster home, Gaensbauer saw this withdrawal process reversing itself as Jenny went from withdrawal to active distress and protest when reunited with her mother. Each of these reactions reflects the early flexibility of the infant's responses. Protest demonstrates discriminatory capacities that allow the infant to adapt to different confrontations. While the protest may not be rewarded with a desired outcome, it is a more active response than withdrawal.

Factors Mediating the Impact of Separation

By now it is well recognized that depression in infancy occurs in many contexts, not just in institutional settings. Nevertheless, studies of institutionalized infants provide some of the best data from which to generalize about the causes and correlates of infant depression. These studies have not only identified the experience of loss as a key precipitating factor in infant depression but have also helped qualify this model. As research in the last 30 years has shown, separation experiences may differ qualitatively as a function of a number of variables; most critically, timing and context affect the infant's developmental status and coping mechanisms, as well as protective factors in the environment.

Compensating for Maternal Deprivation: A Comparison of Institutional versus Noninstitutional Separations.   Spitz and Wolf (1946) hinted at some of these qualifications of the infant depression model when they distinguished between loss of the caregiver and loss of the mothering function. Their implication was that, to some extent, the effects of the latter may be ameliorated while the effects of the former cannot. This distinction was not addressed explicitly and in a controlled way until Robertson (1953; Robertson & Robertson, 1971) examined separation in settings not only free of the adverse effects of institutions, but also adequate in compensatory support. These investigations offer one response to the allegation that the study of separation within an institutional context may confuse the impact of a single event, separation, with the impact of an overall environment, the institution. This criticism, that the study of maternal separation within the institution is not a "pure" study of a specific event, was raised by Yarrow (1964), who argued that

> *Most of the direct studies of institutional settings describe very impoverished environments . . . institutional environments tend to be deviant in many other respects, such as in the amount, the quality, and the variety of sensory and social stimulation and in the kinds of learning conditions provided. (p. 99; David and Appell, 1962; Goldfarb, 1955; Provence and Lipton, 1962; Rheingold, 1960, 1961)*

Robertson and Robertson (1971) studied 13 young children (17 months to 2 years, 5 months) who were separated from their mothers but were cared for in noninstitutional settings by parent substitutes. The Robertsons cared for four of these children. Another nine children were cared for in their own homes by familiar relatives. During the separations, which ranged from 10 to 27 days, none of the 13 children responded with protest and despair. The Robertsons concluded that the difference in results seen with children separated from their parents in institutional settings is a significant one, and that variation in response was qualitative and not simply a matter of degree. Furthermore, they proposed that provision of an adequate substitute for the mother is an essential factor in behavioral outcome. The Robertsons found acute distress to be a common response among children between 6 months and 3 to 4 years on separation from the mother, regardless of circumstance or quality of substitute care. However, in cases where substitute mothering was provided, four young children separated from their natural mothers or usual caregivers for 10 to 27 days did not progress from protest to despair as indicated in the literature. Thus the pattern of protest, despair, and detachment was not observed in this noninstitutional study. The Robertsons found that among these children, attention was transferred to the substitute mother to varying degrees, in part depending on the child's levels of object constancy and maturity. The ability to detect these differences in response was attributed to the absence of the obscuring factors present in the institutional setting.

Over the course of the first days after separation, the investigators noted an increase in laughter and activity, which they interpreted as a defensive reaction to anxiety. On the second, third, and fourth days, the children showed some sadness, a lowered frustration tolerance, and some aggression, but they did not exhibit the characteristics of despair expected to surface at this time.

Impact of Age on an Infant's Response to Separation.   Although Spitz and Wolf's (1946) conceptualization of the course of infant depression highlights the sixth month, by which point a specific caregiver-infant bond has been established, as the earliest point at which the depressive syndromes can surface, many researchers have been eager to determine whether separations at any particular point in early development will have a disproportionate influence on an infant's risk for depression. Most investigations have centered on the period immediately after birth. For example, Rode, Chang, Fisch and Sroufe (1981) studied separation from the mother during this time in an attempt to test the sensitive period hypothesis advanced by Klaus and Kennel (1976), who argue that bonding in the period immediately following birth is critical for later development.

The assumption implicit in this contention is that early deprivation of physical contact beween parent and infant can lead to maladaptive parenting, which, in turn, can diminish the relationship that the infant uses to form its earliest self-representations. Rode et al. (1981) address the theory of this sensitive period in their examination of 24 children who had been parted from their mothers due to premature birth ($N = 20$) or illness after full-term birth ($N = 4$). Mean hospital stay in the neonatal intensive care unit was 26.77 days.

Children were tested using the Strange Situation Paradigm (Ainsworth & Wittig, 1969) at the chronological age of 12 to 19 months (mean age, 14.75 months). No significant differences could be found between the three groups consisting of securely attached, anxiously attached-avoidant, and anxiously attached-resistant infants on measures such as days of hospitalization and parental visiting patterns, which may tap the impact of early separation. Mean Bayley mental and motor developmental index scores (1969), adjusted for gestational age, were, respectively, 104.5 and 99.8. The results of this study matched those of other current investigations that cast doubt on whether separation immediately following birth has adverse effects on attachment. Instead attachment security appears to be a function of interactions over a longer period of time than that encompassed by the sensitive period. Rode et al. (1981) concluded that

Attachment patterns are influenced by maternal-infant interaction over a period of time and provide evidence for the resiliency of infants in their formation of attachment patterns . . . although prematurity and physical separation place stress on the family system, of greater importance to the infant-caregiver attachment relationship may be the length of time that the infant has been at home with the caregiver and the quality of care experienced. . . . The earliest days are important; however, attachment is a process that evolves during the first year of life. (pp. 188-190)

Rode et al. cited two other possible explanations for the seeming lack of significance of early separation. First, parents of the infants observed were encouraged to visit their infants and participate in their care once the infants' condition stabilized; and second, infants were reared in stable family situations. Thus, as in Trause's (1981) study of children separated from their mothers on the occasion of the birth of a sibling, some contact with the parent during the period of separation may have had a significant impact on the child's response.

Field (1977) also addressed the sensitive period and confirmed Rode et al.'s (1981) results in a study that focused on a more specific criterion—face-to-face interactions and their role in separation. Given the theory that interactions between infants and their mothers provide the infant with an arena in which to develop communication skills, and that these skills are generally established during the first few months of life, Field sought to determine whether the early separation from their mothers experienced by many high-risk premature infants contributed to disturbances in their later interactions. Theoretically, interactional dysfunctions may be viewed as a very primitive type of failure that can lead to a sense of loss. Although Kagan's (1983) research suggests that the infant's ability to conceive of his or her own failure does not develop until the second year of life, face-to-face interactional failures may be a precursor that leads to a sense of loss. In a study of the developmental aspects of children's responses to the stress of separation and loss, Garmezy (1986) notes that failure can be considered a type of loss, though an intrapersonal one. As he states:

The threat of failure seems to be something of a misfit among the great loss events, yet there is a linkage to be noted. . . . Depressive feelings often are a consequence of a pervasive sense of failure, and a theoretical link now has been forged between omnipresent attributions of worthlessness as a component of the self-concept of many who develop severe depressive disorders.
Ascriptions of failure are profoundly eroding of self-esteem, and self-esteem remains a key component of competent functioning. Failure experiences, if recurrent, inhibit the development of a sense of efficacy. . . . (p. 313)

Field (1977) focused specifically on the functions of gaze aversion and maternal overstimulation in the interactions examined. According to Brazelton, Koslowski, and Main (1974), Trevarthan (1974), and Tronick, Als, and Adamson (1978) in normal mothers and infants, the infant's gaze indicates a readiness to interact. Conversely, these researchers suggest gaze aversion is a signal to change or end the interaction. The "sensitive" caregiver responds to these visual signals, reserving stimulation for the infant's more attentive periods and reducing or terminating activity when the infant's focus shifts away.

Field (1977) videotaped face-to-face interactions with three types of infants: 12 high-risk premature infants, 12 postmature infants who were born postterm and manifested symptoms of postmaturity, and 12 healthy normal-term babies. The postmature and the high-risk premature infants (i.e., with a mean gestational age of 32 weeks) had received very low Brazelton (1973) neonatal a priori interactive process scores, and Field found little difference in measures of face-to-face interaction between the premature group, which had undergone separation, and the postmature group. She felt that this finding revealed that the effects of early separation, although important, were ameliorated by the infant's compensatory behavior.

The shortage of empirical support for the sensitive period hypothesis does not mean that the time at which separation occurs is unimportant; rather, it indicates that the particular period isolated by Klaus and Kennel (1976) may not be as critical as they hypothesize. Age at time of separation may still be an important determinant of both the short and longer term consequences of separation. A number of investigators have speculated on the long-term effect of separation and the child's resilience in the face of separation experiences. Among them is Robertson (1953), who suggests

> it be left an open question how far such disturbances are really resolved, and how often they leave some scar behind which can cause distress to be reactivated much later by some trivial reminder. (quoted by Yarrow, 1964, p. 97)

More recently Sroufe and Rutter (1984) added a developmental perspective to the discussion. Among infants younger than 6 months of age, these investigators observed no grief reaction during a situation of loss. After this age, the sequential process of protest, despair, and detachment in the face of loss is believed to be in effect, they report, until about the age 4 or 5 years, when disorders with the cognitive and affective elements of depression begin to appear. Children at this later age may be the most vulnerable, according to Garmezy (1986), who reports that

> Groupings of children by age at a time of separation or loss (0-4, 5-10, 11-15) indicate that the 5-10 age bracket seems to be the most vulnerable age of all, particularly if [the loss] occurred for a period exceeding a 6-month separation from both parents, siblings, and the family home. (p. 310)

Sroufe and Rutter (1984) note, however, that anomalous reactions may occur much earlier, in children of 1 year of age. In particular, they point out that some infants react to very brief separations with detachment, a pattern shown normally only following prolonged separations. The work of Schaffer (1958) supports Sroufe and Rutter's findings. Overt behavioral responses to separation, he reports, occur "relatively suddenly and at full force around seven months of age" (quoted by Yarrow, 1964, p. 98).

Research data collected by Yarrow and Goodwin (1963) indicate that separation may affect children at a much earlier age than reported by Sroufe and Rutter (1984). Although they acknowledged that true separation reactions cannot occur prior to establishment of a specific attachment relationship with the mother, Yarrow and Goodwin found evidence of certain antecedent separation reactions as early as 3 months of age in infants who moved from foster to adoptive homes. In infants moved at 4 months, withdrawn behavior, increased apathy, and feeding and sleep disturbances were observed. At 6 months, more overt social disturbances (excessive clinging or definite rejection of the new mother) was seen with increasing frequency. Yarrow (1964) speculates that some of these behavioral disturbances may stem from environmental changes, noting that separation usually causes changes in many areas of the child's environment, including sensory and social stimulation, scheduling, and so on. The concomitant strangeness and loss of predictability may be sufficiently strong stressors to account for many kinds of behavioral disturbances (Trad, 1986).

Yarrow (1964) also calls attention to the implications of age with regard to adoption practices, suggesting "that attempts be made to place infants as early as possible in adoptive homes" (pp. 129-130).

Separation from Peers and Parents

Maternal figures have clearly dominated the literature on depressive reactions to separation. Important evidence suggests, however, that separation reactions can occur in response to many different people in an infant or toddler's environment. Field, Vega-Lahr, and Jagadish (1984) expanded on the study of separation by assessing the play behavior and sleep patterns among a group of toddlers and infants on the occasion of their graduation to new nursery classes. The study group included 12 infants (average age 15 months) and 20 toddlers (mean age 24 months). Behavior of the children was observed during the first and fourth weeks of the month preceding and following graduation. An increase in amounts of fussing, verbal interaction, wandering, fantasy play, and both affectionate and aggressive physical contact was observed immediately preceding the transition. Moreover, activity level was elevated and absenteeism more frequent. Sleep problems emerged with more of the children crying preparatory to sleep and reducing the amount of designated nap time spent sleeping.

The time at which agitation was exhibited appeared to be age-related, with infants displaying less agitation than toddlers just prior to graduation, but more during the first week of their new class. The investigators interpreted this as evidence that, by the end of infancy, cognitive development allows for anticipatory separation stress. The presence of a close friend accompanying the child going into the new class also appeared to be a significant factor. The friend appeared to act as a buffer for the toddler against the dual stress of leaving one environment and adjusting to another.

Several similarities in the constellation of behavioral changes were seen in comparing these results with those found in the mother-child separations of Field, Vega-Lahr, and Jagadish (1984), Field and Reite (1984), and Trause et al. (1981). In all of these studies, behavioral changes included increases in negative affect, activity level, physical aggression, and sleep disturbances. All of these disturbances were interpreted as agitated responses to separation stress.

The age-sensitivity of proximity-maintaining behaviors and the importance of individuals other than the primary caregiver have also been documented in preschool settings, which have served as a backdrop for studies of parents' leavetaking and reunion with infants, toddlers, and preschoolers. In another study by Field et al. (1984), these partings and reunions were observed daily as children were dropped off and picked up at their nursery school. An analysis of the development of distress behavior revealed that, while toddlers were initially more distressed by leavetaking (even those who had experienced leavetaking since infancy), their distress behavior significantly diminished during the second semester. In contrast, infants (3–17 months; mean, 9 months) showed increasing amounts of clinging and hovering. Developmental age, rather than experience with leavetaking, appeared to be the decisive factor in determining the behavior of those observed in the study.

CONCLUSION

As Bowlby (1980) suggests, sadness is a natural reaction to loss. A person suffering great sadness may still have hope; the sense of self-worth is not necessarily diminished. Depression, however, brings with it disorganization and a sense of helplessness and hopelessness. Bowlby attributes this sense of helplessness that is associated with depressive disorders to the experience of loss as an insoluble problem.

Diagnosis of infant depression began with the descriptions of hospitalism and anaclitic depression, formulated by Spitz and Wolf, for infants who were separated from their mothers for prolonged periods of time. Symptoms included crying, withdrawal, weight loss, insomnia, sadness, and an expression that "would be described in adults as depression" (Spitz & Wolf, 1946, p. 316).

The occurrence of the hospitalism syndrome in infants clearly demonstrates the necessity for sufficient coenesthetic stimulation if affective development is to proceed. The emergence of anaclitic depression on separation from the mother or caregiver serves to illustrate the importance of an adequate attachment bond in sustaining normative emotional growth.

As the literature reveals, separation, in various forms and to varying degrees, is a likely common pathway to functional depression in infancy, beginning as early as 3 months of age. The pervasiveness of separation in the etiology of early depression is further evidenced by the finding that separation from peers or siblings is also traumatic.

Despite the etiologic significance of separation trauma in infant depression, the origins of depression are often manifold. As Cicchetti and Schneider-Rosen (1986) contend:

> *Early loss, inadequate maternal care, lack of a secure attachment relationship, an impoverished environment, maternal depression, or a temperamental predisposition to heightened awareness . . . may lead to the formation of depressogenic schemata which make an individual vulnerable to depression. (p. 108)*

The diffuseness of the portrait of symptomatology calls for a broad approach to diagnosis. Such a careful, inclusive perspective will be particularly valuable when it provides developmental data, since signs and symptoms of depression differ at different periods of maturation (Trad, 1986).

CHAPTER FOUR

Regulation and the Development of the Self

The developmental framework provides a reliable and predictable model for assessing the normal course of maturation. By inference, since expected behavior may be charted in this manner, abnormalities or deviations from maturational orientations may also be pinpointed by using the developmental model, and thus incipient infant psychopathology may be identified. Particular developmental milestones, including infant temperamental displays, attachment behaviors, and self-concept formation, serve as landmarks offering the researcher both the tools to probe the evolution of the infant's internal mechanism and the data necessary to extrapolate theory pertaining to psychopathology. But these milestones do not serve only as events or phenomena worthy of observation and analysis; they also represent the dynamic process of maturation from which the infant's ultimate sense of self-identity will emerge.

The prevailing consensus remains that only when the process of self-formation is complete can depression as a full-fledged syndrome be identified. This chapter focuses on the *process* aspect of the developmental milestones. That is, infant temperamental predisposition is discussed not only as a concretized phenomenon capable of evaluation, but the milestone also is interpreted as a continually fluctuating characteristic capable of responding to and interacting with environmental stimulation. In the same way, the infant's cognitive and affective capacities are viewed both as integral elements of the infant's internal mechanism and as dynamic forces that are modulated by interaction. Finally, throughout the discussion, reference is made to the infant's sense of self. Although assiduous efforts have been devoted to pinpointing the precise chronologic point in development when an intact sense of self emerges, the process of development that precedes self-concept formation is vitally significant in shaping the ultimate sense of self. In other words, while an infant of several months may be as yet incapable of articulating affects and cognitions, and of attributing these phenomena to the self or to the environment, his or her perceptual capacities are developed sufficiently so that environmental influences will exert an enduring effect on his perceptions.

To better conceptualize the dynamic process of development, the concepts of "regulation" and "dysregulation" are used throughout the chapter. Indeed, at each phase of development, the infant is engaging in a process of self-regulation. As temperament interacts with environment, as discrepancy and contingency are discerned, and as inchoate capacities in the domain of self-awareness evolve, the infant begins to regulate both the self and interaction with the external world. Regulation, in this context, refers to the comprehensive, all-embracing ability to function in a manner most likely to produce competency, mastery, gratification, and positive affect. As such, a highly functioning regulatory mechanism is one capable of flexibly responding to environmental stimuli and modulating interaction with an optimum of agility. The infant who is performing in a self-regulating manner will be characteristically alert and responsive, displaying mobility and plasticity in each response.

In contrast, examples of "dysregulation" within the infant's internal mechanism will also be discussed. Dysregulation is a response that is characteristically rigid, inflexible, and automatic. Infant reactivity becomes stiffened and reflex-like, so that sensitivity to environmental cues is diminished, and the infant is divorced or detached from the environment. In effect, a dysregulatory response is a stifled response, preventing the infant from engaging the full spectrum of his or her affective and cognitive capacities. Moreover, the phenomenon of dysregulation appears to suffuse all infant response, so that dysregulation transfers across tasks and situations. This dysregulation may affect various domains of infant perception, creating deficits of cognition, affect, and motivation, as well as impinging on the incipient sense of self. The cognitive deficit may be manifested by a characteristic dulling of perception, the affective deficit may express itself via depression or flat affect, and the motivational deficit will reveal itself as an apathetic response to social interaction and environmental stimulation.

This chapter discusses the mode whereby dysregulation may occur—during the period when discrepancy and contingency awareness are developing, during the formation of the caregiver–infant interaction, and during the attachment relationship. Additionally, the discussion of neuroendocrine function indicates that infants, from the first hours after birth, possess a sophisticated hormonal mechanism capable of responding physiologically to stress in a manner similar to adult response. As such, we may inquire whether the neuroendocrine dysregulation encountered in depressed adults and children can also be manifested by infants.

The theme of dysregulation serves as a barometer for gauging the degree of damage that the infant's mechanism has sustained. In essence, infant dysregulation in the domains of cognition, affect, and motivation may effectively be interpreted as symptomatic of depression. Moreover, infant dysregulation may serve as a sign for distinguishing between depression as an affect disorder and depression as a mood disorder. If the dysregulation is pinpointed during early interaction and appears to color response in many domains, such an infant may be primed for experiencing a subsequent mood disorder, whereas dysregulation occurring at a later phase of development may affect development in only one area and may subsequently emerge as an affect disorder.

Any attempt to understand the origins of infant depression, and to understand how the disorder may interfere with ongoing adaptation, must first consider how the self develops. In this regard, many fundamental issues need to be addressed, such as how early a meaningful concept of the self emerges and what constitute the earliest precursors of the self-concept. Genetic and environmental resources that coalesce in the individual to build a strong and adaptive self must also be pinpointed. Insights into these issues will help identify risk factors for depression (Trad, 1986).

The capacity for self-regulation by modulating the transitions between physical, affective, and cognitive states is instrumental in creating the sense of continuity that may underlie the development of the self. Winnicott (1956, 1960) suggests that protection against intrusive external or internal stimuli provides the stability of experience on which ego strength is constructed. According to Winnicott's conception, however, this experience is largely passive; the mother, not the infant, provides this regulation.

The development of regulatory capacities, however, implies a move from external to internal control. This process occurs from birth, partly as a consequence of endogenous processes and partly as an outgrowth of interaction with the mother. It entails the development of a flexible sense of competence without which an individual may fall prey to depression. During the first 18 months of life, most infants develop increased sophistication in regulating themselves. Their growing awareness of their own internal states facilitates their appreciation that others are separate entities with individual perceptions and intentions. This awareness allows infants and young toddlers to accept some forms of necessary regulation from their caregivers. The repertoire of attachment behaviors that is "instinctive" to the infant helps to engage the mother in repeated interactions. These rhythmic, repetitive interactions (reciprocal smiling, babbling, talking, movement) form the matrix from which the infant's awareness of contingency experiences emerges. Interactions of this type are also the basis for the infant's first feelings of efficacy (White, 1959). Contemporaneously with the growth of self-regulation, infants begin to perceive contingencies between their own actions and responses from their environment. Infants at a very early age not only behave intentionally, but are aware of their own intentionality. Not surprisingly, this awareness may be inferred from the particular kinds of affective displays the infant exhibits.

Some tentative evidence of the link between self-regulation and depression may be available from research into infant discrepancy awareness. By comparing infants' responses to novel and familiar stimuli, investigations in this area have enabled researchers to determine how early in life infants move from largely reflexive behaviors to those resulting from their entrance into an interactive relationship—however primitive—with their environment. More important, these studies reveal how well infants perceive the environment and how adept they are at responding to it. Clear patterns of affective response (McCall & McGhee, 1977) associated with different levels of discrepancy suggest a strong link between different qualities of affect and the ability to regulate stimuli from the environment.

Watson's (1966) theory of contingency awareness, presented in greater detail later in this chapter, describes a similar interplay of perception and affect. White (1959) posits that the perception of learned contingency is pleasurable. For the infant, the experience of noncontingency—discrepancy from an expected contingency—is unpleasurable. If the experience is repeated, if the infant fails to perceive contingencies with the primary object in its world (its mother), the infant may suffer a loss of esteem that ultimately hampers the development of the self. This loss parallels the self-esteem deficit seen in adults as outlined by the learned helplessness paradigm (Klein and Seligman, 1976; Seligman and Maier, 1967). Implicit in this deficit is the experience of depressive manifestations. Depression in adults is the affective counterpart of loss of control. It is the prime contention of this chapter that the perception of loss of control also embodies a negative affective component for infants, and that it is the fundamental starting point for depression and depressive disorders. The perception of loss of control in infants necessarily involves the caregiver, and the degree to which the caregiver's behavior is predictable will determine, in part, the degree to which the infant perceives control over its environment. If the environment is noncontingent and untrustworthy, the infant may withdraw and show signs of depression.

Failure to regulate smoothly between affective states may result in other psychopathology besides depression. In all of its guises, this failure to regulate prevents adaptive and flexible response to developmental challenges. The case of depression is particularly illuminating from a developmental vantage point, because it highlights the way in which failure to integrate functions and behaviors at one developmental level can pave the way for subsequent maladaption, thus creating a self-reinforcing situation.

A variety of factors determine how an individual develops a self-regulatory system. This development is shaped partly by innate reactivity (Rothbart & Derryberry, 1981), which may be a function of temperament and biological factors. The course of development is also affected by the responsiveness of the caregiver, who is the infant's main ally in establishing a sense of efficacy during interactions with the environment. This chapter begins by exploring factors endogenous to the infant and then turns to a discussion of how these factors interact with characteristics of the environment.

MECHANISMS OF TEMPERAMENT AFFECTING SELF-REGULATION

Endogenous individual differences in infant reactivity profoundly affect the course of cognitive and affective development and may have a significant impact on a child's ability to acquire the self-regulatory abilities requisite for establishing a secure sense of self. Such differences are highlighted and examined in studies of infant temperament. Several different schemata have been developed to describe these innate or "temperamental" elements of the infant mechanism. Most modern theories of temperament rely on the fundamental definition of the concept formulated by Allport (1937), who wrote:

> *Temperament refers to the characteristic phenomena of an individual's emotional nature, including his susceptibility to emotional stimulation, his customary strength and speed of response, the quality of his prevailing mood. . . ; these phenomena [are] dependent upon constitutional make-up, and therefore [are] largely hereditary in origin. (p. 54)*

Rothbart and Derryberry

Rothbart and Derryberry (1981) defined temperament as differences in reactivity and self-regulation. They stated:

> *We will define temperament as constitutional differences in reactivity and self-regulation, with "constitutional" seen as the relatively enduring biological makeup of the organism influenced over time by heredity, maturation, and experience. By "reactivity" we refer to the characteristics of the individual's reaction to changes in the environment, as reflected in somatic, endocrine, and autonomic nervous systems. By "self-regulation" we mean the processes functioning to modulate this reactivity, e.g., attentional and behavioral patterns of approach and avoidance. (p. 834)*

These researchers defined emotion in terms of the infant's ability to regulate internal states. Through affective tone, the self-regulatory mechanisms are set in motion. These self-regulatory mechanisms are reflected in such behaviors as approach/avoidance, self-soothing, and focusing of attention. Using these behaviors as a vehicle for response, the infant can modulate the effects of stimulation by either accentuating or attenuating stimuli in order to achieve a state of equilibrium.

Rothbart and Derryberry (1984) found that some of their subjects were less vulnerable to negative emotional states than others, because they were able to selectively avert their attention from negative aspects of their environments. The researchers' concept bears similarity to Siever and Davis' (1985) concept of "dysregulation," which stipulates that the maturation of self-regulation is associated with the development of neurotransmitter mechanisms during the first months and years of life. Failure of the neurotransmitter chemicals to emerge on schedule developmentally may leave the infant vulnerable and incapable of controlling new emotional states, thus leading to "dysfunctions" such as depression. Significantly, Rothbart and Derryberry introduce the notion that temperament is not merely the clustering of disparate personality traits; rather, it is the ability to *regulate* or *modulate* these traits. In this sense, temperamental traits represent the behavioral manifestations of an infant's regulatory process. Thus temperament may be conceived of as individual differences in internal regulation.

Thomas and Chess

Thomas and Chess (Chess & Thomas, 1984; Chess, Thomas, Birch, Hertzig, & Korn, 1963; Thomas & Chess, 1977, 1980; Thomas, Chess, & Birch, 1968, 1970), who conducted the preeminent study of temperament development, the New York Longitudinal Study (NYLS), extrapolated nine dimensions of temperament from their operational definition: activity level, rhythmicity (regularity), approach or withdrawal, adaptability, threshold of responsiveness, intensity of reaction, quality of mood, distractibility, and attention span or persistence. It is significant that Thomas and Chess' dimensions of temperament, like Rothbart and Derryberry's (1981), focus on the regulation and reactivity of infant behavior. They define temperament as follows:

> *Temperament is the* behavioral *style of the individual child—the* how *rather than the* what *(abilities and content) or* why *(motivations) of behavior. Temperament is a phenomenologic term used to describe the characteristic tempo, rhythmicity, adaptability, energy expenditure, mood, and focus of attention of a child.* . . . *(Thomas, Chess, & Birch, 1968, p. 4; emphasis in original.)*

In Thomas and Chess' definition of temperament, the "how" of behavioral style represents the modulation of infant behavior, and the outlined traits describe, implicitly, various aspects of a regulatory process.

Throughout their investigations, Thomas and Chess argued that temperament traits must be understood in terms of how they contribute to what Henderson (1982) referred to as "goodness or poorness of fit" with the environment. Goodness of fit suggests that the organism's capacities, motivation, and style of behaving are in harmony with the expectations of the environment. When goodness of fit is present, the potential for optimal development is enhanced, and the individual is said to be in consonance with his or her environment. In contrast, dissonance between an individual's expectations and abilities and the environment's expectations and demands results in poorness of fit, which the NYLS investigators said can lead to distorted development and maladaptive functioning (Thomas & Chess, 1980). According to this interactionist viewpoint, temperament traits alone do not dispose an infant to depression. Instead, these traits interact with environmental factors. The interaction of all these factors may or may not create a vulnerability to depression. Hence the investigators' emphasis on the predictive value of clusters or typologies of temperamental traits, rather than on individual attributes. Temperament may, for example, affect an infant's ability to resolve discrepancies perceived in the environment. Similarly, temperament may be a significant factor in an infant's ability or inability to perceive contingency in its environment or to experience positive affect associated with such contingency.

NYLS Typologies.   Thomas and Chess (Thomas, Chess, & Birch,1968) identified three common temperamental typologies: the "easy," the "difficult," and the "slow-to-warm-up" child. These clusters are based on observations that particular temperamental traits demonstrated consistent relationships or associations with other traits. Correlations among the nine categories of temperament for the total population of children in the NYLS revealed that three of the temperamental variables—intensity, adaptability, and mood—demonstrated the largest number of significant correlations with other categories. For example, high intensity correlated positively with high levels of activity, persistence, irregularity, low adaptability, and negative expressions of mood. Adaptability showed positive correlations with rhythmicity, approach, and mood. Finally, the dimension of mood correlated positively and very highly with adaptability and approach to new situations and negatively with intensity.

"Easy" children, as suggested by these patterns, were characterized by positive mood, regularity of body functions, adaptability, and positive approach. "Difficult" children, on the other hand, tended to exhibit negative mood, irregularity of bodily function, and withdrawal from new stimuli. "Slow-to-warm-up" children had low activity levels, slow adaptation, mild reaction, and a tendency to withdraw from new stimuli.

"Easy" children were strongly self-regulating, moving easily between affective states. They responded smoothly and promptly to caregiver interventions, and contributed significantly to their own goodness of fit. "Difficult" children had more difficulty self-regulating, and consequently responded less flexibly to parental regulation. They were often troublesome to manage and were found to be at greater risk for developing behavior disorders.

COGNITIVE AND AFFECTIVE MECHANISMS AFFECTING SELF-REGULATION

One goal of this chapter is to articulate how the regulatory abilities, which first became apparent in temperament studies, converge over time to result in a sense of "self." The emphasis on "self" is based on the premise, articulated by Abramson, Seligman, and Teasdale (1978), that an infant or child cannot be vulnerable to learned helplessness depression until a sense of self and a capacity for self-attribution are firmly entrenched. That is, only with the emergence of the self does susceptibility to depression become a viable possibility (Trad, 1986).

If we assume that Abramson, Seligman, and Teasdale (1978), as well as other researchers, are correct, it is essential to map out the cognitive and affective prerequisites for the development of the self. Here the self should not be perceived of as a static concept. As Kopp (1982) suggested, affect regulation has been identified as a fundamental requirement for the development of the self. It is perhaps from studying the abilities of regulation, which serve as an internal modulator, that researchers may glean the most data about the infant's incipient sense of self. For now, regulation should be viewed as the capacity to shift between affective states in a manner appropriate to environmental cues, as well as the ability to draw on cognitive skills for adapting to interactive events.

What capacities beyond temperamental predispositions does the neonate possess which enable him or her to regulate behavior? Confirmation of fairly sophisticated visual-perceptual capacities—including the finding that visual acuity in newborns is at least 20/150 (Dayton, Jones, Aiu, Rowson, Steele, & Rose, 1964), and the verification of active neonatal peripheral vision (Harris & MacFarlane, 1974)—has resulted in an increased appreciation of the complexity of the internal sensory and cognitive apparatus that newborn infants possess. In addition, Fantz and Miranda (1975) demonstrated that infants under 7 days of age are capable of selectively fixating on curved contours, rather than on straight patterns, while the capacity to discriminate between two different visual stimulus arrays has been shown in infants under 1 week of age (Antell & Keating, 1983). Four-month-old infants have been found to pay selective attention to a human face, rather than to geometric patterns (McCall & Kagan, 1967), suggesting a measurable preference for one form of stimuli over another. Fagen and Rovee-Collier (1976) report that by 7 months of age the infant has established the capacity to remember and to recognize faces.

In addition to these cognitive capacities, infants, even neonates, have been shown to possess an intricate repertoire of affective responses to environmental stimuli. Indeed, since such young infants are not yet capable of communicating verbally, much of the significance of early infant behavior has been inferred from the spectrum of affective facial expressions displayed. In this regard, Izard et al. (1980) reported that adult evaluators could discern such emotions as interest, joy, surprise, sadness, disgust, anger, and fear after observing infants aged 1 to 9 months old. Moreover, Barrera and Maurer (1981) reported that 3-month-olds could discriminate between smiling (happy) and frowning (angry) faces when these facial expressions were exhibited by their caregivers.

Cardiac response has also been used as an indicator of infant cognitive and affective response. Deceleration of heart rate is generally interpreted as indicating that the perceptual system is becoming more receptive to environmental stimulation (Graham, 1979), while acceleration of heart rate is associated with nonreceptivity to environmental events. Vaughn and Sroufe (1979) demonstrated that cardiac acceleration was associated with crying in infants between 8 and 16 months of age. The researchers suggested that cardiac acceleration was not only a by-product of crying, but was also associated with the negative affect that precedes crying.

Given evidence of this prodigious armamentarium of infant response, it is worth inquiring into the origins of these capacities. First, do the infant's cognitive capabilities coordinate with affective responses? Second, what is the nature of the regulatory exchange between cognitive and affective realms? In other words, do young infants possess some sort of internal regulating process, and if so, how does this process evolve? Finally, and most crucially, how do cognitive and affective capacities mature to create a sense of self and identity?

Discrepancies

Preliminary answers to these questions may be derived from a theory of development called the discrepancy awareness hypothesis, articulated by McCall and McGhee (1977). According to these researchers, neonates draw on capacities from both their cognitive and affective repertoires to respond to new stimuli in the environment. "Discrepancy" is defined as the degree of similarity or disparity between two stimuli. The theory posits that infant response to gradations of discrepancy may be charted on a standard inverted U curve. Thus the perception of a discrepancy that is only somewhat or moderately deviant from a familiar, standard stimulus will trigger an optimal level of both attention and nonpositive or neutral affect, while extreme discrepancy will result in low levels of attention, accompanied by negative affect. Based on this formulation, moderate discrepancy registers on the highest portion of the inverted U model.

In fact, several investigations have verified this pattern of inverted U curve affective and cognitive response in both infants and adults. McCall and Kagan (1967) exposed infants of 3.5 months of age to a standard stimulus until a level of habituation was achieved. Stimulus-experienced infants, as well as a group of nonexperienced control infants of the same age, were then exposed to the standard stimulus and to three other stimuli of graded variations of "discrimination." The conclusions of the study lend qualified support to the discrepancy hypothesis. The researchers found that for the female infants, a stimulus that closely matched a prior stimulus schema elicited less cardiac deceleration than a moderately discrepant event, while a stimulus that was moderately discrepant evoked greater cardiac deceleration than if the same stimulus was completely familiar. In explaining the difference between the male and female infants in the study, the researchers hypothesized that girls may be more perceptually precocious than boys, meaning that they may achieve critical developmental milestones earlier.

Further clinical verification of the discrepancy hypothesis response curve was provided by Parry (1973). Comparing 6-month-old with 12-month-old infants, the researcher familiarized both groups to standard stimuli, and then presented gradations of discrepant stimuli. Using measures of visual fixation, it was found that both age groups perceived differences in the range of stimuli. Interestingly, however, it was found that only the older infants displayed "wariness," and that the greater the discrepancy between the standard and the discrepant stimulus, the greater the wariness.

When Hopkins, Zelazo, Jacobson, and Kagan (1976) explored the presence and characteristics of discrepancy awareness in 7.5-month-old infants, they discovered that reactivity—defined as instrumental responding, fixation, vocalization, and smiling—was maximal to a moderately discrepant stimulus, following a period of habituation to a standard stimulus. The researchers concluded that their findings confirm discrepancy theory, and indicate that stimuli that are moderately different from existing cognitive representations recruit more sustained attention and provoke more sustained excitement than stimuli that are either familiar or completely novel.

Finally, Conners (1964) demonstrated that the response curve outlined by the discrepancy awareness hypothesis achieves its full realization in adults. Using undergraduate volunteers, the researcher found that through both eye-movement fixation and verbal report, greatest preference was expressed for slightly discrepant figures, while the least preference was expressed for the most discrepant figures.

The discrepancy hypothesis assumes that affective displays may be used as artifacts for measuring the level of the infant's awareness of disparate stimuli. Positive affective displays, such as smiling, have been correlated with raised expectancy and increased learning (Masters & Furman, 1976; Masters, Barden, & Ford, 1979). Crying, in contrast, has been associated with the temperamental dimension of "distress to novel stimuli" (Fagen & Ohr, 1985). Thus an infant's temperament, as disclosed by individual differences in affective expression, may exert a significant impact on his capacity to experience discrepancy, and subsequently, to respond to discrepant stimuli.

Haber (1958), investigating the effect of discrepancy on affect arousal in adults, found that affect displays—both positive and negative—fluctuated according to the amount of discrepancy present. Moreover, after subjects had had their hands habituated to a specific water temperature, it was found that immersion of hands in water with a moderately discrepant temperature was preferred over immersion of hands in water that was of an extremely different temperature. Thus positive affect was associated with more minimal discrepancies of a sensory-perceptual event from adaptation level, while negative affect correlated with larger discrepancies from an adaptation level.

Investigating the relationship between cognitive discrepancy and affect in 10-month-old infants, Sroufe, Waters, and Matas (1974) found that novel situations and strangers can activate both strong approach and strong avoidance tendencies, with affective outcome often determined by the environmental setting, sequence of events, and familiarization.

As initially formulated, the discrepancy awareness hypothesis presumes that infants are equipped with adequate memory capacity which allows them to distinguish subtle differences between stimuli. Further, the theory also suggests that a process of retrieval from memory storage is present. Moreover, memory must be of the type labeled "evocative" memory, rather than "recognition" memory. Evocative memory, as defined by Nachman and Stern (1984), implies stored engrams or schemas that can be brought to consciousness in the absence of an external presentation of the stimulus. The presence of such evocative memory retrieval has been confirmed in 7-month-olds (Nachman & Stern, 1984).

Exploring the process of memory retrieval in young children, Loftus and Grober (1973) determined that 6-year-olds use a process of superordinate groupings to retrieve schemas from memory. The researchers noted that semantic development appears to occur in a hierarchical structure, with children first retrieving a category from memory and then retrieving an appropriate member of that category.

A form of complex memory retrieval may also be occurring in very young infants, according to McCall, Hogarty, Hamilton, & Vincent (1973). These researchers presented 120 infants, 12 and 18 weeks of age, with a simple visual stimulus until visual fixation reached a habituation criterion. Infants were then exposed to a discrepant stimulus. It was found that infants who habituated rapidly displayed an inverted U curve of fixation as a function of discrepancy in accord with the discrepancy hypothesis. The researchers noted that the results are in keeping with the notion that the phenomenon of habituation itself may reflect some form of internal processing of a memory engram for the standard stimulus. Infants who habituate engage in this processing and are then equipped to respond to a new stimulus. If a discrepant stimulus is introduced prior to habituation, however, the infant has no opportunity to draw on a memory engram and will not respond positively to the discrepancy. The researchers concluded that within the first year of life sufficient memory capacity has developed to enable the infant to compare an external perception with an associated memory engram.

Although most of the data confirming the existence of discrepancy awareness during the early months of life has involved infants from 2 to 6 months of age, Friedman, Bruno, and Vietze (1974) demonstrated that neonates as young as 28 hours old respond to variations in stimuli on the inverted U curve predicted by McCall and McGhee (1977). Perception of discrepancy triggers the process of subjective uncertainty, whereby the infant attempts to formulate a response to the stimulus. If a discrepant event can be processed internally in a successful manner (most likely to occur with moderately discrepant stimuli) the infant will likely experience positive affect. In contrast, extreme discrepancy will evoke stressful processing coupled with negative affect. Moreover, McCall and McGhee (1977) note that negative affect occurs during difficult processing, whereas positive affect results only when processing is successfully completed. Thus the same stimuli may evoke both negative affect (during processing) and positive affect (during resolution). In essence, the interaction of negative and positive affect during the phase of subjective uncertainty most likely represents the infant's first efforts to regulate his or her internal state in response to an external stimuli and to exercise some degree of control over the environment. Indeed, if the stimulus event is particularly threatening or extremely discrepant to the infant, his or her fragile regulatory capacity may be disrupted, with the result that negative affect will not be controlled and will engulf the infant, creating the diffused experience of helplessness.

The underlying memory processes determining response to stimulus discrepancy were examined by McCall and Kagan (1970) in a study involving 4-month-old infants. The researchers found that the manner in which infants habituated to an initial, standard stimulus, as demonstrated by visual fixation, could be used to predict response to discrepant stimuli. Those infants who habituated rapidly to the initial, standard stimulus showed increasing fixation to increasing amounts of stimulus change in accord with the discrepancy hypothesis. In contrast, infants who failed to habituate did not evince a differential response to the discrepant stimuli. These findings suggest that the theory of memory processing is accurate. Once habituation has occurred, subsequent response to a discrepant stimulus—either negative or positive depending on the degree of discrepancy—may be anticipated.

In sum, as the discrepancy awareness hypothesis stipulates, and as data from these studies suggest, the infant derives highest levels of gratification from, and appears best equipped to process, moderate stimulation. Extreme levels of stimulation result in negative affect, while familiar stimuli evoke a display of disinterest in the infant.

The Impact of Temperamental Factors on Discrepancy Awareness. The type of response displayed by an infant confronted with a discrepant stimulus is not only a function of the attributes of the stimulus, it may also be modulated by the individual temperamental attributes of the infant. For instance, when confronted with a discrepant stimulus an infant with a high level of persistence (a temperamental trait) may be better suited to engage in an assiduous memory scan, in an attempt to retrieve a related engram. At the other end of the spectrum, an infant possessing minimal degrees of innate persistence may become frustrated by an encounter with even moderate discrepancy and may give up memory scanning relatively early. Such an infant may then exaggerate the effect of moderate discrepancy by interpreting it as extreme discrepancy and may experience negative affect as a consequence. Viewed in this manner, the discrepancy hypothesis suggests a mechanism of dynamic interaction between the infant and his external milieu. Just as the stimulus' degree of discrepancy will provoke a particular kind of cognitive and affective processing response in the infant, so too will the infant (primarily through the vehicle of temperament) exert an impact on the stimulus.

Another facet of the infant's ability to perceive discrepancy in his environment involves capacities to attend to the stimulus for a period of time sufficiently long to enable the process of retrieval from memory storage to occur. Thus studies exploring attention span in young infants may provide insight into the mechanisms operating to facilitate discrepancy awareness. Attention, then, may be a key external indicator of internal processing.

McCall and Kagan (1967) investigated attentive perception in 36 4-month-old infants. Infants were presented with solid black random shapes. Shapes contained a variant number of sides (e.g., 5-, 10-, and 20-sided figures) and were of three different sizes. Using visual fixation as their gauge, the researchers found that the number of fixations directly correlated with the size of the figure and was unrelated to the number of sides each figure possessed. The researchers noted that results other than dimensional "complexity" may be at work when infant populations are exposed to random shapes. Moreover, these data suggest that young infants may be better equipped than previously supposed to integrate and process fairly sophisticated visual stimuli.

In a related trial, the same researchers presented another group of 4-month-olds with achromatic slides of regular and irregular faces. Both duration of fixation and magnitude of cardiac deceleration were significantly greater to the regular faces than to the random shapes. These latter results indicate that young infants are not only capable of integrating a face stimulus (as evinced by gaze or fixation time), but also that face stimuli are associated with affective habituation, as demonstrated by lowered cardiac rates.

McCall and Melson (1969), in a similar investigation, tested 5.5-month-old infant boys to formulate the distribution curve for attention to varying magnitudes of discrepancy from a familiarized standard. Relying on cardiac deceleration as their main index of measurement, the researchers found that attention varied as a function of magnitude of discrepancy. Significantly, the pattern discerned was consistent with the inverted U curve configuration predicted by the discrepancy hypothesis. Further, once habituation to a repeatedly presented standard stimulus had been achieved, it was found that fixation time was also a reliable predictor of the extent of infant response to discrepancies. This study, then, corroborates earlier suggestions that infants possess the attentional equipment necessary to perceive discrepancies and, by implication, that they are best suited to incorporate moderate levels of disparity among stimuli.

Probing the relationship between the infant's facial expression, visual fixation, and heart rate in response to stimuli that vary in face relatedness,

Langsdorf, Izard, Rayais, and Hembree (1983) reported that these indicators do, in fact, respond differentially based on the stimulus presented. Four different age groups of infants (2-, 4-, 6-, and 8-month-olds) were presented with a live female face, a female mannequin, and an inanimate object with scrambled facial features. During presentations, visual fixation, heart rate, and facial movements (considered to be indicators of interest) were measured. Significantly different responses were found to relate to the infant's age and to the characteristics of the stimuli. The researchers concluded first that facial expression demonstrating interest, visual fixation, and heart rate deceleration varied in a similar fashion in response to all three stimuli. Second, the researchers found that an infant's facial expression of interest was sensitive to differences in face relatedness of stimuli and was also predictive of visual fixation. These findings further confirm the existence of a complex mechanism of responsive equipment that is designed to acclimate to variant levels of stimulation in the environment.

In a review article summarizing the implications of infant attentive capacity, McCall (1970c) synthesized previous data in this area. He noted that studies of infant attention provide clues to early cognitive development. Moreover, according to McCall, the studies consistently indicate that the infant's perceptual-cognitive system develops during the first several months of life, and that progressively, preferential attention is given to patterns of increasing complexity. Habituation of attention with repeated presentations of a given stimulus may be useful as an index of the extent to which the infant has formed a memory engram of that stimulus.

The various evidential clues from studies involving infant evocative memory capacity, infant temperament, and most pertinently, infant manifestations of attention (as demonstrated primarily through facial expression, visual fixation, and cardiac deceleration), form an intricate portrait of early cognitive and affective development. From these studies, it appears that from the first months of life, the infant possesses a sophisticated set of behaviors for integrating the myriad stimuli emanating from the environment. But, as the discrepancy hypothesis indicates, the infant not only possesses various capacities for integration, but also appears to respond to stimuli in a particular manner. That is, stimuli that are moderately discrepant from stimuli to which the infant is habituated or accustomed will evoke the highest levels of positive response, both affectively and cognitively. In contrast, stimuli that are either relatively familiar or overly discordant from those previously encountered will evoke relative indifference or negative response, respectively.

Given this scenario, researchers have asked how the infant's incipient control mechanism evolves into a system of self-control. Vaughn, Kopp, and Krakow (1984) note that self-control emerges and is consolidated during the second year of life. Kopp (1982) has delved into the concept of self-control and has reported that as distinguished from control, *self-control* represents the ability to modulate behavior in accord with environmental demands. Moreover, she observes that self-control emerges developmentally through childhood and that its cognitive roots lie in the capacities of representational thought and evocative memory. It is significant that Kopp refers to evocative memory, since this ability is a prerequisite for engaging in discrepancy awareness, according to McCall and McGhee (1977). Elaborating on the concept of self-control, Kopp (1982) has written that it is an organizational construct around which many other developmental milestones are orchestrated. That is, self-control is a fundamental regulatory capacity. Finally, Kopp observes that self-control includes the capacity to inhibit responsiveness to compelling stimuli and to defer gratification, qualities that are observed fleetingly in 18-month-old children.

Focusing on the development of control during infancy and the effect of increased mastery on the infant's affective state, Gunnar (1980) examined the effects of control in infants aged 6, 9, and 12 months. The researcher found that control did not reduce distress reactions in infants (including fussing and crying) until the age of 12 months. The infants tested were exposed to a potentially fear-provoking toy. Under the control condition, the toy could be obliterated from view when a wooden tray was touched. Addressing the issue of why control did not reduce distress in the younger infants, Gunnar noted that by 12 months, the infant has developed expectancies regarding the consequences of active and inhibiting behavior. That is, by this age, infants not only conceptualize the concept of control, but they have also formulated a sense of self-control sufficient to understand that they can directly cause an event through action or prevent an event by inhibiting action. The process of individuation whereby infants can attribute causal events in the external environment to their own actions has occurred, at least on a basic level.

The development of control and self-control is also related to the degree of negative affect the infant may experience. For example, since the caregiver signifies security for the infant, it is not surprising that 8-week-olds displayed mild distress when their mothers were told to act motionless and unresponsive. Further, infant distress in the presence of strangers during the first months of life is magnified if the mother is absent. This response may be due to the fact that the caregiver serves as the focal point of control for the infant, who has not yet developed capacities of self-control. However, it has also been reported by McCall and McGhee (1977) that if the infant can control a stimulus it will not elicit fear during the first months of life. Thus control and security—at least until the first year—must be provided primarily by the external force of a regulating caregiver. Without the caregiver, the infant, although capable of understanding the gratification that comes with control, cannot autonomously exhibit sufficient self-control to stave off the negative affect associated with strange or extremely discrepant stimuli.

A distinctive change in the infant's level of exerting control over the environment occurs after the first year of life. Gunnar and Stone (1984), in a study of 48 infants aged 12 to 13 months, reported on the phenomenon of social referencing. The researchers define social referencing as the infant's capacity to use selectively the caregiver's behavior to appraise situations that they are not sophisticated enough to assess on their own. In the study, infants were shown three toys: a pleasant toy, an ambiguous toy, and an aversive toy. Infants had two trials with each toy. On the first trial, mothers displayed positive affect to each toy; on the second trial, mothers displayed neutral affect. Maternal affect resulted in more positive infant response, but only for the ambiguous toy. These findings suggested to the researchers that infants of this age may be processing responses to stimuli on their own and are only using caregivers to gain perspective. That is, the infant's internal self-regulatory system has replaced the caregiver as the key standard for security and for achieving positive affect. This study, in conjunction with the earlier Gunnar (1980) study, indicates the progression from control to self-control during the first year of life and implies processes whereby the infant—if caregiving has been adequate—masters methods for gaining increased competence over discrepant stimuli.

Expectancies

The studies described thus far deal with situations in which stimuli are presented to infants in order to evoke a response. We must ask, however, what happens after the temporal moment of interaction when the infant has husbanded his or her resources to confront the stimulus. That is, what is the residue of interaction? In asking about what occurs to the infant subsequently, we are, in essence, asking about the role of expectancy. Researchers in the area of discrepancy awareness can make reasonably reliable predictions about how the typical infant will respond to a particular stimulus based on the stimulus' level of disparity from previously encountered stimuli. But at what point do infants start to make predictions about their own responses? How and when do they come to expect to encounter a particular kind of stimulus and to anticipate what the response will be to that stimulus? In asking these questions the perspective shifts from that of the researcher, an external observer, to that of the infant. By focusing on the infant's point of view, we are fundamentally inquiring about the incipient stages of self-awareness (Trad, 1986).

Lansman, Farr, and Hunt (1984), exploring the notion of expectancy in adults, found that there are essentially two versions of this phenomenon. First, expectancy can be a consequence of the frequency with which a stimulus is presented. When expectancy is developed based on frequency or repeated exposure, according to these researchers, response is in the nature of automatic activation, similar to a reflex reaction. The second form of expectancy is a more sophisticated, "cueing" form of presentation. Following the cue, subjects attend, and then upon presentation of the "expected" stimulus, display a predictable response. Implicitly, the latter type expectation involves more complex processing and suggests that the subject has assimilated an understanding of cause and effect between two unrelated stimuli.

Stern and Gibbon (1978) investigated expectancy formation in infancy. These researchers posited that even from birth, the infant is capable of forming temporal expectancies. In a study of three mother-infant dyads, with infants ranging in age from 3 to 4 months, the researchers employed a process of repetitive stimuli. All of the infants demonstrated anticipatory response, even when the amount of time between the presentation of stimuli was varied. This study suggests that young infants may be capable of formulating the sort of expectations Lansman, Farr, and Hunt (1984) associated with frequent, repeated exposure to a stimulus.

With regard to the more sophisticated kind of expectancy, which relies on a perception of a cause and effect relationship, it is necessary to turn to another theory of infant cognitive and affective development, the contingency awareness hypothesis.

Contingencies

The contingency awareness hypothesis was articulated by Watson (1966, 1971, 1972). He defined contingency awareness as the ability to formulate a strategy for achieving goals by connecting two or more stimuli and perceiving a cause-effect relationship between them. Moreover, Watson asserted that an awareness of contingencies permits one to experience the cognitive and affective aspects of success and failure. In essence, according to Watson, an organism possessing a high degree of contingency awareness is ready and equipped to learn.

Watson (1972) proposed that infants 2 to 3 months old are capable of perceiving contingencies. Indeed, in the researcher's opinion, whenever such infants perceive the occurrence of a new stimulus, they initiate a process of contingency analysis. Describing the playful interaction that occurs between the infant and caregiver during the early months of life, Watson commented that via such interaction the caregiver consistently presents an identical response to repetitive behavior. Watson termed such behavior "The Game," noting that manifestations of pleasure displayed during this interactive exchange are indicative of contingency awareness.

One possible limitation to Watson's contention that infants are capable of learning contingencies is the fact that contingency awareness requires sufficient memory span to enable the infant to associate one form of behavior with another. For example, an infant might lift an arm and immediately his mother might kiss it. Unless the infant can lift an arm again quite quickly, causing the mother to repeat the kiss, the infant will not learn that lifting the arm and having the arm kissed are contingent. Recent data suggest, however, that even very young infants possess sufficient memory capacities to enable them to perceive contingency relationships. Fagen et al. (1984) demonstrated 24-hour memory retention in 3-month-olds, while DeCasper and Carstens (1981) provided evidence that neonates can learn contingencies and retain learning for 24 hours. Bower, Broughton, and Moore (1970) demonstrated intentionality in the reaching behavior of infants younger than 1 month of age. Most impressively, Davis and Rovee-Collier (1983) taught 2-month-old infants a contingency relationship in two training sessions and established that memory of the contingency could be retrieved nearly 3 weeks after the initial experience.

Issues raised by Watson's theory of contingency awareness (1966) include whether the pleasure infants appear to derive from mastering a contingency relationship facilitates the learning of future contingencies. Further, do infants transfer the learning of contingencies from one situation to another?

Turning to the empirical support for the theory of contingency awareness, Watson and Ramey (1972) conducted a study involving 8-week-old infants. In the experiment, infants were exposed to a mobile for 10 minutes a day during a 2-week period. Head-pressing against the pillow caused the mobile to turn. Control-group infants were exposed to either a stable or noncontingent mobile. Following the 2-week period, the subject infants significantly increased the number of head-presses against the pillow and exhibited distinctive smiling and cooing behavior when the mobile turned. Control infants did not exhibit these behaviors.

DeCasper and Carstens' (1981) investigations of contingency awareness focused on a population of neonates. One group of infants was exposed to a vocal music stimulus that was contingent on their executing appropriately spaced bursts of nonnutritive sucking. A second group was exposed to noncontingent music. When the groups were switched, the researchers found that infants who were first exposed to contingent singing did in fact learn to space their sucking bursts so as to produce more singing. In sharp distinction, infants who were first subjected to noncontingent singing did not learn the subsequent contingency. Equally noteworthy was the fact that the infants who first encountered the contingent singing reacted with negative affect (fidgeting, crying) to noncontingent singing, while noncontingent singing did not upset infants exposed to it first. Ostensibly the disruption of an already perceived contingency was upsetting.

These findings suggest some implications for the earlier discussion on expectancy. It may be argued that unless the infants exposed to contingency singing had come to *expect* future contingency, they would not have responded negatively. Exposure to contingency, generally experienced pleasurably, may facilitate the development of expectancy, which in turn is experienced pleasurably. Subsequent contingent experience, which fulfills the expectation, is also experienced with positive affect. But if the infant confronts subsequent noncontingency instead of subsequent contingency, both the noncontingency itself and the shattered expectation are experienced with distress in both the affective and cognitive realms.

Blass, Ganchrow, and Steiner (1984) supplied further evidence that infants experience contingency, that they come to expect contingency, and that contingency learning and affect response are correlated. Infants as young as 2 hours old, in the study's experimental groups, were stroked gently on their foreheads during 18 2-minute conditioning trials. Following the stroking sessions, these infants received an intraoral delivery of sucrose. One control group was stroked randomly and then sucrose was administered, while another control group received sucrose in each trial, but was not stroked.

After the trials, all infants experienced nine 1-minute extinction trials in which they were just stroked. Only infants in the experimental group presented evidence of conditioning. These infants emitted more head-orienting and sucking responses during the stroking sessions, and exhibited a classic extinction function to head stroking during extinction trials. Moreover, 7 of the 9 experimental infants cried during the extinction trials, whereas only 1 of the 16 control infants cried. Data from both DeCasper and Carstens (1981) and Blass, Ganchrow, and Steiner (1984), therefore, demonstrate that disruption of a contingency relationship—and by implication, of the infant's expectation of future contingency—produces negative affect.

Evidence from the investigations of DeCasper and Fifer (1980) also indicates that neonates are capable of perceiving contingencies, and therefore reacting to noncontingent experiences. The researchers had neonates (younger than 3 days old) suck on nonnutritive nipples that would, depending on the sucking pattern, produce a recording of the mother's voice or the voice of another female. Tests showed that the infants were able to learn the behavior required to produce the mother's voice and that they preferred her voice over other voices. This suggests that infants possess far more powerful discriminatory capabilities than had been generally acknowledged.

In a related study, Fagen and Ohr (1985) studied 110 infants of approximately 3 months of age, who were trained to use foot kicking to control a crib mobile containing 10 objects. Following the learning trials, infants were given a crib mobile containing only two objects. Fifty-five percent of infants cried after exposure to this second mobile. Fagen and Ohr interpreted the crying behavior as evidence of a violated expectancy and postulated that the variation in response might be due to "temperamental differences."

By temperamental differences, Fagen and Ohr, (1985) appear to imply that contingency learning in itself might be a function of "intrinsic motivation," a phrase coined by White (1959). Indeed, the fact that infants have been shown to experience contingency pleasurably and to respond to disrupted contingencies with distress responses suggests that each infant's individual affective proclivities, as manifested in overall temperament, will exert a significant impact on early learning experience. Thus the temperament variations each infant brings to the learning situation will affect his or her ability to learn either contingency or noncontingency and to respond to these experiences with either pleasure or distress. Temperament dimensions may therefore provide a screen through which to assess and to predict infant susceptibility to learning competency and developing a sense of self.

Lewis, Sullivan and Brooks-Gunn (1985) found further evidence indicative of the positive affect associated with contingency experience. Sixty infants divided equally among three age groups (10, 16, and 24 weeks) were exposed to an audio-visual stimulus contingent upon arm movement. During the experiment, particular attention was paid to such signs of affective display as visual fixation, fussing and smiling. The study revealed that irrespective of age, subjects in the contingent condition devoted more time to the experiment and fussed less than controls. Additionally, subjects at age 16 and 24 weeks smiled more than noncontingent controls.

Another important aspect of contingency awareness theory is the degree to which infants can transfer learning across tasks. In other words, assuming that the experience of contingency is pleasurable and creates an expectation of future pleasurable contingency experiences, will an infant who has encountered previous contingency bring expectation to future tasks and situations? That is, will the repeated experience of contingency create an enduring mood of pleasurable expectation? Conversely, since disrupted contingency is experienced with affective distress, will repeated instances of a disrupted contingency create a lingering negative mood? These questions have been the subject of several studies; their answers may shed some light on the infant's earliest susceptibilty to depression and depressive-like phenomena.

Finkelstein and Ramey (1977) investigated the phenomenon of the transference of contingency experience across tasks. Infants with a mean age of 8.5 months were familiarized with an array of colored lights that could be activated by pressing a panel. This phase of the experiment represented an initial exposure to a contingency relationship, or what the researchers referred to as "prior contingent stimulation." This group of infants was then divided in half: One subgroup was exposed to a pleasant audio-visual stimulus that was activated by an arm-pull motion—in other words, a subsequent contingency experience; the second subgroup was subjected to a noncontingent audio-visual stimulus. Measuring the frequency with which the infant executed the correct arm-pull movement, the researchers found that the total number of arm pulls executed by the contingent group of infants increased, while noncontingent infants engaged in substantially fewer arm pulls. The researchers labeled the subgroup exposed to the repeated contingency trial as "more competent and efficient learners," and their findings suggest that this increased competence is a consequence of the phenomenon that prior contingency experience is "transferred" to new tasks and situations.

In another experiment (Finkelstein & Ramey, 1977) designed to evaluate the effect of contingent stimulation on subsequent learning response, infants were presented with a two-phase experiment. In the first phase of the experiment, infants were exposed to a contingency relationship. During the second phase, they were tested for discrimination learning. Using a group of 4.5-month-old infants, half of the infants were first subjected to an audio-visual stimulus contingent upon vocalizations. The control group of infants received no audio-visual stimulus. It was found that only the group receiving contingent stimulation increased the number of vocalizations. During the second phase of the experiment all infants were observed during conditioning and extinction periods. Infants were presented with pleasant audio-visual stimulation that they could control by manipulating a lever. Only infants who previously received contingent stimulation learned to discriminate contingent and noncontingent response during conditioning and extinction periods. This segment of the Finkelstein and Ramey study dramatically revealed that contingency awareness can foster the mastery of complex, unrelated learning tasks. The implication is that contingency training facilitates a transfer to more complex discrimination-learning tasks. The study suggests that infants who receive prior experience learning to control stimulation are subsequently better able to determine the relationship between their behaviors and environmental events.

Contingency and discrepancy awareness may theoretically be viewed as conceptual milestones. Indeed, like discrepancy awareness, contingency awareness represents a fundamentally discrete way in which the infant perceives the world and regulates his or her response to environmental stimuli. With the advent of discrepancy awareness, the infant begins to separate phenomena in his environment and to distinguish among them. The infant is therefore attuned to conceptualizing *differences,* and to responding to them both cognitively and affectively. A different kind of function is at work with contingency awareness. The perception or comprehension of a contingency relationship requires that the infant engage in a process of associating or *linking* two stimuli that very likely have no external connection with respect to physical or visual characteristics.

As noted earlier, discrepancy awareness results in a residue of expectancy that may be characterized as an anticipation that variations on previous stimuli will occur in the future. With contingency awareness, a comparable type of expectancy may be inferred. In the case of contingency awareness, however, the expectancy involves looking for or being attuned to cause–

effect types of relationships that can exist between two stimuli that appear to be superficially unrelated or unconnected. The development of this type of expectancy is more sophisticated in scope and more indicative of complex internal processing than the development of the type of expectancy processing that occurs following discrepancy awareness. Implicit in the changes in internal processing—from the ability to perceive discrepancies to expectations concerning discrepancies to contingency awareness and corresponding expectancies about contingencies—is the infant's ability to integrate affective and cognitive states in a more sophisticated manner. Such integration may be interpreted as a form of regulation, demonstrating the infant's ability to modulate and control transitions between different affective and cognitive states.

Learned contingencies, like certain types of discrepancies, create positive affect (White, 1959). Broucek (1979) refers to this positive affect as "effectance pleasure." White suggests that the motivation for learning, which bestows such pleasure, is intrinsic and calls this type of motivation "effectance motivation." According to White, effectance pleasure is closely related to cognition, and the infant's self-esteem is affected by the experience of efficacy. Indeed, he claims that the internal experience of mastery or efficacy exercises a greater influence on self-esteem development than does social reinforcement.

Behaviorally, the motivation to learn, which Bowlby (1969, 1982) also regards as innate, may be manifested as a desire to explore the environment. However, while Bowlby views the desire for exploration as a counterbalance to the attachment system of proximity–seeking behavior, White (1959) proposed that the innate drive for competence is the primary impetus propelling exploratory behavior. Thus the acquisition of skills by the infant provides a double benefit: The infant achieves enhanced ability to manipulate the environment and derives mastery pleasure from his or her accomplishments.

If White (1959) is correct, from the time of birth onward, experiences slowly accumulate and mold the infant's perception of control over the environment. This sense of control—or lack of it—has been related to depression in the learned helplessness theory articulated by Seligman and others (Maier, Seligman, and Solomon, 1967; Seligman, 1975). Positive affect created by the experience of mastery may serve as a protective factor, while negative affect, stemming from noncontingency and perceived lack of mastery, would constitute a risk factor for depression.

Several empirical studies provide graphic evidence of infants' affective responses to perceived *lack* of contingency. Papousek and Papousek (1975) found that infants who mastered a contingent task and then had the contingency disrupted underwent an aversive reaction to the stimulus. Young infants (2 months and under) became motionless and withdrawn; older infants showed active avoidance. Broucek (1979) suggests that these are defensive regulatory strategies shielding the developing "self" from assaults on the sense of mastery.

> *If the infant's sense of self arises as I propose, from such a basic consideration as "I cause and I intend, therefore I am" then the rudimentary sense of self is vulnerable to traumatization by any failure in the area of omnipotence or to put it differently, by any disturbance in the sense of efficacy. (Broucek, 1979, p. 313)*

Disturbances in contingency, particularly related to the caregiver's behavior, may constitute examples of the serious threats to the infant's sense of efficacy that Broucek describes. Bibring (1953) notes that

> *any condition which forces a feeling of helplessness upon the infantile ego may create a predisposition to depression. . . . the emphasis is . . . on the state of helplessness of the ego confronted with an insolvable problem. (Bibring, 1953, p. 42)*

Lewis (1967) believes that infant motivation for development can be found in the infant's expectations of efficacy and contingency in its environment. Lewis describes a three-stage paradigm of somatic discomfort leading to an action motivated toward the cessation of discomfort. For instance, in an ideal situation, an infant will feel hunger and will cry, and the caregiver will respond by feeding the infant. If this paradigm is followed, the infant learns to expect particular consequences of its behavior, and receives the double reward of being fed while simultaneously acquiring a sense of mastery over its environment. If there is a delay between the action and the cessation of discomfort, the awareness of contingency is reduced, and the motivation for action is reduced.

> *What we have been hypothesizing is that quantity and timing of maternal response to the infant's behavior, and the degree of consistency of her responses have important motivational qualities, developing and reinforcing the infant's belief that his behavior can effect the environment. (Lewis, 1967, p. 33)*

In support of this theory, Lewis describes a study by Provence and Lipton (1962) involving institutionalized infants. Lewis contends that institutionalized infants are more likely to receive responses that are geared to the institution's schedule, rather than to their own. For this reason, such infants would be likely to show deficiencies in their awareness of contingency. Lewis notes that Provence and Lipton found that infants reared in institutions differed from home-reared infants not in the acquisition of skills, but in the use of those skills. That is, they suffered a motivational deficit which we may infer was a deficit in their self-regulatory capacities.

The degree of contingency experienced during an infant's relationship with the caregiver will have an important impact on individual differences in the level of efficacy motivation. It is also possible, however, that indiviudal differences in the level of efficacy motivation may be partially attributed to temperamental differences in such dimensions as intensity of reaction, attention span/persistence, and duration of orienting. Harter's (1974, 1977a, 1978, 1982) and Harter and Pike's (1984) work on operationalizing White's theory attempted to split effectance motivation into two components: one innate, as suggested by White, and one mediated by social reinforcers. They found that both temperament and environmental factors affect effectance motivation and learning. This combination of innate and environmental factors may thus affect not only learning capabilities, but also self-esteem and self-concept. If the experience of contingency is the reward for learning, then differences in efficacy could lead to different rates of development of the self (Trad, 1986).

Control and Controllability

It may be postulated that the facility with which the infant learns to regulate will exert a strong influence on his sense of control over the environment and over the self. Rotter (1966) distinguishes two types of "locus-of-control"—internal and external. He defined external locus of control as the belief by the individual that reinforcements occur by chance or luck, and internal locus of control as the belief that reinforcers and personal skill can be used to master the environment. Several researchers have focused on the concept of locus of control as a variable that may be used to assess the child's sense of competence in interacting with the environment. Weisz and Stipek (1982), for example, reviewed a series of developmental studies in an effort to discern how locus-of-control perception may alter with age. Although no distinctive pattern emerged, the researchers noted that locus-of-control parameters can help tap into perceived contingency of outcome and perceived competence of self.

Although most locus-of-control studies involve adults or children rather than infants, the concept of locus of control is raised here because it may be of value in articulating a theory of infant regulation. Implicit within Kopp's (1982) concept of self-regulation as pertaining to infants, for example, is the notion that the infant begins to distinguish between external and internal domains of control at 24 months. However, in light of the previous discussion of discrepancy and contingency awareness, the formation of expectancies, and the suggestion that each of these capacities carries a concomitant ability to regulate the input of new stimuli, locus-of-control may be a pertinent concept to apply to infancy.

It may be postulated that as the infant gains in ability to embrace discrepancies and contingencies, so too does his regulatory capacity increase. When an infant receives adequate amounts of discrepancy and contingency from the environment, regulatory capacities will in turn progress and become increasingly more sophisticated. Eventually such an infant may acquire a sense of mastery and competence over the environment and may come to perceive the source of this "control" as originating within himself. Such an infant can be expected to develop an internal locus-of-control and an accompanying sense of high self-esteem. In contrast, an infant whose discrepancy and contingency experiences are frustrated— for example, by being subjected to repeated bouts of extreme discrepancy or by being deprived of contingency experiences—may fall prey to a tendency toward dysregulation, in which internal affect and cognition cannot be efficiently integrated with stimuli from the environment. Such an infant may come to attribute the dysregulation to the self, in which case an internal locus of control will evolve with concomitant negative self-esteem. Alternatively, such an infant may come to view the self as helpless in an adverse universe, in which case an external locus of control will evolve, coupled with low self-esteem. The infant's sense of locus-of-control is crucial to the development of his or her incipient sense of self, which in turn will set the stage for either his or her vulnerability to or immunity from depression.

Uncontrollability and Depression

One of the affects accompanying depression is the pervasive feeling of helplessness—the perception that events are uncontrollable and the sense that one's problems are not solvable by one's own efforts. The work of Seligman and others (Klein & Seligman, 1976; Seligman, 1975; Seligman & Maier, 1967) suggests that this affect can be a learned response. Seligman (1975) states that learned helplessness, as simulated in man and other species in laboratory experiments, creates motivational, affective, and cognitive deficits.

Seligman (1975) defines uncontrollability in terms of contingency.

> *If the probability of an outcome when some response occurs is different from the probability of the outcome when that response doesn't occur, then that outcome is* dependent *on that response: the outcome is* controllable. *(p. 17)*
>
> *When the probability of an outcome is the same whether or not a given response occurs, the outcome is* independent *of that response. When this is true of all voluntary responses, the outcome is* uncontrollable. *(p. 16; emphasis in original)*

Perceptions of contingency and controllability are believed to alter with age, and thus vulnerability to learned helplessness depression may have a strong developmental component. Weisz (1980) demonstrated that during the course of development the perception of contingency becomes more realistic and that illusory contingency, defined as a misappraisal of the control one can exert over events, declines. Kindergartners in Weisz's study perceived chance-related outcomes (drawing cards from a deck) as contingent on competence-related factors, while fourth graders were better able to identify the outcomes as resulting from luck. However, Langer (1975), in studying the perception of contingency in adults, found that most adults retain some confusion about differentiating chance-related and nonchance-related events. She found that most adults tend to behave as if chance events were under their control. She refers to this fallacy as "illusion of control"—which may be viewed as being at the opposite end of the spectrum from learned helplessness depression. Illusion of control was defined as "an expectancy of a personal success probability inappropriately higher than the objective probability would warrant" (p. 313). This perception is related to the "just world hypothesis," which is a belief that people get what they deserve (i.e., "good" things happen to "good" people; "bad" things happen to "bad" people). Langer found that in situations involving skill-related factors (choice, stimulus or response familiarity, passive or active involvement, or competition), subjects tended to view the outcome as being contingent on those factors even when such outcomes were clearly determined by chance, such as lotteries. Langer points to both the positive affect associated with control and the negative affect associated with lack of control as causes of illusions of control.

Alloy, Abramson, and Viscusi (1981) induced mood states in students and found that artificially depressed students gave more objective assessments of personal control than did artificially elated students, who demonstrated more instances of illusions of control. Pervin (1963) performed an experiment in which adult males were given either unpredictable or self-controlled electric shocks. Although there was no difference in the amount or intensity of the shocks, the subjects showed a preference for the controlled situation. In a similar study, Gunnar (1980) examined infant control over an arousing, potentially fear-provoking toy. The researcher found that although predictability did not reduce fear responses or increase positive approach responses in 1-year-olds, control did reduce fear responses in 1-year-old males and increased positive approach responses in both sexes. Further, control of a toy was found to produce positive affect. However, control did not reduce distress in infants younger that 1 year. Thus it appears that a positive response to control develops only after the experience of positive affect resulting from contingency awareness.

The developing infant maintains a balance between the illusion of total control, in which the caregiver's behavior is perceived as contingent on infant desires, and the ability to accept regulation from the caregiver. If the caregiver is perceived as being entirely noncontingent (e.g., a mother who is depressed), the infant has little foundation on which to base feelings of efficacy and concomitant self-esteem. If, on the other hand, the caregiver's behavior is sensitively modulated, the developing infant is allowed to gain control over self and environment in such a way as to foster a strong sense of self. The mechanisms for such infant-caregiver interaction are examined in the next section.

MECHANISMS OF CAREGIVER-INFANT INTERACTION AFFECTING SELF-REGULATION

The discussion until this point has focused largely on "nature" variables—the infant's innate equipment and the products of maturation—that contribute to the infant's capacities to self-regulate. In turn, depending on the efficacy of self-regulation, the infant will either move in the direction of a stable sense of self, relatively immune from depression, or will be vulnerable to depression. Factors that might be seen as a function of "nurture" variables affecting self-regulation may also offer important insights concerning the pathogenesis of infant and childhood depression. Attempts to develop objective measures of the impact of potentially pathogenic environments have yielded reasonably conclusive evidence relating insecure attachment to risk for depression. Efforts to capture the subjective elements of an infant's interactions with his or her caregiver, and to explore how such interactions might be implicated in depression, have also produced compelling evidence of the importance of these interactions in the etiology of depression. Studies of face-to-face interaction have illustrated the complexity of affective exchanges between caregiver and infant. These studies provide one way of tapping into the intimate process of nonverbal communication and self-regulation occurring almost from birth between caregiver and child. Such communication may not, however, be limited to face-to-face signaling, but may extend to other forms of communication. These interactions inform the infant of his or her success in relating needs and feelings to the caregiver, and provide the first opportunities to experience a sense of competence. Such experience has a profound impact on the early development of the self, and thus on the child's vulnerability to depression (Trad, 1986).

The infant-caregiver relationship develops in tandem with the development of self-regulatory capacities in the infant and contributes significantly to the evolution of the internal self-concept. It is apparent that the infant needs interaction with a significant nurturing figure in order to formulate a mature self-concept. Viewed in this way, it may be said, metaphorically, that the mother gives birth to the child again. Shields (1978), Newson (1977), and Vygotsky (1962), among others, have suggested that the caregiver aids this process by attributing meaning to the infant's acts from birth. During this process, the caregiver reinforces some chance behaviors and creates meaning for others. That is, by responding as if the infant were behaving with intention, the caregiver serves as the definer of intention, as well as attention and affect, for the infant.

Emde and Sorce (1983) point out that exposure to a wide range of emotional expressions helps the infant by broadening the possibilities for communication. Caregivers are "pretuned" to interpret primitive emotional signals that would be unclear or abstruse to an outside observer. Thus the caregiver invests the infant's behavior with affective meaning, while the infant is in the process of creating such meaning. At the same time, the infant learns to use the caregiver's affective signals to regulate its behavior.

When the infant is in a receptive state, the caregiver is commonly the agent who can supply the simple, repetitious stimuli needed to optimize the infant's learning capacity (Papousek & Papousek, 1979, 1983). These researchers suggest that parents have instinctive behaviors designed to maximize successful dyadic interactions. They label these intuitive behaviors "primary parenting" (1983) to distinguish them from conscious tactics. Papousek and Papousek suggest that parents tend to maximize quiet waking or quiet sleeping states and to minimize transitionary states. Other ways in which the caregiver helps facilitate learning include modification of speech, exaggeration of sounds and facial expressions, and modulation of the speed and pitch of speech. In this manner the caregiver makes the speech recognizable, repetitive, and predictable. These three elements are particularly important for the structuring and awareness of contingency. Parents make analogous modifications in their visual interactions when they present consistent expressions to the child. One familiar expression consists of a wide-eyed, open-mouthed, or smiling face which facilitates recognition, imitation, and synchronous interaction.

Researchers have suggested a number of mechanisms by which affects (which fortify or threaten the emerging self) are shared by mother and infant. These include reciprocity, rhythmicity, affect attunement, intersubjectivity, and empathy. Empathy may be considered an example of how affect is transferred from mother to infant and may explain, in part, how depressive affect is communicated over the course of a child's development.

Simple rhythmical reactions allow the caregiver to act as a mirror for the infant (Kernberg, 1984). The experience of reciprocity (Brazelton, Koslowski, & Main, 1974) prepares the infant for experiencing contingency, while affect attunement helps the infant recognize his or her own internal states. The more smoothly and successfully these interactions occur, the more securely are self-regulatory capacities reinforced. In contrast, however, interactional failures in these domains may impose deleterious effects on the evolving skills of self-regulation, and ultimately, result in a "damaged" sense of self.

Reciprocity

In normal development, the caregiver-infant interaction appears to undergo four major stages of evolution that affect the infant's increasing ability to regulate its own attentional states (Brazelton & Als, 1979). The first stage in this development is the infant's innate ability to control its physiological system—its breathing, heart rate, and bodily temperature. Along with aspects of physiological control comes a parallel control of the infant's states of consciousness, that is, waking, sleeping, and transitions between the two. By the second stage, the infant learns to prolong its attention and to use social cues to focus attention. As early as 4 weeks of age, the infant is able to engage in a cycle of attention and withdrawal with the caregiver. As each partner becomes acquainted with the responses of the other, the cycles of looking and smiling become more rhythmical and more reciprocal. The dyadic "conversation" lengthens. The third stage witnesses a further development of the infant's capacity to incorporate or assimilate information. An infant in the fourth stage (about the fourth or fifth month) can select objects autonomously and initiate games with his parents.

Perhaps the first observable social interaction in which the child engages is smiling. Wolff (1969) comments on the immensely attractive power of an infant's smile, and Bowlby (1969) notes its importance in the attachment process. Wolff (1969) observes that what is initially a reflex movement becomes differentiated in the first two weeks of life into a vocabulary of expressions that can be elicited by a wide range of stimuli. Only in the third week do human stimuli elicit smiles more frequently than other stimuli, such as bells or bird whistles. At 3 to 4 weeks, Wolff noticed that the infant's eyes become involved with smiling manifestations. The smile seems specifically directed at someone or something. Wolff quotes mothers as saying of their infants at this time "now he can see me" and "now he is fun to play with."

Brazelton, Koslowski, and Main (1974) describe the origins of reciprocal interaction between infants and mothers at 3 weeks of age. Prior to this age, they postulate, like Wolff, that the infant does not possess the requisite physical skills necessary to focus attention sufficiently for engaging in social interactions. The authors filmed face-to-face interactions between mothers and their 3-week-old infants. They found that the interactions consisted of alternating states of attention and withdrawal on the part of the infant. During the attentional phase, the infant became increasingly excited and agitated, waving his or her arms and legs, smiling, and sometimes vocalizing. After building to a peak of excitement, the infant decelerated into a state of withdrawal when he or she turned his or her attention away from the mother. After a certain period of time had elapsed, the cycle would begin again. The authors theorized that the infant used the period of withdrawal to process the information received during the attentional phase. Another theory was that the infant withdrew in order to protect itself from overstimulation.

The mothers in this study showed routinely characteristic modes of interacting with their infants, particularly in dealing with the infant's withdrawal of attention. The infant demonstrated that he or she could withstand only a limited amount of stimulation. The mothers usually had a greater tolerance for interaction, and therefore it was incumbent upon them to modulate the interaction. Sensitivity to the infant's tolerances led some mothers to reduce their attention in synchrony with the infant. Other mothers were insensitive to their infant's withdrawal and kept up a steady stream of stimulation. Still another group of mothers responded by increasing their attention and stimulation, but they were out of phase with the infant. The authors found that "sensitive" mothers increased the frequency and duration of interactions with their infants in comparison to more intrusive mothers. In regard to one infant, the authors state:

> *This baby has learned "rules" about managing his own needs in the face of an insensitive mother. He has learned to turn her off, to decrease his receptivity to information from her. (Brazelton, Koslowski, & Main, 1974, p. 60)*

The infants demonstrated four different strategies for dealing with intrusive, unpleasant stimuli: turning away, pushing away, decreasing sensitivity (i.e., yawning, sleeping, generally withdrawing to a dull state/ and crying).

Rhythmicity

Researchers have found that infant-caregiver interactions usually occur in rhythmical, as well as cyclical, patterns. This implies that interactions are structured and regular, with both factors aiding the infant's appreciation of the contingency of the interaction.

Lester, Hoffman, and Brazelton (1985) conducted microanalytical studies of face-to-face interactions in term and preterm infants with their mothers, similar to the analyses conducted by Brazelton, Koslowski, and Main (1974). Their purpose was to compare the attentional periodicities of each member of the infant-mother dyad, and the occurrence of synchrony between them. They point out that the rhythms of social interaction "provide the infant with the structure to form temporal expectancies that organize cognitive and affective experiences" (Lester, Hoffman, & Brazelton, 1985, p. 15). These authors found that "temporal patterning is a fundamental property of early face-to-face mother-infant interaction" (p. 22). They felt that these rhythms were a major regulating factor in mother-infant interaction. Moreover, a higher degree of synchrony of interaction was identified in full-term than in preterm infants. The researchers attribute this to differences in infant rhythmicities that make it more difficult for preterm infants to regulate themselves. Such temperamental differences affect interactions with the mother by making it more difficult for the infant to adjust to the mother's rhythms, and by making the infant less predictable, and therefore more difficult for the caregiver who seeks to adjust to the infant. The ultimate result is a lower incidence of synchronous exchange, coupled with shorter, less successful interactions.

Affect Attunement

The process of developing synchrony encompasses affective states, as well as shared physical interactions, between caregiver and infant. The infant's growing self-regulatory capacities and sense of self are facilitated by interaction with the caregiver, and the interaction of affective states helps to define the infant's awareness of an internal self. Stern, Hofer, Haft, and Dore (1985) have called this process "affect attunement." They believe that affective sharing helps the infant to perceive how he or she is perceived by others.

Affect attunement involves the caregiver responding to the infant's behavior in such a way that the response is reflective of the infant's inner experience. The response may be cross-modal (e.g., the infant moves in a particular way, and the caregiver responds with a vocal interpretation), intramodal, or mixed. A caregiver watching the infant going down a slide may respond with the vocalization "wheee." The mother interprets the infant's affective state, and in so doing reinforces the internal feeling and helps the infant to recognize itself as the entity who is experiencing this affect. In essence, the infant recognizes the feeling reflected in its caregiver and has an internal response of "That's me!" This process differs from mirroring in that the caregiver's response is not simply an imitation of the action or sound of the infant, but is rather a shared feeling state with a different behavioral expression. Affect attunement is a virtually automatic process entailing a complex "matching" between the infant's internal state and the caregiver's internal state.

Stern et al. (1985) distinguish between attunement and imitation by noting that attunement allows reference to the internal state while imitation does not. Although physical mirroring and rhythmic caregiver-infant interactions can be found in infants as young as 3 weeks of age, Stern et al. felt that in the first 6 months of life modifying imitations take precedence over attunements. That is, modifying imitations are not strict mirroring but represent patterns of reaction that correspond to overt behavior. At 9 months, according to Stern et al., the self is sufficiently developed to be aware of self and others' subjectivity. By imitating the infant's movements, the caregiver makes the infant more aware of his or her physical self, but only through attunement does the infant gain awareness and appreciation of his or her mental states.

Stern et al. (1985) studied a group of infant-caregiver pairs in order to examine these phenomena. The mean age of the infants was 11 months. To focus on attunement behaviors with cross-modalities, the researchers first defined the characteristics that constituted a "match." They identified three types of match. A match could occur if caregiver and infant behaviors resembled each other in intensity, timing, or shape. For example, if the infant performed an action at a given level of intensity and the caregiver's response was at that level, it was considered a match. Similarly, if the curve of the intensity of behaviors was identical, it was considered a match. Timing matches included beat, rhythm, and duration matches. Shape matches occurred when the physical shape of the behaviors was similar. For example, the infant shakes a rattle up and down, and the caregiver responds by shaking her head up and down.

Stern et al. (1985) suggested that the functions of attunement were:

To commune. To be with the infant, either in a positive sense as in participating in the child's experience or in a negative sense, as in parodying or mocking.

To respond, by reinforcing, acknowledging, approving, or disapproving.

To adjust or tune the child's experience. To attempt to increase or decrease the level of arousal.

To restructure the interaction, including the teaching of word meanings.

To engage in play routines.

Both observers and caregivers rated over 75 percent of the observed matches as either communing or responding. Interestingly, when the attunement is effective, the infant generally gives no acknowledgement of the process. The authors observed that when the caregiver has made a communing attunement, the infant frequently continues his or her activities with no response or change in activity or expression. Mismatched attunements, however, such as changes in rhythm or intensity, commonly produce a response or change in behavior from the infant.

As the foregoing discussion indicates, the significance of infant-caregiver interaction has been underscored by numerous researchers and the behavioral manifestations evinced during such interaction have been probed in depth. But the form of interaction established by the dyad has implications beyond those that can be inferred from overt behavior. Bell (1970) has suggested that the interaction may be viewed as a dynamic paradigm from which the infant's incipient sense of object permanence and self emerge. The researcher noted that infants in whom person permanence develops before object permanence were more interactive with their caregivers and achieved object permanence more rapidly than those in whom object permanence preceded person permanence.

Tronick and Gianino (1986) noted that the infant-caregiver interaction provides an opportunity for the infant to learn and master various coping behaviors. In effect, coping behaviors, according to these researchers, may be defined as the infant's continual attempts to overcome subtle mismatches of response with the caregiver. In this sense, through the process of continually devising behavioral mechanisms of coping, the infant may be viewed as striving for the type of harmony or "affect attunement" referred to by Stern et al. (1985).

Tronick and Gianino (1986) also hypothesize, however, that if the infant encounters too many obstacles to coping with environmental mismatches, genuine coping behavior may eventually be abandoned and may degenerate into "defensive" behavior. The researchers define defensive behavior as the use of coping behavior in an automatic, inflexible, and indiscriminant fashion and suggest that such defensive mechanisms are adopted to preclude episodes of interactive stress. Based on this formulation then, defensive behaviors represent a form of adaptation in an environment hostile to the infant's achievement of mastery and competence. In this respect, they are a preservation mechanism. However, defensive strategies may similarly be viewed as a form of dysregulation. The infant has, in effect, ceased to engage in the ongoing dynamic with the caregiver necessary to achieve an integrated sense of self. Significantly, Tronick and Gianino note that such defensive strategies may be employed by the infant *before* self-integration has occurred; that is, before a distinction between self and others has been achieved. Implicitly, therefore, defensive behavioral responses may become ingrained during the first months of life, and the infant's increased rigidity and inflexibility with regard to discrepancy and contingency in the environment will likely color his or her sense of self (Trad, 1986).

Intersubjectivity

The term "intersubjectivity" refers to the developmental milestone in the evolution of self-regulation that occurs when the infant is approximately 9 months old. Intersubjectivity represents the momentous emergence of the self from its undifferentiated state. Both Stern (1985) and Trevarthen and Hubley (1978) describe this emergence as being intimately connected with the awareness of an internal reality existing in others. At this time, the infant shows evidence of an awareness of the caregiver's intentions, perceptions, and affects. Awareness of the possibility of a shared internal reality, which includes both awareness of an internal self and an awareness of an internal reality in others, is a prerequisite for intersubjectivity. These types of awareness develop simultaneously and interdependently, fostering new types of sharing as well as new dimensions of the self. Stern (1985) wrote that "both separation/individuation and new forms of experiencing union (or being-with) emerge equally out of the same experience of intersubjectivity" (p. 127). Trevarthen and Hubley describe the onset of what they call "secondary intersubjectivity" [which Stern (1985, p. 134) refers to as "intersubjectivity"] at around 40 weeks of age. Developing concurrently with affective sharing, secondary intersubjectivity involves the connection of a partner in object interactions. Although by the age of 2 months, the infant is able to engage in reciprocal mirroring interactions, not until approximately 9 months will the infant engage in reciprocal interactions involving an object, that is, giving and receiving objects, or sharing enjoyment resulting from a manipulation of an object.

Several researchers (Stern, 1985; Trevarthen & Hubley, 1978) have catalogued behaviors that first occur at approximately 9 months, all of which involve the infant's awareness of the caregiver's intention and internal response. The first of these behaviors, according to Stern, is pointing and looking, which is indicative of shared attention. Looking in the direction where the mother is pointing requires that the infant be able to change its frame of reference to the mother's point of view. Other infant behaviors that indicate intersubjectivity include performing simple tasks on instruction, playing "pretend" games, invoking adult help in a task, and pointing to objects that are unreachable (Trevarthen & Hubley, 1978). At this age, concurrent with the infant's growing awareness of self, adults cease to be animated objects in the infant's eyes and become other "selves." It appears that the growth of the infant's sense of intentionality is accompanied by the infant's awareness of intentionality in others.

Trevarthen and Hubley (1978) made a detailed study of the interactions of one caregiver-infant dyad over the course of the infant's first year. Although the infant and her mother routinely played with toys during these videotaped sessions, a qualitative change was observed at the age of 40 weeks. At that time, the infant began to engage in giving and receiving objects and began to respond to the names of toys. These behaviors were accompanied by evidence of affect attunement, with mother and daughter sharing responses to the infant's manipulations of toys. The researchers noted that

> In contrast to her earlier reactive *regulation of [the infant's] behavior, reflected in a questioning and coaxing manner of speaking, Tracey's mother now regulated in a* directive *manner, issuing instructions and asking rhetorical questions. Tracey, for her part, acted as if she happily accepted the leadership of her mother in a joint definition of experience. (p. 205; emphasis in original)*

The infant's acceptance of regulation from her mother expands the range of her experience over her earlier self-regulation. In light of Lewis, Brooks-Gunn, and Jaskir's (1985) findings that insecurely attached infants develop earlier self-recognition than securely attached infants, it seems likely that an early development of the self places undue reliance on self-regulation, leading to a lessening of shared affective experiences such as affect attunement and intersubjectivity.

Empathy

Empathy is an important vehicle through which developing infants gain an awareness of the affective states of others, particularly their caregivers. Zahn-Waxler et al. (1984) and Radke-Yarrow (1983) have called attention to the role of empathy, and its derivatives such as prosocial behavior, in shaping children's social interactions. Empathy, which Hoffman (1982a) described as "affective response . . . more appropriate to someone else's situation than to one's own" (p. 281), enables children to share a wide range of affects experienced by those in their environment. Among the most significant of these shared affects may be the distress of their caregivers. As infants mature, empathic distress will vary in the way it is experienced, in the types of cues needed to evoke it, and in the manner in which it is expressed. An infant's vulnerability to empathic distress is a function of overall empathic development which is, in turn, a function of cognitive development.

Hoffman (1982a,b) delineates four stages in empathic development. During the first year of life, infants act as if what happens to others happens to them. In a distressing situation, they will interpret the distress of others as their own. Since cognitive immaturity prevents infants from identifying the source of distress correctly, during this stage they may be more vulnerable to another's distress than at subsequent stages.

The stage Hoffman (1982a,b) calls "egocentric empathy," which lasts through the third year, follows the first stage. By this time, infants have begun to differentiate themselves from others and can share the emotional distress of another while being aware that the direct emotional experience is occurring to the other person. Once toddlers can accept the separate physical and psychological existence of others, they enter into a third phase of empathic development in which they can assume another person's perspective. They can also empathize through symbolic expression, as well as through facial and somatic distress. At this stage, it is within the child's capacity to respond empathically to more complex emotions, such as another's disappointment or sense of betrayal, or even conflicting emotions. By the final stage, which develops in late childhood, children can experience empathic distress for someone's general life condition rather than for specific events. They can understand that immediate behavior may be at variance with another's general condition and make sympathetic allowances for outside factors in a person's behavior. According to Hoffman's model (1982a,b), increased cognitive capacities sensitize infants to a far broader range of possible distress cues, thereby increasing their exposure to empathic distress arising from the depressed affect of another. Empathic distress may also predispose the infant to depression in indirect ways, through the production of guilt. According to Hoffman (1982a), guilt is a normal byproduct of empathic distress and generally finds an outlet in prosocial behavior aimed at alleviating the distress of others.

MECHANISMS OF ATTACHMENT AFFECTING SELF-REGULATION

It is by now generally agreed that the infant has needs beyond those for simple nutrition and physical protection in order to develop into a well-adapted adult. For example, the infant also requires stimulation and contact with a caregiver. This need, identified by numerous researchers in the early twentieth century, was probed in depth by Bowlby and Robertson (Bowlby, 1969, 1973, 1980; Robertson & Bowlby, 1952). Bowlby refers to the relationship designed to satisfy these needs as the "attachment relationship," and this seminal interaction has generally been viewed as a paradigm for later interpersonal relationships (Ainsworth, 1979; Bowlby, 1969; Freud, 1938; Main, Kaplan, & Cassidy, 1985; Sroufe, Waters, & Matas, 1974).

In a 1985 study, Main, Kaplan, and Cassidy reconceptualized the attachment relationship, emphasizing the representational rather than the behavioral aspects of the relationship. According to their reconceptualization, individual differences in attachment organization evolve as a function of individual differences in internal working models of attachment relationships. Thus the infant's temperament will implicitly impinge on and indeed help to shape the attachment relationship.

Equally significant in shaping the attachment relationship are maternal personality and environmental factors. As the infant progresses from simple reactivity to interactive social regulation, he or she learns behaviors primarily from one caregiver. Main, Kaplan, and Cassidy (1985), elaborating on the implications of the infant-caregiver attachment bond, have noted that the infant develops an internalized schema of the relationship—an internal model—based on the inner representation of experienced outcomes and on subsequent expectations derived from these outcomes. That is, the infant's skills in discerning discrepancy and contingency, as well as his or her growing ability to formulate expectations, congeal within the framework of the attachment relationship to create an internal dynamic of interaction.

The researchers note that the basic dimensions of this internal working model may assume form during the first months of life. By the age of 1 year, the internal schematic is structurally intact, and the individual variations that emerge during the Strange Situation, revealing security or insecurity of attachment relationship, may be conceived of as a reflection of the infant's internalized conception of the interaction. Moreover, the internalized model does not merely govern behavioral response but also incorporates a diverse array of feelings and ideations. Significantly, the researchers also note that patterns of interaction emerge between the infant's working model and the external attachment dynamic. These patterns, once established, become actively self-perpetuating.

It may be suggested, then, that if the attachment bond forged between the infant and caregiver is one of mutual responsivity, the infant's internal working model will serve as a flexible tool for achieving a sense of mastery and competence over the environment, as well as for contributing to the evolution of a fortified sense of self at a later stage of development. However, if the attachment forged within the dyadic relationship is one of nonresponsivity, the self-perpetuating nature of the patterns of the internalized schema will become rigid and inflexible, and the infant will become increasingly less adept at responding sensitively to environmental stimuli. This insensitivity has two main effects. First, it serves a self-preserving function. By immunizing the self from a nonresponsive environment, the infant avoids the distress associated with repeated assaults of noncontingency from the caregiver. Second, the increased rigidity and inflexibility of the internal working model represents a form of dysregulation. That is, since the patterns of the internal schema tend to be self-perpetuating, the infant may gradually lose the ability to modulate affective and cognitive responses to the environment. This dysregulatory response may not only affect infant behavior within the parameters of the attachment relationship, but may also extend to other aspects of infant behavioral manifestation. In other words, the rigidity of the internal schema will likely transfer across situations and tasks. Moreover, since the skills acquired during the attachment relationship are among the prerequisite building blocks in the construction of an intact sense of self, an infant whose internal schema has become "crystallized" into a pattern of nonresponsiveness will probably develop a damaged sense of self-esteem and an impaired self-image during subsequent stages of development.

The writings of Greenspan (1981) are pertinent if we consider the internal working model of the attachment relationship as an introjected schema or representation. Greenspan noted that when representations are first being organized, they are particularly fragile and susceptible to regression and fragmentation under the stress of internal affect states. Thus if the caregiver provides sustained noncontingent response, the infant may experience affective distress that in turn will impinge on the internal representation, potentially disrupting or shattering the schema. Greenspan has also hypothesized that during the consolidation phase of representational capacity (30 to 48 months), various stressors, such as separation, may activate regression, anxiety, depression, and other forms of impairment.

If the process of representation is subjected to repeated instances of disruption, it may be difficult for the infant to establish the sense of permanence necessary for differentiating object from self. That is, the development of both object and self-constancy requires a sufficiently stable set of internalized schemas which function as points of reference to which the infant can continually return. Bemesderfer and Cohler (1983) have noted that without object constancy, the infant may evolve a defective self-concept characterized by an inability to resolve inner tensions. The infant, unable to cope with tension, may experience negative affect in the form of unworthiness and depletion. These affects, if pervasive, may be integrated into the self-concept and, according to Bemesderfer and Cohler, may be a critical factor in the development of a matrix from which depression later emerges.

Thus Main and Goldwyn's (1984) research suggests the possibility that the maturing infant who perceives rejection from the caregiver is at an increased risk for the subsequent development of depression. If the attachment relationship is broken or disorganized, then the infant's subsequent representation of "self" must suffer, and damage to the self-concept is one of the precursors to and correlates of depression. Both Zahn-Waxler et al. (1984) and Radke-Yarrow et al. (1985), in their studies of children of depressed parents, found that depressed parents may transmit a picture of low esteem to their children, thereby fostering a reflective form of poor self-image in the child. Such a transmission may occur during early infancy.

In contrast, if the attachment provides the infant with consistent, positive caregiving, the infant is given a nurturing environment for developing confident self-regulatory abilities with a concomitant rich range of affective response. However, if the attachment is noncontingent, or if the caregiver is absent, the infant does not receive the advantages of maternal regulation in development. When the attachment bond is severed, as during a separation from the mother, the infant commonly reacts by exhibiting "protest" behavior. If the separation is prolonged, the infant will react with symptoms similar to those manifested by adults who are in mourning (Bowlby, 1958, 1969). If the infant passes through this stage of "despair" while still separated from the mother, it is probable that he or she will enter a stage labeled "detachment." At this point the infant will evince superficial signs of recovery, but may actually suffer permanent emotional damage. The infant who experiences a noncontingent or absent caregiver may also respond with "avoidant" behavior (Ainsworth, 1973), including precocious development of self-regulation and a tendency to withdraw from the caregiver. Another possible reaction to an inconsistent or absent caregiver is "resistant" behavior, whereby the infant displays poor self-regulation and a narrow, poorly controlled range of affects. These affective disorders, stemming from failures of both self and maternal regulation, can culminate in depression and depressive disorders. Such a phenomenon may be particularly likely if dysregulation is accompanied by poor social relationships, as Zahn-Waxler et al. (1984) noted.

Description of Attachment Behavior

Bowlby's original formulation of the attachment relationship (Bowlby 1958, 1960) drew heavily on ethological studies to demonstrate that attachment behavior is derived from natural selection, and is not an offshoot of another drive, such as the feeding instinct. He postulated that among the higher primates, the need for frequent contact between mother and infant protects the infant from predators. Any disturbance in the environment would alarm either the mother or the infant and bring them into physical proximity for the protection of the infant. Bowlby (1969, 1973, 1980) later theorized that the *attachment system* was merely one of several instinctive systems of behavior that were interconnected and interactive. A parallel *exploratory system* tends to lead the infant away from the mother and serves the adaptive function of providing enhanced experience for the infant. The infant's desire to explore and the mother's desire to maintain a secure knowledge of the infant's whereabouts are kept in a constant dynamic equilibrium. When the infant strays too far, the mother becomes alarmed and calls it to her or makes efforts to retrieve it. Similarly, if the infant feels that the mother is not within easy access, it engages in behaviors geared to regain contact.

Attachment behavior in the neonate and young infant includes a number of instinctual responses such as sucking, smiling, looking (at the caregiver), listening, calling, crying, babbling, reaching,and following. Bowlby (1969, 1973, 1980) divides these behaviors into two main categories: signaling behavior, which has the effect of bringing mother to infant, and approach behavior, which has the effect of bringing infant to mother.

In the neonate, attachment behaviors serve to mediate the first relationship with the caregiver. Smiling, looking, sucking, and reaching are all ways of creating and maintaining contact. Bowlby (1969), Brazelton, Koslowski, and Main (1974), and others have described the familiar dialogue of back and forth smiles, coos, and babbling between infant and mother. Such reciprocal conversations are the basis for the infant's first experiences of contingency (Trad, 1986).

Just as the notion of self-regulation was implicit in the temperamental traits discussed earlier, so too does regulation play a key role in attachment theory. As the attachment relationship develops, the infant tends to surrender higher regulatory functions to the mother. Emde and Sorce (1983) observed the "maternal referencing" that occurs when infants are presented with situations that create uncertainty. Sorce et al. (1985) presented 1-year-old infants with a "visual cliff" and found that infants routinely looked to the mother before venturing across it. After observing her affective response, the infant proceeded across the cliff if the mother smiled, and retreated from the edge if the mother presented a fearful expression. Thus the infant used the mother's nonverbal emotional signaling as a form of regulation.

The Strange Situation Procedure

The most widely accepted instrument for assessing attachment is the Strange Situation Procedure developed by Ainsworth and Wittig (1969). The Strange Situation consists of eight episodes which progressively tax an infant's ability to cope with the stress of separation from the caregiver. The episodes involve separation and reunion with the mother, exposure to a new environment and to an unknown adult. The infant is assessed in terms of reactions to the separation and the reunion—the reunion behavior being considered the most important in categorizing infants. The eight episodes are described below.

The subjects for Ainsworth and Wittig's (1969) initial study were 23 white, middle-class mother–infant dyads. The infants were all 51 weeks old. On the basis of observed behavior during the Strange Situation episodes, particularly during the reunion episodes, the infants were classified into three groups: A, avoidant; B, securely attached; and C, resistant. A infants showed little desire for contact with the mother after separation. They tended to show little distress at separation, and treated the stranger very much the same as the mother. B infants actively sought contact with the mother on reunion, showing reactions that ranged from smiles to tears. They also showed a wide range of distress during separation. The C infants were a heterogenous group that shared a general quality of maladaptiveness. They were unable to use the mother as a secure base for exploration, showing either distress throughout the separations or general passivity.

The Strange Situation Procedure

Episode	Participants	Duration	Behavior Highlighted by Episode
1	Mother, baby, experimenter	Approximately 30 seconds	(Introductory)
2	Mother, baby	3 minutes	Exploration of strange environment with mother present
3	Stranger, mother, baby	3 minutes	Response to stranger with mother present
4	Stranger, baby	3 minutes	Response to separation with stranger present
5	Mother, baby	Variable	Response to reunion with the mother
6	Baby	3 minutes	Response to separation when left alone
7	Stranger, baby	3 minutes	Response to continuing separation, and to stranger after being left alone
8	Mother, baby	Variable	Response to second reunion with mother

Source: From Ainsworth, M. D. S., Bell, S. M., & Stayton, D. J. (1971). Individual differences in strange-situation behavior in one-year-olds. In H. R. Schaffer (Ed.), *The origins of human social relations* (p. 20). London/New York: Academic Press. Reprinted by permission of © The Development Sciences Trusts.

The original three groups were later broken down into subgroups by Ainsworth and her associates. The subgroups are divided as follows (see Ainsworth, Bell, & Stayton, 1971, p. 22-25):

A. Avoidant infants.
> A1. Avoidant reunion behavior. These babies tended to resist being picked up, did not approach mother at reunion, or wanted to be put down after a short time.
> A2. Ambivalent reunion behavior. These babies first approached and then turned away from the mother, or approached and then ignored the mother. When picked up, they may cling momentarily and then show signs of wanting to be put down.

B. Securely attached infants.

> B1. Smiled at reunion, seemed interested in establishing interaction, but did not especially seek proximity. Little or no distress during separation.
> B2. Approached on reunion, desired contact. Showed little or no distress during separation.
> B3. Strong response to reunion, may cry. The babies in this group may or may not show distress at separation, but at reunion they definitely seek physical contact more than those in subgroups B1 or B2.
> B4. Seeks proximity throughout all episodes. Babies in this subgroup showed some insecurity even before separation episodes and showed little exploratory behavior. They tended to cling to the mother. Clearly distressed during separation.

C. Ambivalently attached infants.

> C1. Ambivalent contact with mother, perhaps marked by clinging, pushing, hitting, and so on. Distressed throughout separations. Exploration mixed with anger or anxiety.
> C2. Very passive, both in lack of exploration and in reunion behavior. May or may not show distress at separation.

Other researchers, such as Radke-Yarrow et al. (1985) and Main, Kaplan, and Cassidy (1985), have isolated yet additional attachment categories. Radke-Yarrow et al.(1985) describes an *A/C* category, of mixed avoidant and resistant characteristics, that is strongly associated with the children of depressed parents.

Stability and Correlations of Behavioral Patterns

Several researchers (Bowlby, 1982; Sroufe, 1985) have pointed out that although specific behaviors are mutable during development, attachment patterns may be expected to demonstrate consistency through the years. Waters (1978), for example, demonstrated stability of attachment from 12 to 18 months. Others have established strong correlations between attachment and various types of competence. Matas, Arend, and Sroufe (1978) showed correlations between attachment at 12 months and autonomy in preschoolers. Sroufe (1983) established correlations between secure attachment at 1 year and self-esteem and positive affect in a preschool environment.

Factors Affecting the Development and Display of Attachment Behaviors

Many researchers have focused on the fact that attachment is a phenomenon of a dyadic system, an interactional relationship between caregiver and infant. As such, it is affected by both parties. Primarily genetic endowments of the infant, such as temperament and physiology, have an effect on the quality of attachment, just as the innate characteristics of the caregiver have an impact on the relationship. However, attachment theory has demonstrated that the caregiver exerts a greater influence on the attachment relationship than does the infant.

Ainsworth (1979), for example, found that mothers of securely attached infants demonstrated more "sensitive response" toward their infants than mothers of A or C babies. Sensitive response was described as consisting of awareness of the infant's demands, acceptance of the infant's affective expressions, respect for the infant's autonomy, accessibility to the infant, and promptness of response to the infant's demands. Such response allows the infant to develop a sense of mastery over the environment and an awareness of contingency between its behavior and resulting outcomes. By contrast, mothers of avoidant babies were found to be high on scales measuring rejection or interference. Mothers of resistant babies were found to be highly ignoring or nonrejecting and highly interfering. Neither of these latter patterns permits the infant to formulate a relationship between its behavior and positive consequences.

The Function of Avoidant Behavior

Ethologists have shown that avoidant behavior actually serves a biological function in many species. Tinbergen and Moynihan (1952) suggested that visual avoidance (turning away) serves to present a less threatening posture so that the organism can approach an attachment figure without frightening it away. Chance (1962) suggested that avoidant behavior also serves to quell the fight or flight response in an organism, allowing it to approach an otherwise threatening situation.

If Bowlby is correct in noting that the need for proximity to a caregiver is an instinctual drive in a human infant, then in threatening situations the infant will be driven to the caregiver to quell its fears. The need to achieve proximity is still present whether the attachment figure is responsive and comforting or abusive or rejecting. If the caregiver is rejecting, avoidant behavior may function to give the infant an opportunity to reach an acceptable level of proximity. Similar avoidant behavior has been observed in human infants. Significantly, researchers such as Main and others (Gaensbauer & Sands, 1979; George & Main, 1979; Lewis & Schaeffer, 1979; Main, 1977; Main & Stadtman, 1981; Main, Tomasini, & Tolan, 1979; Main & Weston, 1981) have found avoidant behavior common in infants who experience rejection by their caregivers.

Main and Stadtman (1981) observed that reunion behavior exhibited by some of the infants in the Strange Situation resembled the behavior of infants who had been separated from their parents for prolonged periods of time. They theorized that infant's avoidant behavior may stem from a perception of caregiver rejection. This behavior may actually serve an adaptive function, according to the researchers, who concluded that "in the stressful separation situation avoidance may function to modulate the painful and vacillating emotions aroused by the historically rejecting mother" (p. 293). Main, Kaplan, and Cassidy (1985) observed that infants who were classified as insecurely attached (*A, C,* or *A/C*) demonstrated a variety of avoidant behaviors during a reunion with the mother, including gaze aversion, moving away from the mother, or shifting their attention to inanimate objects. Many normal attachment behaviors were dampened or were exhibited at a minimal level and many such infants did not cry on separation. Generally, a low level of affect was displayed—a symptom related to depression in adults.

Mothers of insecurely attached infants tended to show low affect also, either masking hostile feelings (in the case of avoidant babies) or simply not responding to the infant (in the case of insecure/avoidant infants). Many expressed an aversion to physical contact with their children.

RELATION BETWEEN TEMPERAMENT AND ATTACHMENT

Kagan (1982) and Chess and Thomas (1982) have suggested that rather than measuring the quality of the relationship between the infant and caregiver, the Strange Situation measures certain infant temperamental traits such as "susceptibility to stress" or "approach/withdrawal." Rothbart and Derryberry (1982), another team of temperament researchers, have also speculated that Strange Situation classification may be influenced by temperament. They hypothesize that infants who fail to exhibit strong attachment behaviors, and are thus classified as insecurely attached when evaluated in the Strange Situation, may actually be temperamentally equipped to tolerate separations without experiencing the intense levels of stress exhibited by those classified as securely attached.

Frodi and Thompson (1985) point out that this view is incompatible with the evidence that measures of attachment appear to be less context-sensitive than are measures of temperament. For example, attachment categories generally remain consistent when measured in the home and in the Strange Situation laboratory setting, while measures of behaviors indicative of temperamental qualities do not show comparable stability across settings. Kagan's argument for a temperamental basis for attachment classifications is equally inconsistent with the findings (Main & Weston, 1981; Ainsworth et al., 1978) that infants frequently have different attachment classifications with different caregivers.

Moreover, Bates, Maslin, and Frankel's (1985) study of the interaction of temperament and attachment on behavior problems found that measures of temperament did not predict attachment classification. Sroufe (1985), who also reported on the failure of early measures of temperament to predict subsequent attachment, further observed that children classified similarly in the Strange Situation may still be temperamentally, and therefore behaviorally, quite heterogeneous. In a letter to the American Journal of Orthopsychiatry (1982), Sroufe and Waters state that

> *Various discrete behaviors, which might be presumed to reflect temperament, are not indices of attachment. Moreover, these discrete behaviors* are not stable over time. *The attachment assessments, which may* not *be reduced to temperament were highly stable across a six-month period.* (emphasis in original).

Considered together, these findings strongly suggest that attachment is not simply a reflection of temperamental traits, although attachment may interact with and be affected by these traits. It is equally apparent that not all infant characteristics can be ascribed to external experience. Sroufe's (1985) description of temperament and attachment as "orthogonal"—shaping the developing personality in distinct ways, yet with influences that ultimately converge—may offer a useful way to conceptualize the relationship of these milestones. He proposed that attachment and temperament interact in the following fashion:

1. Temperament may influence discrete behaviors but not overall behavioral organization, that is, attachment classification.
2. Temperament may influence subcategory classification (*B1, B4,* etc.), but not major category placement.

3. Quality of care may influence security of attachment (*B* or Non-*B* Classification), and temperament may determine the pattern of insecure attachment (*A*, *C*, or *A/C*).

Goldsmith and Campos (1982), positing a more determinant role for temperament, outlined the following ways in which temperament could be seen to influence attachment categories:

1. The infant's temperament may influence the caregiver's degree of responsiveness, thus influencing attachment and Strange Situation classification.
2. The caregiver's social responsiveness may influence both attachment and temperament expressions.
3. Temperamental differences may directly influence attachment categories. If this is the case, then the Strange Situation is not measuring attachment at all.

A number of studies have identified specific areas of interaction between temperament and attachment. Thompson and Lamb (1983) investigated the contribution of temperament to stranger sociability, a type of behavior also examined in the Strange Situation. The researchers examined infants' responses to initial encounters with an unfamiliar adult, measured when the infants were 12.5 and 19.5 months. During this procedure, the stranger engages in a series of social overtures of gradually increasing intrusiveness. After each assessment mothers completed questionnaires, including the Infant Behavior Questionnaire (IBQ; Rothbart, 1981), which measures temperament dimensions such as fearfulness, activity level, and distress to limitations, as well as behaviors such as smiling and laughter. Thompson and Lamb found that at 12.5 months stranger sociability correlated negatively in a significant way with the infants' reported fearfulness. At 19.5 months sociability correlated negatively not only with fearfulness, but also with activity level and distress to limitations. This study attests to the contribution temperament makes to stranger sociability.

Other investigators have also documented specific correlations between temperament and attachment measures. Paradise and Curcio (1974) found that infants 9 to 10 months of age who displayed fearful reactions to strangers were rated by their mothers as being more cautious when approaching a wide variety of new social and nonsocial situations. This finding may be construed as relating to the temperament dimension of "approach/avoidance" described by the NYLS investigators (Thomas, Chess, Birch, Hertzig, & Korn, 1963).

Harmon et al. (1977) observed that 1-year-old infants who reacted with avoidance to a stranger had a high rating for the temperament trait of "fussiness." Observing a sample of 42 infants, the researchers found that of the infants who were classified as being "unusually fussy" ($N = 9$), 89 percent avoided the stranger. This finding contrasted with the "unusually fussy" babies ($N = 23$), among whom only 35 percent avoided the stranger. Furthermore, it has been noticed by Scarr and Salapatek (1970) that 2- to 23-month-old infants showed negative correlations between the temperament dimension of approach and fear of strangers.

The data reported by Belsky, Rovine, and Taylor (1984) support the contention that both maternal care and stable innate characteristics of the infant account for differences in attachment among infants. In their study, 60 mother-infant dyads were observed when the infants were 1, 3, and 9 months of age. These findings were correlated with an attachment classification when these same infants reached the age of 1 year. Analysis indicated that infants who were classified as "insecurely attached" were also found to be more "fussy" than their counterparts at 3 and 9 months of age. The finding that maternal stimulation accounted for less than 10 percent of the variance in "fussiness" revealed that the degree of maternal involvement predicted infant "fussiness" more consistently than "fussiness" itself predicted the degree of maternal involvement. In this sense, the contribution of "fussiness" to attachment appeared to be "direct, organismic, and temperamental rather than transactional" (p. 727). That is, "fussiness" does not appear to contribute to attachment by lessening the mother's desire for contact; instead, "fussiness" may serve as the infant's direct contribution to the attachment relationship. The authors summarized by stating that individual differences in attachment reflect both the factors of maternal care and the infant's temperament, as manifested by potentially enduring characteristics.

Gaensbauer, Connell, and Schultz (1983) demonstrated strong correlations between affective states and attachment behavior. They attempted to show that affective states, which may have a significant temperamental component, motivate attachment behavior. The authors correlated their studies of facial expression in infants, as indicative of affect, with observations of infants in the Strange Situation. Their work included rigorous microanalytic studies of facial expression that evaluated the presence and intensity of six different emotion categories: pleasure, interest, fear, anger, sadness, and distress. These emotion categories were compared with the traditional measures outlined by Ainsworth, Blehar, Waters, and Wall (1978) for attachment/affiliative behavior during separation and reunion episodes. Findings of the study clarified the relationship between the events of the Strange Situation and the infants' affective states. The authors found that when an infant was highly distressed, he or she was motivated to maintain close contact with the caregiver. Infants who displayed low ratings for the emotions of pleasure and interest concomitantly with high ratings for the emotions of distress, fear, anger, and sadness during the separation episodes tended to demonstrate high degrees of proximity-seeking and contact-maintaining behavior during subsequent reunion episodes.

Along the same lines, high degrees of pleasure and toy interest during separation correlated positively with low intensity avoidant behavior during reunion. Similar correlations between emotional states and behaviors were documented in other episodes. For example, if the infant showed anger during the stranger approach episode, the same infant showed high intensity avoidance ratings toward the caretaker during the reunion episode. In contrast, stranger interest predicted low intensity avoidance during reunion. Gaensbauer et al. (1983) remarked that

> The findings suggest that certain attachment behaviors are highly related to the preexistence of a negative emotional state and that avoidance behavior, especially low-intensity avoidance, may be due in part to the decreased motivation to renew close contact with the mother—characteristic of an infant who is not highly distressed. (p. 823)

Furthermore; "it may be that *A1* children do not stop experiencing and expressing anger once reunited with their mothers whereas *B1* children do." (Shiller, Izard, & Hembree, 1986,p. 382)

Another interesting finding with respect to the interplay of temperament and attachment was reported by Frodi, Bridges, and Grolnick (1985). The study involved 41 dyads observed during the Strange Situation at both the first and second year. The researchers found that infants categorized as avoidant manifested an apparent persistence at object-related activities when tested at 1 year of age. These avoidant infants, in other words, appeared to be as persistent as secure infants. Despite the seeming similarity between the two groups on measures of persistence, however, avoidant infants were the least competent during play, despite persistent attempts. This study suggests, then, that the effects of an insecure attachment can, in certain instances, override such temperament dimensions as persistence, and may undermine the infant's efforts toward mastery motivation.

If temperament is seen as expressive of infant self-regulation, and the attachment relationship is viewed as indicative of developing social regulation, then it is apparent that the two milestones are inextricably intertwined. Each contributes to the infant's growing abilities to modulate the impact of its environment.

Historically, temperament studies have focused on endogenous characteristics, while attachment investigations have concentrated on the environmental contributors to infant behavior. As the above studies demonstrate, the current mode of thinking for both constructs encompasses an interactive framework. As Plomin (1983) has noted,it is a "truism" that behavior takes place in a social and environmental context. Currently, most researchers would agree that both the infant's endogenous traits and the environmental milieu contribute to the expression of genetic and evolutionarily determined behavior.

Caregiver's Social Responsiveness Influencing Expression of Temperament and Attachment

Thomas et al. (1963) identified irritability as a temperamental trait lying within the dimension of "quality of mood." A high level of irritability is one of the traits common to infants typed as temperamentally "difficult" at age 3 months. In 1984, the NYLS investigators (Chess and Thomas, 1984) reported that "difficult" children appeared to be at greater risk than other children for behavior disorder.

Several investigators have questioned whether typologies such as "difficult" or "easy" are reflections of endogenous characteristics of the infant—that is, temperamentally determined—or actually are a function of interactions with caregivers—that is, a product of the attachment relationship. Data reported by Bell and Ainsworth (1972) showed that any stability demonstrated by an infant to manifest a crying response may actually reflect the caregiver's degree of responsiveness to the infant's needs. Following this line of inquiry, several attachment researchers have observed and recorded overt acts of physical rejection by the caregiver and have concluded that a caregiver's rejection of the infant contributes to behavior problems in the infant (Fraiberg, 1982b; Main & Stadtman, 1981).

Still, many observations of avoidant behavior recorded no overt acts of rejection on the part of the caregiver, leading researchers to conclude that infant resistance and anger may be endogenous to the infants exhibiting them. Ainsworth and associates (1978), however, speculated that mothers of avoidant infants may manifest physical rejection of their infants almost imperceptibly; for example, they may pick up their babies less often than do mothers of ambivalently and securely attached infants. These implications of the effects of subtle rejection were supplemented by data reported by Tracy and Ainsworth (1981). They reported that mothers of avoidant infants exhibited a greater number of affectionate behaviors of all types toward their infants than did mothers of ambivalently attached infants—an observation appearing to run counter to the popular notion among attachment investigators that the degree to which an infant exhibits avoidant behaviors reflects the degree to which the infant has been rejected by the mother. While it is possible to interpret infant anger toward nonrejecting mothers as temperamental "uncuddliness," Tracy and Ainsworth's data suggest that the infant's behavior may be related to maternal behavior. If the caregiver's affection is unrelated to infant desire for stimulation or comfort, the infant may respond with rejection. The realization that a caregiver need not actually reject the infant in order to contribute to the infant's avoidant behaviors should caution investigators not to overlook nuances of the infant-caregiver relationship in which the caregiver is playing a vital role.

Lewis, Brooks-Gunn, and Jaskir (1985) suggest that there is a proper balance to be struck between too much and too little responsiveness on the part of the caregiver. They found that insecurely attached *A* infants actually had more responsive environments and more maternal stimulation at 3 months than infants later classified as *B*. Ambivalently attached, or *C* babies, received the least stimulation.

The researchers also found that insecure attachment appeared to promote visual self-recognition. Insecurely attached infants were more likely to recognize themselves at 18 months than securely attached infants. They suggested that whether due to individual differences in temperament or attachment, insecurely attached infants tend to rely more on self and less on mother than securely attached infants, thus precipitating an earlier development of self-recognition.

Finally, Weber, Levitt, and Clark (1986) examined the relationship between attachment classification, infant temperament, and caregiver responsivity. These researchers found that temperament indeed is a factor in attachment classification, but that the mother's temperament is at least as significant a factor as the infant's. They found that mothers of *A* infants perceived themselves as more highly reactive than mothers of *B* or *C* infants, and that mothers of *A*, *B1*, and *B2* infants rated themselves as more adaptable than mothers of *B3* or *C* infants. This finding correlates maternal adaptability with infant distress on separation.

The researchers demonstrated that insecure infant-mother attachments and avoidant behaviors exhibited by infants may not simply reflect the mother's sensitivity and flexibility. Rather, they may be largely a function of the interaction of the mother's and infant's temperaments. If Rothbart and Derryberry (1982) are correct, experiments such as the Strange Situation, which supposedly assesses the security of infant-caregiver attachments by introducing the infant to a series of progressively threatening stresses, may inadvertently measure the infant's innate susceptibility to stress. If so, infants who don't exhibit strong attachment behaviors on reunion may be scored as avoidant when they simply haven't experienced intense stress on separation. Mothers who fail to comfort their distressed infants may be assessed as rejecting when they simply have a clear understanding that their infant can quite adequately calm him or herself.

NEUROENDOCRINE CORRELATES AFFECTING SELF-DEVELOPMENT

Temperamental factors, cognitive and affective capacities, and attachment behaviors, which are major contributors to the infant's incipient sense of self, emerge through the nuances of regulation. These nuances, in turn, have been interpreted as the orchestration of the infant's increasingly sophisticated internal mechanism with the external world. Despite the clinical evidence that permits these theoretical inferences to be drawn, however, no researcher has yet defined precisely what an "affect" is composed of or has identified the ingredients of cognitive processes. One area of psychopathogenesis, neuroendocrine analysis, does permit researchers to identify specific measurable substances which have been demonstrably linked to affective states and their regulation.

Hypothalamic-pituitary-adrenal (HPA) axis dysfunction has been documented as a key correlate of major depression. Among the manifestations of this dysfunction are adrenal cortisol hypersecretion, flattened cortisol circadian periodicity, and inability to suppress plasma cortisol levels following administration of dexamethasone. This evaluation of cortisol response is referred to as the dexamethasone suppression test (DST) and is considered a measurement of the pituitary adrenal interface (Matthews, Akil, Greden, & Watson, 1982). The rationale behind the DST is that dexamethasone (a synthetic glucocorticoid) inhibits cortisol secretion in humans for as long as 24 hours. Thus failure to suppress plasma cortisol after dexamethasone administration suggests hyperactivity along the HPA axis (Carroll, Curtis, & Mendels, 1976).

Irregularities in cortisol secretion are prominent in large numbers of endogenously depressed patients and are considered highly specific markers for a wide range of primary affective disorders (Risch, 1982). Researchers have also found that changes in cortisol production can be artificially induced in animals when they are subjected to situations of stress, such as maternal or peer separation. Kalin and Carnes (1984), for example, reported that after 4 days of peer separation, 4 out of 11 juvenile rhesus monkeys failed to inhibit plasma cortisol levels normally following administration of dexamethasone.

In addition, the DST has been found to be a fairly reliable marker in children with diagnostically confirmed depression or separation anxiety disorder. In a study involving 15 prepubertal children, aged 6 to 12 years, Livingston, Reis, and Ringdahl (1984) found that 7 of the children studied had high serum cortisol levels. Two of these children had a diagnosis of schizoaffective disorder; three suffered from separation anxiety disorder. Two of the children in the study had "borderline" cortisol levels. One child was depressed and the other had separation anxiety disorder. Of the six children whose cortisol levels were normal following DST evaluation, only one displayed the signs of depression, and symptomatology in this instance was less intense.

Commenting on the findings, the researchers noted that the DST may have limited specificity in diagnosing psychiatric disorder in prepubertal children. Moreover, findings suggest that separation anxiety and major depression may appear similar physiologically or that separation anxiety may be a physiologic "depression equivalent."

Recent studies have shown that the HPA axis is also operative in neonates and, as with adults, children, and infant monkeys, changes in cortisol level have been found to correlate with stress in young infants. For example, cortisol levels become elevated following circumcision. It remains to be shown, however, whether cortisol response in connection with separation and other kinds of depression-evoking stimuli in infants is similar to cortisol secretion in adults (Trad, 1986).

Changes in infant cortisol level as a response to stress have been reported by Anders, Sachar, Kream, Rolfwarg, and Hellman (1970) and Tennes and Carter (1973). The Anders et al. study found that in infants aged 1 to 20 weeks of age, cortisol levels were elevated after crying episodes. In contrast, cortisol levels during other states (quiet wakefulness, rapid eye movement, and nonrapid eye movement sleep) remained at a baseline level. These findings were interpreted as meaning that the adrenocortical response to distress is functional by the age of 1 week. Tennes and Carter found significant adrenocortical response to distress in 3-day-old infants.

Changes in cortisol levels in response to circumcision were documented in newborns by Gunnar, Malone, Vance, and Fische (1985). Blood samples taken before and after circumcision revealed a rise in cortisol levels following the operation. Cortisol levels returned to normal baseline levels within 3 to 4 hours of the procedure. According to these authors, "The pituitary adrenocortical system thus appears to respond sensitively and discriminatingly to aversive stimulation during the newborn period" (p. 825).

Tennes et al. (1977) designed a study exploring the relationship of physiologic response to psychological stress. Focusing on cortisol levels, the researchers found that when infants (aged 11 to 13 months) were separated from their mothers, cortisol levels rose. Significantly, however, infants who responded with fear or anxiety on separation had higher cortisol levels than those who did not react fearfully. Moreover, the fearful/anxious infants had chronically higher levels of cortisol, implying that innate individual differences in biochemistry may affect reactivity to stress. In addition, two measurably different fearful/anxious groups of infants could be identified from this study. One group, which responded to separation from the mother by active affective displays, such as crying, had high chronic and high separation cortisol levels. A second group of infants, who became immobilized and withdrawn upon being separated from their caregivers, had lower cortisol levels both chronically and in association with the stressful event of separation.

We may hypothesize that definite correlations can be made between Tennes' high cortisol groups and specific attachment subgroups. The *B3*, *B4*, and *C1* subgroups, which are highly distressed during separation, might be likely to show high cortisol levels. In contrast, the *C2* subgroup, noted for reacting to separation by withdrawing, might be expected to show low cortisol levels during separation.

Okuno, Nishimura, and Kawarazaki (1972) provided evidence that the HPA axis is already mature in the neonatal population by testing the stress response and negative feedback system in newborns. To investigate the status of HPA function at birth, the researchers used an acetycholine (ACTH) stimulation test, an insulin administration of these tests, and measured plasma 11-hydrocorticosteroid (11-OCHS; corticosterone and cortisol) levels. Subjects included infants aged 1 to 5 days. A control group, consisting of children aged 4 to 15 days was used for purposes of comparison. Prior to testing, it was determined that resting levels of plasma 11-OCHS in the subject infants were similar to resting levels in the control group. Subject infants were then given ACTH and regular insulin. After administration of these substances, plasma levels of 11-OHCS were found to be elevated. In contrast, after administration of the DST, plasma 11-OHCS levels were reduced.

Commenting on the results of the study, Okuno et al. (1972) noted that the insulin tolerance tests revealed that 1- to 5-day-old infants were able to respond to insulin stress. Findings derived from the DST suggest that the negative feedback mechanism, which indirectly results in cortisol inhibition, is also functional in neonates. According to the researchers, these results strongly indicate that both the stress response and the negative feedback inhibitory mechanism of infants is essentially comparable in regulatory response to that of children. Neonates thus appear to possess an internal capacity for regulating both inhibitory and secretory mechanisms with respect to the HPA axis.

Moreover, Vermes, Kajtar, and Szabo (1979) reported that maternal adrenocortical activation during vaginal delivery, as determined by 11-OHCS measurements, is paralled by a comparable fetal response, as evidenced by high 11-OHCS levels in cord blood and amniotic fluid.

Further substantiation for the efficiency of the pituitary function in neonates was provided by Cacciari, Cicognani, Pirazoli, Dallacasa, Mazzaracchio, Tassoni, Bernardi, Salardi, and Zappulla (1976). These researchers assayed growth hormone (GH) levels in 14 newborn infants. Samples were collected from infants at the second, sixth, twelfth, and twenty-fourth hour of life, then daily for 7 consecutive days. During the entire first week of life, plasma GH levels were significantly higher than those found in subjects over 4 years of age. Although GH levels at the second hour of life were similar to those found on the fifth, sixth, and seventh day, these values fluctuated greatly while maintaining overall high levels.

Studies probing the effect of ACTH administration in newborns include one conducted by Gutai, George, Koeff, and Bacon (1972), who found a substantial elevation of cortisol plasma concentration in normal neonates during the first 3 days of life, following intramuscular administration of 5 units of soluble ACTH. Cacciar et al. (1976) assayed ACTH levels in 14 newborns. In their study, the highest mean plasma value was measured at the second hour of life; ACTH then dropped significantly beginning at the twelfth hour, with minimum values reached on the seventh day. Serial determinations of ACTH in pooled fetal blood obtained during labor showed that the average hormone levels increased significantly from the first to the second stage of labor, achieving peak levels at delivery, according to Arai, Yanaihara, and Okinaga (1976). Moreover, these researchers reported that the pituitary gland of the fetus at midtrimester contains ACTH.

Arai et al. (1976) concluded that ACTH concentration in fetal blood significantly increases as labor progresses, giving further credence to the theory that the fetal pituitary adrenal axis is functional during delivery and that steroid production responds to the secretion of fetal ACTH.

Considered cumulatively, these studies provide a plethora of data demonstrating that the newborn infant enters the world with a regulated, adaptive, intact HPA axis equipped to respond to stress and other stimuli appropriately. These studies indicate that neonates respond to physiological stress by reregulating or adjusting inhibitory and secretory mechanisms along the HPA axis. However, future studies must investigate whether infants respond to psychological stress (e.g., maternal depression) with comparable adaptability. Such studies are particularly important, because abnormally high levels of cortisol (a well-known marker for depression) are also encountered in infants during periods of stress. Thus neonates secrete cortisol during the stress of delivery, circumcision, and so on, and appear capable of inhibiting production back to normal levels when the stress factor is removed. The vital issue that remains is whether there are stress factors to which the infant is susceptible that either alone or through repetition cause dysregulation of inhibitory and secretory function along the HPA axis.

Another category of neuroendocrine function in adults that responds to stress and correlates with depression is the endogenous opioid system. The key endocrinologic substrate of this system is [B]-endorphin, which is secreted by the pituitary. "Both [B]-endorphin and adrenocorticotropin (ACTH) derive from a common precursor, pro-opiomelanocortin" (Rose, 1985, p. 663). The secretion of both hormones is stimulated by corticotropin-releasing factor (CRF) (Vale et al., 1981). "[B]-endorphin operates to regulate ACTH secretion, and participates along with ACTH itself via either short or long feedback loops to inhibit hypothalamic CRF secretion"(Rose, 1985, pp. 663-664). According to Guillemin, et al. (1977), [B]-endorphin and ACTH are secreted concomitantly in increased amounts by the adenohypophysis in response to acute stress, as well as in vitro in response to purified CRF. Moreover, both hormones possess common and identical regulatory mechanisms.

Plasma [B]-endorphin secretion has been found to increase in adults subjected to conditions of stress, such as imminent surgery (Cohen, Pickar, & Dubois, 1981). It has also been demonstrated that depressed patients have a lower ratio of plasma endorphin to cortisol than normal subjects, and that patients with nonmajor depression have a lower plasma [B]-endorphin level than patients with a diagnosis of major depression (Cohen et al., 1984). Thus, as with cortisol, depressed adults may be hypersecreting or "disinhibiting" their release of [B]-endorphin.

Concurring with and elaborating on these findings, Risch, Janowski, Judd, Gillin, and McClure (1983) reported that morning plasma concentrations of [B]-endorphin immunoreactivity were significantly higher in a group of depressed patients and patients with affective disorders than in age- and sex-matched normals and psychiatric patients without affective disorders. Using a radioimmunoassay technique designed to measure [B]-endorphin response, Matthews et al. (1982) found that dexamethasone may be ineffective in suppressing [B]-endorphin-like material in depressed patients. After administration of the DST, it was discovered that a control psychiatric population inhibited [B]-endorphin-like material, whereas suppression was less likely in endogenously depressed patients.

Agren and Terenius (1983), reporting on endorphin evaluation in 92 patients with major depression, found clearly elevated endorphin levels in this population as compared to normal controls. Additionally, higher levels of endorphin secretion were found in unipolar depressed patients. The researchers were also able to pinpoint seasonal rhythms for endorphin elevation, with high concentrations peaking in early fall for unipolar depressed patients and in late fall for bipolar depressives.

As revealed by several researchers, production of endogenous opioids, including [B]-endorphin, is merely one manifestation of a complex system of neuroendocrinologic regulation. However, the endogenous opioids may function as significant catalyst substances that trigger release or inhibition of a number of other substrates. In this sense, the endogenous opioids may be viewed as modulators or stimulators of hormonal response. Thus, as Risch et al. (1983) report, the endogenous opioids appear to modulate response to such physiologic stimuli as stress, suckling, and lactation. Evidence also suggests that endogenous opioids suppress function along the thyroid axis and activate function along the adreno-cortisol axis. Preliminary studies have found that endogenous opioids specifically may decrease concentration of dopamine. Since dopamine is a prolactin inhibitor, by suppressing dopamine, the endogenous opioids may indirectly stimulate prolactin production and ACTH release.

Endogenous opioids have also been found to increase serotonin turnover, which in turn stimulates a release of prolactin, GH, and ACTH and a reduction of norepinephrine turnover, which inhibits ACTH release. Increases in ACTH have also been tied to endogenous opioid production, and increases in plasma concentrations of [B]-endorphin and other endogenous opioids have been found to increase plasma concentrations of cortisol. This finding is most significant, since, as noted earlier, hypersecretion of cortisol, as measured by DST, is correlated with major depression.

To what extent, however, are these complex mechanisms of endogenous opioid interaction functional in infancy? Facchinetti, Bagnoli, Bracci, and Genazzani (1982) examined plasma opioid production during the first hours of life and determined that fairly sophisticated neuroendocrine function of endogenous opioids does, in fact, exist in neonates. The researchers determined that ACTH plasma levels are raised during the first 6 hours of life and decline to normal adult levels approximately 18 hours later. High plasma cortisol levels were also reported during the first 3 hours of life, but cortisol abated to normal adult levels by the second day of life. The researchers also found evidence of a highly sophisticated neuroendocrinologic feedback mechanism present during the neonatal period, which consisted of interaction between corticotropin-releasing factor, mediated cortisol, and ACTH. This mechanism was inferred from the ability of neonates to secrete cortisol in response to ACTH stimulation or during insulin-induced hypoglycemia coupled with ACTH suppression, after administration of dexamethasone. Significantly, in adults, ACTH and [B]-endorphin are secreted concomitantly in stressful situations.

To derive their findings, Facchinetti et al. (1982) took umbilical blood samples in 27 neonates. Further, blood samples were obtained from the jugular vein of the infants at 30 minutes, 6 hours, 12 hours, and 24 hours after birth. It was found that [B]-endorphin concentration during all these time periods was consistently higher than normal adult levels. Thus the data clearly demonstrate that neonates are able to release [B]-endorphins during the first hours of life. The researchers noted that these data are in accord with previous reports of raised ACTH levels during the first 6 hours of life and support the concept that ACTH and [B]-endorphin are released in parallel fashion during stressful situations. However, the researchers commented that the significance of the elevated levels of [B]-endorphin during the first few hours of life remains unclear.

Pohjavouri, Rovamo, and Laatikainen (1985) investigated [B]-endorphin and cortisol levels in newborns, and compared levels of these hormones in neonates born by caesarean section with levels in neonates born by spontaneous vaginal delivery. Of the 27 newborns studied, 10 were delivered by caesarean and 17 experienced spontaneous vaginal delivery. In the caesarean group, it was found that mean plasma concentrations of cortisol rose significantly from 2 hours after birth and then remained high, while mean [B]-endorphin remained at a stabilized high level 2 hours after birth. In the infant group that experienced spontaneous labor, plasma cortisol was also high at birth and remained high after 2 hours, although a slight decline in cortisol levels did occur. However, plasma [B]-endorphin levels declined in this latter group at two hours after birth. Investigating [B]-endorphin levels in neonate cerebrospinal fluid, Burnard, Todd, John and Hindmarsh (1982) found higher levels in preterm than in term infants.

Activity along the HPA axis with respect to cortisol has also been confirmed in newborns, with evidence indicating that the neuroendocrine mechanism is functioning prenatally. Furthermore, discrepancies in the mechanism of metabolism, as reflected by the DST, have been documented between preterm and full-term infants.

In a study by Kauppila, Simila, Ylikorkala, Koivisto, Makela, and Haapalahti (1976), prenatal dexamethasone therapy was administered to 33 mothers with threatened preterm labor. Mothers were given dexamethasone on 3 consecutive days. A control group consisted of 56 mothers who experienced normal vaginal delivery. At birth, maternal venous and mixed umbilical cord blood samples were taken. Venous blood samples were also obtained from newborns periodically during the first 24 hours after delivery. Findings revealed lower ACTH in the mothers and infants within the dexamethasone group than in the control group. ACTH levels in both groups of newborns fell during the first 24 hours after delivery, but the fall was significantly greater in the dexamethasone group than in the controls. The researchers noted that since the mean gestational age for the dexamethasone group was approximately 3 to 5 weeks less than for the controls, the observed differences may signify that premature newborns are less able to synthesize ACTH.

Growth hormone irregularities have also been tied to affective states, specifically in relating emotional abuse with inhibited growth. One disorder, referred to as psychosocial dwarfism or nonorganic failure to thrive, typically begins at approximately 8 months of age. Failure to thrive is one of the clearest and most readily detectable signs of depression in early life. Indeed, Spitz's (1946) study of anaclitic depression in infants presented such compelling evidence of growth retardation that failure to thrive has sometimes been deemed synonymous with depression. It appears from the research of Powell, Brasel, and Blizzard (1967a,b) that there may be some biological link between emotional abuse or neglect and failure to thrive. Powell observed a specific absence of GH release in emotionally abused or deprived children.

Another theory pertinent to depression is the permissive amine hypothesis. This theory posits that abnormally deficient levels of catecholamines are associated with depression (Van Praag, 1978). To validate this hypothesis, Van Praag and de Haan (1980) treated 20 depressive adult patients suffering from recurrent depressions, with 5-HTP, a precursor of serotonin. Patients were randomly divided into two groups. One group received the serotonin precursor, while the other group received a placebo. Findings revealed that the patients receiving the 5-HTP significantly improved and did not experience further depressive episodes, while patients receiving the placebo experienced virtually the same recurrent pattern of their illness.

Siever and Davis (1985) proposed that the biogenic amine theories of depression may tap into a defect in the neurotransmitter systems involved in regulating the body's neuroendocrine production. That is, a dysregulated mechanism, which either overreacts or underreacts in the production of neuroendocrine substances, may be a key etiologic factor in depression. These researchers proposed six criteria that can be used to detect dysregulation;

1. Impairment of one or more regulatory or homeostatic mechanisms.
2. Erratic patterns of basal output in the neurotransmitter system.
3. Diminished selective responsiveness of the system to external stimuli.
4. Disruption in the normal periodicities of the system, including circadian rhythmicities.
5. Sluggish return of the system to basal activity following perturbation.
6. Restoration of efficient regulation by pharmacologic agents demonstrating clinical effectiveness.

These criteria are consistent with the emphasis of temperament researchers on individual differences in reactivity and the regulation of reactivity (Derryberry & Rothbart, 1984). These researchers' concept of self-regulation encompassed procedures whose purpose is to modulate the reactivity state of the somatic, endocrine, autonomic, and central nervous systems.

Attachment behaviors may provide yet another well-documented means for studying the developmental neuroendocrine correlates of affect and depression. The attachment bond between infant and caregiver regulates the infant's neurochemical and hormonal activity through such means as sensory stimulation, affection, and nutrition (Papousek & Papousek, 1984). When this intimate bond between infant and caregiver is disrupted, a number of serious biological alterations have been noted to occur. Among these alterations are changes in sleep patterns, immune function, monoamine systems, heart rate, body temperature, and endocrine function. In contrast, infants who have been labeled as securely attached are frequently observed to be more cooperative, persistent, and enthusiastic than those more insecurely attached.

Specific reactions to separation from the caregiver provide a good operational model for assessing infant neuroendocrine response. In 1-year-old infants separated from their caregivers for 1 hour, for example, increased amounts of cortisol were noted, particularly among infants displaying external signs of distress (Tennes & Mason, 1982; Bliss, Midgeon, Branch, & Samuels, 1956). Alterations in the level of GH have also been noted in cases of separation. In fact, Green, Campbell, and David (1984) proposed that psychosocial dwarfism may be wholly attributed to a highly stressful, negative relationship between infant and caregiver. Thus the dysregulation theory of neuroendocrine function may be integrated with hypotheses concerning the role of regulation in temperament and attachment manifestations.

These studies in the area of neuroendocrine function yield several pertinent pieces of evidence of value in deciphering the origins of depression and depressive-like phenomena in infancy. First, the investigations strongly suggest that the infant, even at birth, possesses finely honed neuroendocrinologic mechanisms that operate at a level of sophistication and intricacy reminiscent of function at an adult level. Thus infants respond to "stressful" situations such as delivery itself and circumcision with elevated levels of both cortisol and endogenous opioids, and the high "stress" levels of these substances abate within several hours once the stressful stimulus is removed. Moreover, as the studies reveal, infants respond by suppressing cortisol upon the administration of dexamethasone. We may infer, then, that infants are capable of regulating their neuroendocrinologic system appropriately in terms of environmental stimuli and that they possess an exquisitely sensitive mechanism of response to stress. Second, abnormalities of response in neuroendocrine function have been documented among adults and children with diagnosed depression and separation anxiety disorder. That is, certain psychopathologic populations appear incapable of reregulating endocrine concentrations back to baseline levels when the imminent stress stimulus is removed. Indeed, the acute sensitivity of response that in a normal population is evident upon administration of dexamethasone is distinctively absent in diagnosed depressives.

It is appropriate to inquire, then, whether a subgroup of infants also evinces this dysregulatory response. In other words, is the HPA axis dysfunctional in some infants, in the sense that adrenal cortisol is hypersecreted, circadian periodicity of cortisol is flattened, or cortisol levels are not suppressed following dexamethasone administration? Further, the mechanisms of neuroendocrinologic response in infants known to fall within particular risk categories, such as maternal depression, maternal separation, or infant abuse and neglect, need to be examined to ascertain whether these infants evince the form of neuroendocrine dysregulation apparent in depressed children and adults. If, in fact, such dysregulation is apparent within a particular population of infants, researchers may be provided with new markers for diagnosing infant depression or incipient depression. The studies of Pohjavouri, Rovamo, and Laatikainen (1985) and Kauppila et al. (1976) are particularly noteworthy in this regard, because they suggest that the stress of a caesarean delivery may provoke a form of neuroendocrinologic dysregulation in neonates.

ATTACHMENT AND TEMPERAMENT CHARACTERISTICS THAT CORRELATE WITH DEPRESSION

DSM-III describes several categories of "affective disorder." The primary symptoms of "major depressive episode" are dysphoric mood and loss of interest or pleasure in all or almost all usual activities. Other symptoms include irritability, sad expression (in children), lack of appetite (or, in children, failure to gain weight), sleep disturbance, listlessness, affectlessness, anxiety, and hypoactivity. With depression defined in this manner, both temperament and attachment studies reveal emotions and behaviors that can be interpreted as expressive of a depressed affective state (e.g., sadness, affectlessness, and irritability). The results of several studies suggest that DSM-III criteria for depression are appropriate for children (Chess and Thomas, 1984; Earls, 1982). Many of these symptoms have been described in infants by various researchers (e.g., Gaensbauer, 1980). Some symptoms, however, are obviously transformed in child and infant populations. For example, failure to gain weight is a variant of the adult symptom of weight loss. Other symptoms may vary to a less obvious degree in children. It may also be suggested that the DSM-III enumeration fails to encompass the full spectrum of depressive symptomatology in children. This mutability of psychopathological symptoms is not surprising in light of observations by both temperament and attachment researchers who have acknowledged that behavior undergoes developmental transformations in the course of maturation.

Temperament Correlates of Depression

Goldsmith and Campos (1982) describe temperament as emotional in nature, and they have correlated the temperament dimensions defined by Thomas and Chess (1963, 1980), Buss and Plomin (1975), and Rothbart and Derryberry (1981) with specific affects. Included in this list are the depression-related affects of fear, anger, distress, listlessness, and irritability. Of the NYLS's (Chess & Thomas, 1984; Thomas, Chess, & Birch 1968) nine temperament dimensions, three in particular relate to negative affect. A negative measure of "intensity of reaction" corresponds to the symptom of affectlessness. A negative score in "quality of mood" may be understood to describe the negative affect of sadness. The symptom of irritability may correspond to a low score in the dimension "threshold of responsiveness."

The NYLS investigators found that although no constellations of traits were identified as descriptive of depression, infants typed at age 3 months as "difficult"—that is, infants for whom the traits of irregularity, intensity, propensity to withdraw, slowness to adapt, and negative mood were clustered—were found to be more susceptible than others to developing adjustment disorder (Thomas, Chess, & Birch, 1968). Slow-to-warm-up infants—infants for whom low activity, propensity to withdraw, slowness to adapt, negative mood, and mild intensity were clustered—were also identified as relatively susceptible to adjustment disorder. While only 4 (7%) of the 56 subjects of the NYLS who were classified at age 3 months as temperamentally "easy" developed childhood behavior problems, 10 (71%) of the subjects classified as temperamentally "difficult" subsequently developed behavior problems in childhood (Chess & Thomas, 1984). Approximately 50 percent of the sample's "slow-to-warm-up" children presented clinical disorders during childhood (Chess & Thomas, 1984). The fact that some children of each temperamental type developed behavior problems led the NYLS investigators to conclude that no individual temperament dimension or type was an infallible predictor of disorder.

One specific trait, negative mood, which might have been thought to correlate with depression, did not, in fact, demonstrate any consistent pattern in the six NYLS cases with depressive pathology. Out of the two cases with recurrent major depression, one case manifested preponderance of negative mood and one did not. Two out of four of the cases with secondary depression showed mild tendency to negative mood; the other two cases of secondary depression showed preponderance toward positive mood.

Each of the cases of secondary depression showed at least one pronounced temperament trait, however. One case displayed extreme persistence; another exhibited marked distractibility along with short attention span. The two other cases showed a difficult temperament pattern which included extreme trait preponderances in several dimensions. This common element among the NYLS cases of depressive psychopathology tends to support Chess and Thomas' (1984) incorporation of the concept of "goodness or poorness of fit." According to this view, a temperamental trait or cluster assumes significance if extremes of the trait cause some imbalance with the child's environment, leading to the experience of "poorness of fit." Thus it is not so much individual traits or clusters that dispose to pathology, but rather these traits in interaction with the needs and behavioral style of those with whom the infant has most frequent contact (Henderson, 1982; see Tables 2 and 3).

Attachment Correlates of Depression

In comparison with studies of infant temperament, attachment studies have generated much clearer evidence of depressive symptomatology, ranging from anger and affectlessness to despair and detachment. Perhaps most dramatically, Main's studies (including Blanchard & Main, 1979; Main, 1983; Main & Stadtman, 1981; Main & Weston, 1981) showed that

Table 2. DSM-III Criteria for Major Depression and Corresponding Dimensions of Temperament

DSM-III (APA, 1980, p. 213-1) Major Depression	Thomas, Chess, Birch, Hertzig, and Korn (1963)— Temperamental Dimensions	Buss and Plomin (1975)— Temperamental Dimensions	Rothbart (1981)— Temperamental Dimensions
Dysphoric mood	Adaptability Approach/withdrawal Mood	Emotionality Impulsivity	Smiling & laughter Fear Distress to limitations Soothability
Eating disturbances Sleep disturbances	Rhythmicity Rhythmicity		
Psychomotor agitation/ retardation	Activity level Approach/withdrawal Intensity Attention span/persistence	Activity	Activity level
Loss of interest/pleasure in usual activities	Approach/withdrawal Mood Attention span/persistence	Emotionality Sociability	Duration of orienting Smiling & laughter
Loss of energy or fatigue	Activity level Intensity Attention span/persistence	Activity	Activity level Duration of Orienting
Feelings of worthlessness Cognitive disturbances Suicidal ideation or behavior			

146

Table 3. Six Cases of Child Depression in the NYLS

Temperamental Dimensions	Cases
Preponderant negative mood	Case 1. Recurrent major depression, first evident at 8 years
Preponderant positive mood	Case 2. Recurrent major depression, first symptoms at 13 years
Extreme persistence	Case 3. Dysthymic disorder, with onset of behavior disorder at 5 years, and first appearance of depressive symptoms at 10 years
Marked distractability Short attention span	Case 4. Dysthymic disorder, with onset of behavior disorder at 30 months, and first appearance of depressive symptoms at 17 years
Difficult profile Low rhythmicity Intense reactions Negative in mood Withdrawal from new stimuli Slow to adapt to changes	Case 5. Dysthymic disorder, with onset of behavior disorder at 13 years and first appearance of depressive symptoms at 16 years
Difficult profile Low rhythmicity Intense reactions Negative in mood Withdrawal from new stimuli Slow to adapt to changes	Case 6. Adjustment disorder with depressed mood, with onset of behavior disorder at 13 years, and first appearance of depressive symptoms at 16 years

Source: Chess and Thomas, 1984.

> *rejection by the mother in normal samples leads to the development of a syndrome of avoidance, hostility and little feeling for others in the infant, a syndrome which is also seen in abusive parents and their toddlers. The hallmark of this syndrome is the infant's early, strongly affectless avoidance of its mother. . . . (Main & Goldwyn, 1984, p. 210)*

Main and Goldwyn (1984), relying on interviews with adult women who, as infants, had experienced their mothers as rejecting, revealed that these women tended to reject their own infants. Main and Goldwyn identified a cluster of depressive-like symptoms—affectlessness and irritability—present in maternally rejected infants, and they determined that avoidance among such infants remained stable until 6 years of age.

Among the most striking parallels with the symptoms of major depression as described in DSM-III are the descriptions of children separated from their parents offered by Spitz and Wolf (1946) and Bowlby (1969). Bowlby describes the process of detachment as paralleling the process by which an adult mourns the loss of a loved one. For a child, an extended separation is not dissimilar to the death of a loved one. Bowlby describes the process that the child undergoes in separation as consisting of three stages: *protest, despair,* and *detachment.* The advent of the initial "protest" phase is distinguished by high agitation and attempts to return to the caregiver. During the phase of "despair," the symptoms described by Bowlby include loss of interest in usual activities, loss of appetite, crying, and hopelessness. Finally, "detachment" occurs when the infant generally withdraws from activity and rejects the caregiver's attempts to reestablish contact upon reunion.

Gaensbauer, Connell, and Schultz (1983) demonstrated correlations between affective states and attachment behavior. These observations have to some extent been replicated in the offspring of manic-depressive parents. In a longitudinal study, Gaensbauer et al. (1984) compared the affective regulation and attachment behavior of these infants with a control group. The investigators noted that by the age of 12 months, the proband group showed significantly more fear during the maternal reunion episode. By 15 months, when the second measure took place, they were less distressed during the maternal separation episode. Finally, when the last observation took place at 18 months, they showed both less pleasure and less interest than did the control group during the reunion episode. The authors concluded that the proband group appeared to be showing a generalized disturbance in their capacities to regulate emotions adaptively.

Higgins, Klein, and Strauman (1985) have presented a model for discerning how distortions of self-concept may contribute to depression and anxiety disorders. The researchers suggest that self-concept is actually comprised of three distinct, internalized schema. First, the schema of the "actual" self is a representation of the attributes the individual believes he or she possesses. Second, the "ideal" self consists of qualities the individual aspires to possess. Finally, the "ought" self is a representation of those characteristics the individual believes he or she should possess. The reseachers suggest that discrepancies between any two of these self-concepts induces a state of discomfort. They note that discrepancy between actual and ideal self-concepts results in dejection-related and frustration-related symptomatology that is indicative of depression, whereas agitation-related emotions are associated with actual-ought discrepancy and are manifested by anxiety symptomatology.

Significantly, for a self-concept discrepancy to be present, the individual must possess capacities to engage in discrepancy analysis and must possess an intact sense of self. With respect to infant psychopathology, infant capacities in the area of discrepancy awareness were discussed earlier in this chapter. The infant's incipient sense of self was charted through various stages of development, and the effect of temperament and attachment behaviors on the inchoate self-concept were noted. It may be argued that since the infant is capable of discerning discrepancy in the environment from the earliest months of life onward, he or she may also be capable of engaging in a process of internal discrepancy awareness. Thus as schema are internalized, the infant may exert analytic capacities upon such schema. If, for example, the infant is temperamentally "difficult" and the caregiver responds inadequately to his or her needs, a discrepancy may be created and logged internally. Or if an infant is frustrated by a nonresponsive caregiver, the discrepancy encountered in the environment may be internalized, creating a distortion and causing affective distress. The key point here is that although the young infant may not possess a fully intact sense of self, damage to the incipient sense of self may occur relatively early such that negative affect—dejection, frustration, or agitation—may become part of the internal schema from which the sense of self evolves.

Conclusions

Symptomatology relating to DSM-III criteria for depressive disorders is shown by Goldsmith and Campos (1982) to be related to the affective expressions of dimensions of temperament. Almost all of the DSM-III symptoms can be accommodated by one or more temperament dimensions. However, there are as yet no adequate descriptions of common temperament clusters or typologies that relate to depression. The typology of the "difficult" child has been shown to be at greater risk for behavioral disorder than either the "easy" or the "slow-to-warm-up" child, but the risk is not specifically related to depression. One significant fact, although in too small a sample to be statistically significant, is that both cases of major depression found by the NYLS had a history of depressive illness in their families. This suggests that, for cases of primary depression, hereditary factors may be involved.

The attachment construct has been more fruitful in producing full scenarios for infants at risk of depression. The behavior of insecurely attached infants, both avoidant (A) and anxious (C), shares many characteristics with the symptomatology of depression. Also, the literature on children undergoing separation from their caregivers is filled with poignant descriptions of depressive-like phenomena. The studies of Radke-Yarrow et al. (1985) and Belsky, Rovine, and Taylor (1984) on the children of depressive parents indicate a clear correlation between maternal and child depression.

ATTACHMENT AND TEMPERAMENT CORRELATES AS PREDICTIVE OF DEPRESSION

Since the patterns of correlation between measures at one time with measures at another time define stability, one challenge for researchers has been to develop appropriate research methodologies that can identify continuities and discontinuities of traits across developmental stages. The predictive validity of such a methodology is shown when similar patterns of a correlation among measures can be demonstrated.

The attempt to isolate factors contributing to depression and depressive-like symptoms in children and infants is divided into the examination of infant, maternal, and environmental influences. It is postulated that all three of these elements interact in shaping behavior, and that the expression of one element is influenced by the other contributing factors.

Both temperament and attachment studies have grouped commonly observed sets of individual behaviors into clusters or typologies. In some cases these clusters show greater stability than the individual traits.

Stability of Infant Characteristics

The researchers of the NYLS (Thomas et al., 1963) described nine temperament dimensions that they delineated from their observations of infants. These are activity level, approach/withdrawal, regularity, adaptability, threshold, intensity, mood, distractibility, and attention span/persistence. As noted, the NYLS researchers also clustered these dimensions into three common patterns of temperament that they termed the "difficult," "easy," and "slow-to-warm-up" temperaments. Carey (1970) was able to identify two additional clusters that fall between difficult and easy—the "intermediate-high" (more difficult) and the "intermediate-low" (more easy). These two clusters, in conjunction with two of the original model, provide temperament classifications that range from difficult to intermediate-high to intermediate-low to easy. This procedure allows classification of (approximately) 40 percent of the children who did not fall into any of the three original clusters.

Stability of Typologies.   The applicability and benefit of using the NYLS classification was assessed by Carey and McDevitt (1978), who rated 187 children (100 males and 87 females) twice. The first rating took place during infancy (4 to 8 months) and the second rating took place in early childhood (3 to 7 years). Comparison of both ratings showed that 26.1 percent of the children classified as difficult and 39.1 percent of those classified as easy remained within their same categories. Significantly, those children who remained in the difficult or intermediate-high categories during both ratings had two striking differences from those who started out in the difficult or intermediate-high categories and transferred into other clusters at the 3 to 7 year rating: (1) 15 of 17 were above the mean in activity levels, and (2) 11 of 17 had very negative mood ratings. On the other hand, individuals who shifted into the difficult or intermediate-high categories during early childhood differed significantly in one particular way from those with stable easy temperaments: The former were likely to be more withdrawn.

   Stability of Individual Behaviors.   The stability of individual temperament variables has proven more limited than the stability of typologies (Thomas et al., 1963). By 1963, the NYLS researchers had reported the data collected on 80 of their subjects. These 80 children were those in the group who had passed their second birthday. The average age at the time of the first parental report was 3.3 months. Subsequent histories were taken at approximately 3-month intervals for one year, then at 6-month intervals. This method provided data that was collected at five different age periods during the first 2 years of life.
   Since researchers investigating childhood depression have been interested in when infants and children can first experience the persistent negative mood often found in adult depressives, the stability of the temperament dimension "quality of mood" (Thomas, Chess, & Birch, 1968) is particularly important. In the first period (average age 5.9 months), 55 infants had preponderantly positive mood rating and 17 infants had preponderantly negative ratings. When these ratings are compared with those of the fifth period (average age 27.3 months), 67 infants showed preponderantly stable mood ratings. Nine of the 17 infants who showed predominantly negative mood during the first period remained stable in their ratings through the fifth. Of all of Thomas and Chess' temperament dimensions, quality of mood was the fourth most stable. Infants also showed stability for other dimensions. Intensity showed the greatest stability, with 77.7 percent of the infants showing the same rating from the first to the fifth period. High threshold of response was the second most stable dimension, with more than two thirds of the infants maintaining the same rating. Nondistractibility, the third most stable dimension, remained stable in 64.7 percent of the cases.

   Stability of Attachment Classifications.   Studies have generally shown attachment dimensions to demonstrate greater evidence of stability than temperament dimensions. Waters (1978) found attachment patterns to be stable from 12 to 18 months. Matas, Arend, and Sroufe (1978) demonstrated stability in attachment patterns throughout infancy, through the end of the second year. Arend, Gove, and Sroufe (1979) and Waters, Wippman, and Sroufe (1979) found attachment patterns to be stable from 15 to 18 months.
   As part of a longitudinal study, Egeland and Farber (1984) examined data on 189 infant-mother dyads who were tested in the Strange Situation at both 12 and 18 months of age. Other behavioral and temperamental data were collected throughout the first 2 years of the infants' lives. Sixty percent of the sample remained in the same attachment classification from the first to the second test. Stability of attachment classification appeared greater among securely attached infants than among insecurely attached infants. Seventy-

four percent of the securely attached (B), 45 percent of the avoidant (A), and 37 percent of the resistant (C) infants remained stable from the first to the second measure.

Infants who changed from secure (B) to insecure attachment (A or C), showed a number of significant characteristics. Those who changed from B to A cuddled less during their feedings than infants who were stable Bs. Infants who changed from B to C were rated as being less temperamentally easygoing during feedings and less satisfied and attentive during play than B babies who remained stable. The only common measure among infants who changed from resistant (C) to secure (B) attachment was a higher overall developmental level at 9 months than infants who remained resistant at both assessments.

Maternal Characteristics as Predictors

The stability of certain observed attachment behaviors—particularly those which may be precursors to, or symptoms of, depression—is explainable, in part, by the stability of specific maternal characteristics. Not surprisingly, given the high incidence of depression among offspring of depressed parents (Cytryn et al., 1982; Kashani, Burk, & Reid, 1985), many of these maternal attributes are strikingly depressive. In the foregoing discussion of Egeland and Farber's (1984) study, maternal aggression and suspiciousness was noticeably more common in the dyads where the infant changed from secure to avoidant attachment. In comparison with those mothers whose infants remained securely attached, these mothers scored lower on scales of social desirability. Infants who changed from avoidant attachment to secure attachment, by contrast, had mothers who responded to them, spoke to them, looked at them more, and were more effective in responding to their crying than were mothers of infants who remained avoidant at both assessments. Egeland and Farber sought to examine the impact of a range of maternal characteristics considered to place infants at high risk for infant maladaptation. Mothers in the study ranged in age from 12 to 37; 62 percent were single. Well over three quarters (86%) of the pregnancies were unplanned. Forty percent of the mothers had not graduated from college by the time their children were born.

In addition to the maternal contributors mentioned above, mother-infant separation was presumed to account for changes from B to A (N = 3) as well as for stability in 7 resistant (C) infants. Separation in both groups of infants took place anywhere from 0 to 18 months.

Maternal-depressive illness also tends to promote avoidant and withdrawing behavior in offspring, particularly between the ages of 12 and 18 months, as revealed by a longitudinal study performed by Gaensbauer et al. (1984). During the first observation the probands (N = 7) and the control group (N = 7) had the same breakdown of attachment groups: five were classified as securely attached and two as avoidant in each group. When they were reevaluated at 18 months, six of the probands were classified as avoidant and only one was classified as securely attached. In the control group, four were classified as securely attached, two as avoidant, and one as insecurely attached.

The effects of maternal depression on attachment behavior have also been studied by Radke-Yarrow et al. (1985), who found that maternal bipolar disorder, in particular, correlated with infant insecure attachment. These researchers observed children who ranged in age from 16 to 44 months. Fourteen children of 99 in the total sample were offspring of mothers with bipolar depressive disorder, while 42 children in the sample had mothers with major unipolar depression, and 12 had mothers with minor depression. Thirty-one children had mothers with no history of affective illness. The investigators assessed infant attachment behavior and also directly observed maternal affective states, including "cheerful–happy," "tender–loving," "tense–anxious," "irritable–angry," "sad–tearful," "neutral–positive," and "neutral–negative."

Insecure attachment was relatively frequent in families with major affective disorders, as compared with families with no such history of psychopathology. Notably, more than three quarters (79%) of the bipolar offsprings were classified as insecurely attached. Almost half (48%) of the children of unipolar depressives appeared insecurely attached. In contrast, the normal group and the minor depression group had 25 percent and 30 percent respectively of infants who were insecurely attached.

Radke-Yarrow et al. (1985) noted significantly greater incidence of depression among the mothers of those infants who fell into the fourth category of attachment behavior, which they designated A/C. These infants (N = 20) showed moderate to high avoidance and moderate to high resistance during reunion episodes. The authors noted that the maternal emotional expression displayed in interactions with their infants, undoubtedly a function of overall emotional state, also predicted patterns of attachment. That is, the mothers of insecurely attached infants expressed more negative and fewer positive emotions.

Attachment studies conducted in other countries demonstrate the influence of different mothering styles on attachment status. However, measures of attachment are likely to be equally sensitive to cultural norms and to maternal behavior. Miyake, Chen, and Campos (1985) found a much higher incidence of C babies, and no A babies at all in a sample of Japanese infants who were given the Strange Situation Test. A similar test sample taken by Grossmann, Huker, and Warner (1981) in Germany found a much higher incidence of A babies than American norms. Noting that Japanese infants are rarely separated from the mother during the first year, Miyake, Chen, and Campos felt it likely that these babies might find the separations of the Strange Situation paradigm more stressful than American babies.

This does not imply that these babies are necessarily less securely attached, nor that they are more temperamentally prone to distress. However, the finding does imply that attachment measuring devices are likely to be affected by cultural norms as well as by maternal behavior.

Correlations of maternal attributes with infant temperamental characteristics have also been identified. Wolkind and De Salis (1982) identified maternal factors that predicted certain temperamental clusters as early as 4 months and also predicted behavioral difficulties at 42 months. The researchers' measurement scales, which were based on the conceptualizations of the NYLS, focused on the temperament dimensions of mood and regularity. Three groups of children were identified: those with good mood/regular ($N = 24$), those with negative mood/irregular ($N = 24$), and the majority of the infants ($N = 54$), who fell in between these two clusters. Comparison of the maternal psychiatric histories before and after birth showed prepregnancy psychiatric difficulties, mostly depression, in 25 percent of the mothers of the negative mood/irregular group. No such histories were present in the mothers of children in the good mood/regular group during this stage in the study. At the fourth month after birth, 37 percent ($N = 9$) of the mothers of the negative mood/irregular group had psychiatric disorders (mostly depression) in contrast to 29 percent ($N = 7$) of the mothers of the good mood/regular children. When temperament groups were correlated with maternal psychiatric histories at 14 months, it was found that the mothers of negative mood/irregular babies were more likely to develop a disorder during the 10 months following the initial temperament assessments. In the same study, children who at 42 months scored highest (high score indicating greater behavioral difficulty) on the Behavioral Screening Questionnaire (BSQ; Richman & Graham, 1971) demonstrated negative mood/irregular temperament. Maternal depression was also evident.

Maziade et al. (1984) have found clear correlations between temperamentally difficult children at age 7 years and other psychopathologic diagnoses at 12 (e.g., oppositional disorder and deficit disorders). This association was mainly found in "dysfunctional" families where there is a low degree of consensus in terms of parental control (see Tables 4 and 5).

Environmental Predictors

In previous studies we have identified examples of both infant and maternal factors that predict individual differences and psychopathology. In recent years, there has been an increasing recognition that certain environmental factors may also play a crucial role in contributing to the stability of behavioral characteristics of infants and children (Trad, 1986).

Social support may play an important role, especially with infants of particular temperaments. Crockenberg (1981) correlated mothers' per-

Table 4. *A/C Classification Versus Depressive Symptomatology*

	Main and Weston—(1981)	Main, Kaplan and Cassidy—(1985)	Crittendon—(1985a)	Radke-Yarrow, Cummings, Kuczynski, and Chapman—(1985)
Nomenclature	Unclassifiable	Insecure-Disorganized/ Disoriented	A/C Classification	A/C Classification
Affective Sphere	Affectless Dazed behavior: Odd or atypical body posture or movement suggestive of depression	Undirected affective expressions Apprehension		Affectless Sad, with signs of depression
Social Sphere	Proximity seeking in stressful situations and in repeated separations in otherwise "avoidant" infant Low relatedness in play session Strong conflict in play session	Strong avoidance following Strong proximity seeking Characterized behavior as an attempt to control the parent either through directly punitive behavior or through anxious 'caregiving' behavior (i.e., inappropriate role reversal.)	Avoidant High resistance Suggested ambivalence was a manifestation of anxiety, and these 'A/C' infants were most anxious	Avoidant
Physical Sphere		Incomplete movements	Disturbed behaviors (e.g., head cocking, huddling, rocking, etc.)	Odd or atypical postures
Cognitive Sphere		Confusion		

Table 5.

DSM-III Criteria	Main and Weston (1981)	Main, Kaplan, and Cassidy (1985)	Crittendon (1985)	Radke-Yarrow (1985)
Major depressive disorder		Insecure-disorganized/ disoriented		
Dysphoric mood	Unclassifiable		A/C classification	A/C classification
	Affectless	Dazed behavior: Odd or atypical body posture or movement suggestive of depression, confusion, or apprehension	Avoidance	Affectless Sad, with signs of depression
Eating disturbances				Avoidant
Sleep disturbances				
Psychomotor activity		Incomplete movements	Disturbed behavior, head-cocking, huddling, rocking, etc.	Odd or atypical body posture or movement
Loss of interest				
Loss of energy				
Attentional disturbances		Undirected affective expressions		
II. Dysthymic disorder				
Social withdrawal	Low relatedness in play session	Strong avoidance following Strong proximity seeking	Avoidant Resistant	Avoidant
Irritability/anger	Strong conflict in play session			
Loss of pleasure	Affectless			
Less active/talkative				
Tearfulness/crying				
III. Additional symptoms	Proximity seeking in high stress situations and in repeated separations in an otherwise "avoidant" infant	Characterized behavior as an attempt to control the parent, either through directly punitive behavior or through anxious 'caregiving' behavior (i.e. inappropriate role reversal). p. 85	Suggested ambivalence/ avoidance was a manifestation of anxiety, and these 'A/C' infants were the most anxious.	

156

ceived levels of social support with neonatal temperament measures (Brazelton's Neonatal Behavioral Assessment Examination; Brazelton, 1973) and Strange Situation classifications for 48 infants. She found that low social support was associated with insecure attachment, but only in those infants who showed high irritability on the temperament assessments. When social support is low, maternal unresponsiveness can lead to insecure attachment, according to this study. Thus an irritable infant raised by a mother who experiences low social support is prone to develop insecure attachment. However, the findings are ambiguous due to the subjective nature of the measure of social support. It may be that the mother's unresponsiveness and her perception of her support may be functions of another personality variable, and unrelated to objective measures of social support. Nevertheless, the study shows clear evidence of maternal contributors to insecure attachment.

According to a study by Egeland and Farber (1984), stressful living arrangements were a contributing factor in infants who changed attachment classifications from secure (*B*) to resistant (*C*). Seventy percent of these infants were children of single parents. Stressful living arrangements were also a factor when comparing infants who remained avoidant (*A*) at 12 and 18 months with those who changed from avoidant to secure attachment. These authors concluded, in a manner similar to Crockenberg, that a developmentally delayed infant from a low socioeconomic background tended to be at greater risk for forming anxious-resistant attachment.

Factors such as past social experiences also contributed to sociability in infants (Thompson & Lamb, 1983). Lack of social experience might then contribute to lack of sociability. Thompson and Lamb also observed that those infants who had experienced changes in family circumstances, especially those that involved changes in parental employment status, showed lower sociability scores at 19.5 months than those who experienced no remarkable changes in family circumstances.

Another example of the type of effect that the environment may impose on both caregiver and infant is provided by the study done with the offspring of families with major maternal depression by Radke-Yarrow et al. (1985). Anxious attachment characterized seven out of eight of the subjects where no paternal figure was present. That is, infants of affectively ill mothers who were without a husband in the household were noted to be at a higher risk for developing insecure mother-infant attachment (see Table 6).

Summary

Thus far it has been established that stability can be demonstrated from both the temperament and attachment constructs. Further, it has been shown that the stability of negative mood can predict stability of difficult temperament.

Table 6.   Attachment Classification Compared to Temperament Typologies

Ainsworth, Bleher, Waters, and Wall (1978)	Thomas, Chess, Birch, Hertzig, and Korn (1963)
Class A: Avoidant	Slow to warm up
Low proximity & contact seeking	Low activity level
Low contact maintaining	Low approach withdrawal
Low resistance	Low adaptability
High avoidance	Low intensity
Low distress/low search	Mild mood
Low distance interaction	
Class B: Securely attached	Easy
High proximity & contact seeking	High approach/withdrawal
High contact maintaining	High rhythmicity
Low resistance	High adaptability
Low avoidance	Low or mild intensity
Low distress/high search	Mild or positive mood
High distance interaction	
Class C: Resistant	Difficult
Mild to high proximity & contact seeking	Low approach/high withdrawal
Mild to high contact maintaining	Low rhythmicity
High resistance/anger	Low adaptability
Low avoidance	High intensity
High distress/low search	Negative mood

In contrast to temperament characteristics, attachment classifications seem to show far greater stability than any discrete attachment behaviors. This is consistent with attachment theory (Bowlby, 1969; Sroufe, 1983) which suggests that the expression of attachment will be labile, and constantly reregulate to fit the changing configurations of the infant-caregiver relationship. In addition, it has also been demonstrated that expressions of both temperament and attachment characteristics are affected by the environment.

CHAPTER FIVE

Social Support as a Risk Factor for Infant and Childhood Depression

The link between mental health and family relations is well accepted, perhaps even self-evident (Bengston & Treas, 1980). In recent years researchers have become increasingly interested in how broader social support systems may be linked to both psychological and physical well-being. At the same time, they have also turned their attention to how certain social, political, and economic trends—in particular, those that lead to social fragmentation and isolation—may affect mental health.

The investigations of social psychiatrists have shed some light not only on how social conditions can illuminate the origins of diseases, but also on how the origins of certain diseases can elucidate social conditions. Durkheim's classic study of suicide in 1897 demonstrated that suicide rates reflect the nature of social integration. Many social scientists consider this work to be the first in modern sociological epidemiology and, as such, one of the theoretical landmarks that shapes the current understanding of social support and related concepts.

Other classic studies that build on Durkheim's seminal work include Faris and Dunham's 1939 study of the ecology of mental disorders in urban areas, Hans Selye's physiological study linking environmental stressors to disease (1956), Hollingshead and Redlich's study of social class and mental health in New Haven (1958), and numerous other studies over the past decade and a half involving life-event scales (e.g., Holmes & Masuda, 1974; Holmes & Rahe, 1967), which conclusively connect life-events and stressors to a wide variety of physical and psychiatric disorders (Myers, Lindenthal, & Pepper, 1971, 1975; Myers & Pepper, 1972). Life-events have also been shown to correlate positively with depression (Paykel, 1974; Paykel, Prusoff, & Tanner, 1976) and suicide attempts (Paykel, 1974).

Studies examining the role of social support in health maintenance and disease etiology indicate that individuals with stronger psychological and material resources enjoy better health than those with fewer supportive social contacts and less access to material support systems (Caplan, 1974; Dean & Lin, 1977; Lin, Dean, & Ensel, 1986; Mitchell, Billings, & Moos, 1982). In a 1985 study examining the ways in which social support buffers life stresses, Cohen and Wills (1985) reported that numerous studies conclusively link social support to psychological and physical health outcomes. Several prospective epidemiological studies relate social support to mortality (Berkman & Syme, 1979; Blazer, 1982; House, Robbins, & Metzner, 1982) as well as to mental health (Henderson, Byrne, & Duncan-Jones, 1981; Lin, Dean, & Ensel, 1986; Williams, Ware, & Donald, 1981). Other research has associated the lack of close social bonds and poor interpersonal relationships with both adult and child psychiatric disorder, especially depression (Henderson, 1981; Paykel, Emms, Fletcher, & Rassagy, 1980; Puig-Antich, Lukens, Davies, Goetz, Quatrocle, & Toback, 1985).

As we shall see in the chapters on specific populations at risk for depression (e.g., the abused/neglected, the handicapped, the offspring of the affectively ill), one factor that looms especially large as a risk factor for infant or childhood depression is psychopathology or symptomatology in a parent. Varying degrees of parental disorder can lead to parental deprivation, the impact of which has been implicated in many different models of childhood depression (Trad, 1986).

Parental psychopathology, like child psychopathology, has multiple roots. Moreover, to the extent that the causes of parental disorder are nonbiological—that is, psychological—they are undoubtedly the product of social influences as well as personality characteristics. The maternally depriving conditions that ultimately can lead to infant and childhood depression are mediated by conditions and structures within the macrosociety. This chapter analyzes some of the major social, economic, and political conditions fostering parental disorder and deprivation, and ultimately increasing the risk for infant and childhood depression. It is not the contention of this chapter that these macrolevel trends alone explain how parents come to deprive their children of adequate parenting and thus increase their risk for depression. However, the social, economic, and political pressures confronting parents do interact with personality characteristics and family dynamics to create stresses with which parents are differentially equipped to cope. As this chapter demonstrates, one critical determinant of parents' success in meeting these demands is their access to various types of social support.

Social support can be viewed as an instrument created by society to interface between the family and society, the parent and society, and the parent and the child. It is "the perceived or actual instrumental and/or expressive provisions supplied by the community, social networks, and confiding partners" (Lin, 1986a, p.18). By definition, social support mediates disruptive and stressful macrosocietal conditions from which psychopathologic and affective disorders may emerge. Dynamically, social support depicts a moment by moment representation of the historical transitions taking place within American families. It reflects the social trends in American society and thus has direct implications for child-rearing practices. Furthermore, it responds to, and also functions as a gauge of, the tension between the family and society, parents and children, and society and children. As the push and pull of each tension unmasks a new need, new social–support systems and programs are often implemented to meet that need. In this manner, social support, and the systems that emanate from it, can buffer life stresses both directly and indirectly. They can buffer stressful conditions *directly* to the parent and/or child and *indirectly* to the child via the parent or the parent via the child.

The developmental framework, which is essential for understanding many facets of depression (its origins, expressions, clinical course, and prognosis), is equally valuable for understanding how social support may affect an individual's risk for depression. Not only can parents define and reflect their interactions with social support systems, but children, also, can report and reflect their own interaction with social support. The way in which children perceive this interaction will be influenced by their sex, age, the family context within which they operate, and the type of stress they experience (Bryant, 1985). Thus the developmental approach allows researchers to assess social support from the child's perspective and to predict long-term socio-emotional functioning (Bryant, 1985).

This theoretical possibility notwithstanding, most research still analyzes social support primarily from the perspective of adults under high-stress conditions. If, however, sources of support are understood to derive from the self as well as from others, and to involve experiences and occasions for both autonomy and relatedness, then researchers need to assess who or what provides "casual and intimate social exchanges in children's lives" (Bryant, 1985, p.3) and how these, in turn, predict social-emotional functioning. From a developmental standpoint, it is important to explore social support from both adult and child perspectives and in low-stress as well as high–stress conditions. This means allowing children opportunities to speak directly for themselves rather than relying solely on adults (parents, teachers, social workers, etc.) to assess their personal and social experiences (Achenback & Edelbrock, 1978, 1981; Brim, White, & Zill, 1979; Bryant, 1985; Kogan, Smith, & Jenkins, 1977; Zill, 1977).

Description of Social Trends

The period following World War II has witnessed sweeping changes in both macrolevel phenomena such as international political and economic organization and microlevel phenomena such as the structure of family life. It is virtually impossible to remain remote from the repercussions of such developments as escalating international terrorism, the nuclear arms race, changes in the nature and structure of the workplace, and the disintegration of traditional family life. The erosion of social values through crime and the new emphasis on personal fulfillment over social responsibility has undermined trust and diminished cooperation between individuals and groups. All of these trends converge to isolate families and individuals. Isolation, in turn, can lead to psychiatric and physical disorders, particularly depression.

One trend that is especially significant in relation to the child-rearing climate, and ultimately to the risk for infant and childhood depression, is the spiraling divorce rate documented in the United States since 1962. This phenomenon particularly warrants study because single-parent households are increasing and are expected to do so into the next two decades. In 1978, 18.1 out of every 1000 children under 18 were involved in a divorce.

This statistic is more than double the rate in 1965 and close to three times the rate in 1955. In the 12-month period from June 1979 to June 1980, 5.4 out of every 1,000, or 1,184,000, marriages ended in divorce. Currently, the average length of a marriage before divorce is 6.6 years, an indication that many of the children involved in these divorces are very young "and particularly vulnerable to the disruptive effect of divorce on family cohesion" (Jellinek & Slovik, 1981).

Most research on the impact of divorce on family life has focused on how it influences children and women/mothers (Jellinek & Slovik,1983; Kelly & Wallerstein, 1976; Kurdek, Blisk, & Siesky, 1981; Wallerstein, 1984; Weintraub & Wolf, 1983). More recently, however, researchers have begun examining how divorce exerts an effect on all family members, including fathers (DeFrain & Eirick, 1981; Fine, Moreland, & Schwebel, 1983; Jacobs, 1982).

Indeed, numerous studies correlate divorce to depressive symptomatology (Paykel, 1974; Wortman, 1981) for both women and men. The increased prevalence of parental disorder is especially significant given the well-established connection between depression in a parent and depression in the child (see Chapter 6 for a detailed discussion of this relationship). Such investigations have revealed that divorced men are even more vulnerable to psychiatric disorders than are divorced women. Men from broken marriages are nine times more likely to be admitted to a psychiatric hospital than those from intact homes, while divorced women experience a threefold increase in admissions (Jacobs, 1982). Men, however, are less likely to be disturbed in their primary roles and socioeconomic status. After a divorce, the average income for fathers is reduced by 10 percent, whereas the average mother suffers a 50 percent reduction in income (Jellinek & Slovik, 1981). This reduction occurs for many reasons, two primary ones being that women do not command the same earning levels as men and that less than one half of all divorced or separated women receive any type of alimony or support (Duncan, Coe, Corcoran, Hill, Hoffman, & Morgan, 1986). Most recently, the Albany Area Health Survey conducted by Lin, Dean, & Ensel (1986) confirmed previous findings concerning marital-status differences in depression. The researchers found that married people are significantly less depressed than never married or formerly married persons.

Any marital disruption has a substantial effect on depressive symptoms because it constitutes an adverse life event and also causes the disintegration of the previous network of intimate and confiding ties. This double jeopardy endemic to marital disruption causes more prolonged and pronounced depressive symptomatology in women (Lin, Dean, & Ensel, 1986). Indeed, parenting patterns in single-parent families may closely resemble Zussman's (1980) description of "minimal parenting." The researcher, as well as MacKinnon, Brody, and Stoneman (1982), found that parents forced to perform tasks that competed with child care for their attention (in this case, work outside the home and, at the same time, the role of the only authority figure within the home) were slower to respond to their children, showed fewer positive responses, and interacted with them for much shorter periods of time.

The investigations of MacKinnon et al. (1982), revealed the strain of parenting without a spouse. They conducted studies comparing the home environments of children whose mothers fell into one of three groups: married/working, married/nonworking, and divorced/working. The researchers administered the HOME (Home Observation for Measurement of the Environment; Bradley & Caldwell, 1979), in order to assess the amount of cognitive and social stimulation in single-parent versus intact households. Children in the study were 3 to 6 years of age. Half were male and half were female. All were middle-class Caucasians. The median income for the married families (with both working and nonworking mothers) exceeded $25,000, while the median income for divorced/working mothers was $10,000 to $15,000.

Overall, the researchers discovered that the home environments of children from divorced/working homes were substantially less stimulating cognitively and socially than those of married homes. Both the quantity and quality of stimulation for social and cognitive growth differed. Even when family income was controlled through a covariance analysis these differences in level of stimulation remained. That is, regardless of family income, the divorced households had much less of the stimulation related to intellectual growth and academic performance than did intact households. From this observation, the researchers hypothesized that income per se does not cause the behavior of the parents. Instead, the stresses and lack of social support that generally accompany low income probably produce the notable modification in parental behavior. As MacKinnon stated, "Unfortunately, mother-headed divorced families have to contend with the reality that they live at or near subsistence levels" (p. 1397).

The stresses arising from the multiple conflicting demands placed on a parent in a single-parent household are not, however, necessarily unique to homes in which divorce has occurred. Cleary and Mechanic (1982) found that even among married women, the stresses associated with working and being responsible for children simultaneously were primary factors in increased levels of depression. Warr (1982) and Parry (1982) found that role pressure, stemming from conflicting demands, is related to depression in employed mothers. It is not surprising, then, that another important variable to be considered concerns how the child responds to the mother's working life. As Lerner and Galambos (1986) emphasize, it is important to view the mother-infant interaction as a bidirectional relationship in which the mother affects the child's adjustment equally as much as the child's attitudes influence maternal perceptions.

It is important, however, not to be overly simplistic in correlating the phenomenon of marital status with maternal depression, poor mother-child interaction, or impaired infant development. One must look at the mediating variables—for example, how supportive the father is of his working wife, how career-oriented and ambitious the mother is, how much satisfaction the woman derives from her work, how much strain she is under because of her need to juggle many roles, whether her philosophy of childrearing is consistent with the amount of time she has available to spend with her child, and how much contextual support in the form of child care and household help the mother receives (Lerner & Galambos, 1986).

Divorce may lead to less than optimal parenting not only by diverting parents' emotional attention, but also by causing economic strain in the family. The mother who is subject to stress because of poverty can have difficulty viewing her infant as a high priority. Lichtenberg (1971) states that economically deprived parents "engage in social relations in all areas of their lives" that can be characterized as "authoritarian, punitive, inconsistent, arbitrary, frustrating, and infused with a minimum of playfulness and pleasure" (p. 1432). It is not surprising, therefore, that the child's individuality is not valued, and is not responded to in such a way as to foster the child's initiative, self-esteem, and sense of productive responsibility. Thus the children of the extremely poor are likely to "lack self-control based upon security in one's own autonomy, and lack the means for cooperating with others, including trust and hope" (p. 1432). These conditions, without proper intervention, make social class a factor in the etiology of depressive symptoms.

Poverty and social class may be a significant factor in determining depressive symptoms. Evidence for this was found in a study by Parmelee, Beckwith, Cohen, and Sigman (1983), who compared the mother-infant attachment and bonding between 35 preterm infants and 35 full-term infants from similar family backgrounds and showed—unlike the Albany Area Health Survey, where no clear-cut linear relationship was established between social class and depression—that social class did relate significantly to depressive symptoms. As in the Albany Area Health Survey, Parmelee et al. found that mothers who received strong social support in both emotional and financial terms from their husbands, friends, and family and also had a history of adequate mothering, recovered from the stressful life event of divorce better and with less depressive symptomatology than those who did not receive strong social support. As a result, a healthy mother-infant dyad was formed. In addition, they found that nursery personnel can provide emotional and social support which increases the chances of favorable mother-infant interaction. However, the researchers also found that when economic factors associated with low socioeconomic status contributed to the infant becoming a low priority in the family, medical intervention and social support typically failed to mitigate depressive symptoms. These findings coincide with Beckwith's (1979) study, which revealed that by the time the infant was 8 months old, economically deprived mothers were less able to maintain a pleasurable, responsive relationship with their offspring than were middle-class mothers.

Not only is poverty implicated in the development of depressive illness in families, but it has also been found to be a significant barometer of the probability of chronicity of depression. Keller, Lavori, Rice, Coryell, and Hirschfeld (1986) found a 22 percent probability of chronicity, with a long prior episode, older age at relapse, and low family income as key predictors of a lengthy depressive episode.

The impact of poverty on family health must be considered in light of the fact that women and children today comprise a disproportionate number of our nation's poor. Although children are 27 percent of the population, they make up 40 percent of those living in poverty (Moynihan, 1986). The "feminization of poverty" has seen the proportion of the poor who are members of female-headed and single-person households rise from 30 to 60 percent between 1959 and 1979 (Bane, 1986). In 1970, 13 percent of all families were single-parent families; today, 26 percent are, and of these, 89 percent of the single parents are women (Moynihan, 1986).

Families need not be shattered by divorce and pressed by poverty for major social change to lay the seeds for depression. Indeed, families may remain intact, but still have deviant interactional styles, such as those often found among the families of alcoholics. Rising levels of alcoholism, another major social trend, should alert clinicians to the presence of subtle family interactional patterns that can proven as damaging to all family members as the marital breakdowns that alcohol often occasions. (For a discussion of the epidemiology of alcoholism, see "Parental Psychopathology as a Risk Factor for Infant and Childhood Depression," Chapter 6.) Although Adler and Raphael (1983) reported that 40 percent of judicial separations in Australia were the result of alcohol problems, Steinglass (1981) has observed that families with alcoholics often remain structurally intact but develop different interactional patterns. These patterns affect selected aspects of family interactions, particularly what Steinglass refers to as "distance regulation," and not all behavior across the board. Steinglass has observed that families with alcoholics adopt rigid interactional patterns and are especially inflexible in their use of shared and independent space.

Researchers disagree about the factors contributing to the disruptive trends in family structure and economic status. Some see these trends as a consequence of the frequent dissolution of family structures per se. Others, such as Bane (1986), maintain that the feminization of poverty, especially among blacks, is actually the result of the "reshuffling" of existing poverty, while among whites, the "split" from high-income to low-income status does play a major role in 80 percent of such cases.

Social support for families of the poor has not kept pace with the original goals of the War on Poverty. When this assault on chronically low socioeconomic status began in the 1960s, 19 percent of the population was poor. After a decline to 11.5 percent in the 1970s, the percentage of poor in the population figures rose to 15.2 percent in 1983. Government programs—notably Medicaid—have displayed a strong institutional bias, with hospitals and nursing homes receiving far more money than ambulatory and community services (Starr, 1986). Such programs have, in some ways, isolated the poor from the mainstream of medicine and linked medical services to means tests that are far below the poverty line, rendering only 60 percent of the poor actually eligible for service (Starr, 1986). Community health centers and other service programs, with their emphasis on primary and preventive care and community participation (once the "key initiatives" of the War on Poverty) have not achieved the numbers of patients originally anticipated, and today their future is fiscally "tenuous," despite the fact that a series of studies show that community health centers have had a significant impact on the health of their communities (Davis & Schoen, 1978).

Thus the proliferation of single-parent families and the economic circumstances in which they are enmired, along with prevailing attitudes about funding for social programs, create unusual environmental stresses for child-rearing. Isolation, lack of self-determination, helplessness, and reduced expectation may cumulatively interact to create depressive disorders in such families (Trad, 1986).

DEFINITIONS OF SOCIAL SUPPORT

Lin (1986) broadly defines social support as "forces or factors in the social environment that facilitate the survival of human beings" (p.17). This definition encompasses all aspects of social relations and interaction. We require a narrower, more focused definition that deals specifically with the aspects of social relations and interaction relevant to mental health. Lin proposes two such definitions. The first represents an inductive synthesis of the numerous definitions given by researchers over the past ten years, and the second is a deductive definition resulting from the theoretical perspective of social resources.

The synthetic definition of social support deals with the way the community, social networks, and confiding partners provide both perceived and actual support to individuals and families. With this definition, Lin identifies three layers of social relations that offer the individual sources of support: the community, social network, and confiding partner(s). The community represents the most general type of social relationship the individual has and offers him or her a sense of *belonging* in the larger social structure. The social network is comprised of substantively specific relations, erected through kinship, shared working environment, and friendships. This network provides the individual with a sense of *bonding*. The third and innermost layer, "confiding partners," consists of relationships that tend to be *binding* "in the sense that reciprocal and mutual exchanges are expected, and responsibility for one another's well-being is understood and shared by the partners" (Lin, 1986).

In this definition, both the perceived and actual support—what Caplan (1979) refers to as the objective and subjective dimensions of support—are highly significant to the individual. The objective aspects of this definition of social support are independently observable and verifiable, in that they do not require verification from the individual receiving the support. Conversely, subjective aspects are dependent on the individual's personal evaluation and understanding of support, and, as such, reflect the subject's own perception of reality. Subjective aspects may or may not be objectively verifiable.

The second definition of social support that Lin proposes draws on the theory of social resources, maintaining that "mental health reflects expressive needs that can best be met by access to and use of ties that are close and homophilous [similar] to ego" (p.30). In this sense, social support is defined *operationally* as access to and use of strong, homophilous ties.

Caplan (1974) perceives social support as attachments among individuals or between individuals and a group that serve three purposes: to further emotional mastery, to provide guidance, and to offer feedback about one's identity and performance. Cobb (1976) focuses on three other constructs in defining social support: emotional support (being cared for and loved), esteem support (being valued and esteemed), and network support (belonging to a network of mutual obligation). Dolgoff and Feldstein (1984) define social support as "those non-profit functions of society, public or voluntary, that are clearly aimed at alleviating distress and poverty or at ameliorating the condition of the casualties of society" (p. 93). They add that social welfare is, in fact, "the collective supply of resources, a sharing of the burden or the risk" (p.341).

SOCIAL SUPPORT AND STRESS

Social support serves many functions with the potential to reach into many areas of an individual's life. Various kinds of formal and informal social support have proven effective in ameliorating the many stresses of ordinary life-events (e.g., the demands of parenting and earning a living), adverse life-events (e.g., death of a loved one, or loss of a job), as well as the more structural changes in social organization. Many researchers stress the importance of social attachment and social bonds for the development of a well-adjusted and regulated psyche (Bowlby, 1969, 1973; Weiss, 1973, 1974), while others focus on intimacy as a major dimension fostering the psychological stability of support (Brown, Bhrolchain, & Harris, 1975;

Brown & Harris, 1978). In their analysis of the social sources of depression, Brown et al. (1975) singled out the presence of an intimate, confiding relationship with a husband or boyfriend as the strongest mediator between adverse events and psychiatric disturbance in women. Lin, Dean, and Ensel (1986) assign a preeminent role to such relationships. Opposite-sex confidants, they found, were more effective than same-sex confidants in protecting against the development of depressive symptoms. They comment that, to a large extent, this "reflects the intimate and confiding nature of the relationship between marital partners" (p. 334).

Weinraub and Wolf (1983) reinforce these findings in their study of the differences between single and married mothers. They report a "significant difference" in the lives of single mothers, who experience greater stress from a greater number of lifestyle changes and longer work hours, and who, at the same time, receive "substantially" less social support, particularly in their roles as parents. Consistent with this theme, Cassel (1974) asserts that the primary group, that is, the group that the individual considers to be most critical to daily life, provides the strongest social support. Cotterell (1986) views the mother's social support network as "a buffer against the stressful intrusions of the workplace into the family" (p. 362). This researcher studied 96 Australian working-class families in terms of how social support, such as companionship, encouragement, and useful advice influenced the quality of childrearing. The investigation revealed that the availability of social support was a powerful factor in improving the quality of the childrearing. As he states, "The prominence of the relation between support and effective parenting was widespread: mothers with higher levels of support in both absentee-father households and in homes where fathers worked normal hours displayed parenting behavior closer to the optimal levels specified by experts in child development" (p. 371).

Given these general findings with respect to the role of social support in parental adjustment, it is not surprising that the degree of social support for the parent has been linked directly with successful parent-child interactions. Crockenberg (1981) investigated how the mother's social support network influenced the security of attachment in infants and revealed that the availability of social support was a strong predictor of secure child attachment and that social support was particularly important for mothers whose babies were irritable. Each of these perspectives on social support thus converges at a single point: the presence of a strong, well-functioning social support system promotes, protects, and solidifies mental health.

Conversely, the absence of a viable, fortified support system has an adverse effect on mental health. Lack of social support has been implicated in a number of major social trends, not the least of which is child maltreatment. Although Fontana (1985) believes the primary causes of maltreatment to be economic and social pressures, a lack of social support appears to reinforce the stress. According to Fontana, social and economic factors produce "a complex, confused, insecure parent without human support [who] is at the mercy of the surrounding social environment and intrafamilial pressures" (1985, p. 6). Concomitant with this lack of social support, research reveals, is often maternal strain and depression which, in turn, may cascade into maternal deprivation and, subsequently, infant and childhood depression.

To test the relationship between social support and psychiatric disorders, Lin, Dean, and Ensel (1986) designed the Albany Area Health Survey. Specifically, the survey measured the correlation between depression, stressful life-events, psychological resources (self-esteem and personal competence), and social support. The project began in the fall of 1977 and was carried out in a tricounty area of upstate New York, approximately 150 miles from New York City. Albany County was the largest of the three counties, with a 1980 population of approximately 286,000. The proportion of males to females in the study was 48 to 52, with an overall median age of 32. Fifty-five percent of the population studied was married, 30 percent were single, slightly less that 5 percent were divorced, and 2.5 percent were separated. The median household income was approximately $16,000, with 61 percent of the population in the work force.

The researchers employed a panel design as their survey method, interviewing the sample group of respondents repeatedly over time. The first interview occurred during the spring of 1979 and the second during the spring of 1980. (A third interview has also taken place and the results are currently being evaluated.) Lin, Dean, and Ensel (1986) discovered that social support—particularly an intimate, confiding relationship—significantly mediates the effect of undesirable life-events. At the same time, they found that psychological resources did not mediate the effects of undesirable life-events. According to this line of thought, certain personality features play a secondary role to the availability of social support in predisposing individuals to depressive episodes.

Why certain individuals should enjoy greater support than others is obviously a complex and controversial matter. Access to social support is clearly a function of social structure and an individual's disposition to seek such support. Exactly what personality type seeks and benefits from social support is still not clear. On the one hand, Richman and Flaherty (1985) found that the personality characteristic entailing a high level of interpersonal dependency appeared to motivate the search for and satisfaction with external supports, rather than inhibiting the successful development of these relationships (p. 594). Thus dependency has a certain self-corrective function which prevents it from leading to isolation and introversion, and ultimately to depression. Because of the overriding importance of interpersonal dependency needs, they found that personality characteristics were stronger predictors of depressive symptomatology than were social supports.

Hirschfeld, Klerman, Clayton, and Keller (1983), on the other hand, found that interpersonal dependency did not promote social engagement but rather led to depression, because it inhibited the individual from seeking out others and thus functioned as a form of introversion. They found introversion to be one of the most powerful personality characteristics associated with primary nonbipolar depression. In 31 females with primary nonbipolar major depressive disorder, personality scale scores, based on standard self-report inventories taken when symptom-free, showed introversion, submissiveness and passivity, and increased interpersonal dependency, but normal emotional strength. The same results were obtained from never-ill relatives who had scores reflecting extraordinary emotional strength.

Parents' understanding of the role of relationships may be another important factor in determining the nature and extent of their social support. Evidence of this comes from studies of maltreating families who experience isolation and ineffective use of resources in addition to high stress. These studies provide an opportunity to investigate hypotheses concerning the effect of social support on parents, and its relation to the quality of their child-rearing methods and to aspects of their children's development (Crittenden, 1985a). Crittenden reported that maltreating families appeared to be "a source of drain, discouraging others from forming long-term relationships with them, and remaining isolated from such relationships" (p. 1310) and that the "mothers' approach to relationships of all kinds was reflected both in their relationships with their children and in their relationship with network members" (p. 1311). Abusing mothers maintain internal models that lead them to nonreciprocal interactions aimed at coercing others to meet their own needs. Models of neglecting mothers also incorporate the idea of scarcity, but it is combined with a sense of helplessness and despair. It is important, therefore, to recognize that the contributions of a whole "nexus of relationships" to the development of children results largely from a single process. Maltreatment thus serves as an appropriate paradigm for evaluating the efficacy of social support systems; relationships between mother-network, mother-professional, and child-mother relationships can be observed.

Thus far we have reviewed research on the role of social support for adults. Recently researchers have begun to explore social support from the perspective of children, rather than from the way adults believe children to perceive social support. Zill (1977) discovered that 60 percent of the parents he interviewed concerning the general environment in which their children lived (e.g., family life, friends, schools, health, and community activities) rate their surroundings as "very good" or "excellent" while only 30 percent of the children he interviewed agreed with this assessment. Zill's study highlights the fact that the way children and parents perceive of social support may vary greatly.

Bryant (1985) built on the work of Zill (1977) and other researchers in an effort to determine how children perceive social support and how this perception predicts social-emotional functioning. Bryant approached the study from a developmental perspective, arguing that it is impossible for children "to be open, free and caring within oneself and within the family while remaining emotionally insulated from the wider world outside" (p. 6). According to this view, social supports are crucial to healthy psychological functioning and their importance increases proportionately with the amount of stress being experienced by the individual (Conger & Farrell, 1981; Garbarino & Gilliam, 1980). She further argued that "stress in conjunction with appropriate support is critical to enhancing social-emotional development" (p. 6). Bryant predicted that age, sex, and family context would factor into the child's perception of social support.

Bryant (1985) employed a variety of affective and social development measures to document information about the sources of social support in children's lives and their relation to child development. Equal numbers of 7- and 10-year-old children from 168 families residing in nonmetropolitan, rural northern California participated in the study. Equal numbers of large and small families, and male and female children, as well as equal numbers of older brothers and sisters were tested. All of the children lived in low-stress conditions.

Bryant (1985) discovered that the child's perception of available social support correlates positively with the social-emotional functioning of children growing up under generally secure, low-stress conditions. She found that selected networks of support are predictive of social-emotional functioning under these specific conditions. She also found age and sex to be a factor, with the same support variables functioning differently for the 7- and 10-year-olds as well as for boys and girls. Bryant interprets these findings as showing that "parental support may be more critical in the early years, while parental distance in later middle childhood may facilitate one's productive involvement with other sources of support." She concluded that no matter how one interprets the data, they show that children in middle childhood can assess the social support affecting their lives and that there is a great need for further research of this type.

Social support has even been shown to play an important role in determining an individual's response to major disasters. In a study of reaction to the Three Mile Island nuclear accident, Bromet, Schulberg, and Dunn (1982) found that those individuals who showed the greatest distress after the accident were those with the poorest perceived support.

Bromet, Schulberg, and Dunn (1982) studied 215 mental patients from three community health centers serving the area in central Pennsylvania most affected by the Three Mile Island nuclear accident, which occurred on March 28, 1979. They chose to study this population in order to discern the role of social support networks in mediating the stress-illness relationship. The researchers began with the assumption that individuals who integrated into a large number of well-functioning support systems, with ample psychosocial resources available to them, would have less need for psychiatric intervention following the disaster than those who lacked these vital resources and were marginal participants in community life. Bromet et al. based this assumption on previous research that found that individuals with fewer interpersonal linkages may experience a long-term inability to manage stress following a disaster that impairs natural support systems. From their investigations, the researchers concluded that

> *Precise cause-effect relationships in the etiology of psychiatric symptoms evident after a disaster are yet to be demonstrated, but it is widely believed that interventions could be particularly directed to various high-risk populations. Persons with inadequate coping skills are considered vulnerable to disaster-induced stress, and crisis intervention is best directed toward them. (p. 725)*

From these studies it is clear that social support operates on many levels. It affects the family, which influences the macrosociety, and, conversely, it influences the macrosociety, which in turn influences the family as well as individuals. Thus social support has a direct and an indirect influence that children and adults perceive differently. These studies show that when put into operation by adequate, functioning interpersonal relationships, social systems, and programs, social support alleviates stressful life conditions as well as enhances social-emotional functioning experienced under less stressful conditions.

CONCLUSIONS

Researchers have been able to establish a relationship between depressive symptomatology and stressful social and environmental factors, as well as adverse life-events. They have also been able to document that strong social support mitigates this depressive symptomatology and the other negative effects of stressful life events. The social support may be provided by the community, friends, or family. The more intimate and confiding the relationship, the more it compensates and offsets the adverse factors and their resultant ongoing effects.

The relationship of these findings to caregiver deprivation and subsequent infant depression is highly significant. If the caregiver at risk for depression and, therefore, for poor caregiver-infant bonding, can be identified, he or she can then receive the type of social support mandatory to counteract any predisposition. Psychosocial epidemiology, with its study of constitutional, social, and environmental factors, provides us with the tool for identifying those caregivers predisposed to psychiatric disorders.

Intervention, through social support, can then be used to prevent caregiver deprivation, which leads to infant and childhood depression.

Changes continuously take place within families and societies. Many of these changes are extremely positive, bringing about a higher quality of life, better social conditions, and support systems, as well as increased options and activities. Unfortunately, some of these changes also have negative consequences: The modern family's isolation from the wider social structures that could provide support when necessary has proven to be extremely disruptive.

There is no question that the dimensions of the family of the future are changing. We have yet to discover how we will adjust to the increasing number of working women, the shifting roles within the family, and to the way we utilize our leisure time once the children are gone (Dolgoff & Feldstein, 1984, p. 340).

To date, social welfare in American society has developed "piecemeal and incrementally," attacking problems one by one, unsystematically, and without a view to their social context. The future of the family may depend to a great extent on the outcome of the argument between the hedonism or self-fulfillment of adults and the cause-oriented, dependent existence of children.

Although our society has significant abilities to anticipate problems and to solve them, most significant problems are not simple to solve, and solutions may bring problems of their own. Society's great complexity is focused on the issue of whether social welfare will expand or not, and this issue, in turn, will have an important impact on how families develop and survive in the future (Dolgoff & Feldstein, 1984).

Thus the ongoing challenge for the mental health community and for society as a whole is to support the individual family unit and, at the same time, integrate this unit into the wider community. This wider community can then provide the social support that mitigates the life stressors that lead to psychiatric disorders in general and depressive symptomatology in particular. In this manner, the community can intervene and interrupt the debilitating process which often leads to infant depression and childhood suicide.

CHAPTER SIX

Parental Psychopathology as a Risk Factor for Infant and Childhood Depression

Of all of the infant and child populations that are susceptible to the experience of depression, in no other is the risk so carefully delineated and well documented as in the case of the offspring of depressed parents. Indeed, within this group it may be argued that there is a preponderant likelihood that depression will erupt (Trad, 1986).

It is not difficult to understand why this group is at such high risk. If the primary caregiver—the person who serves as the infant's first mediator with and representative of the external world—is depressed, this symptomatology will be incorporated with virtual certainty into the dyadic interaction and eventually may be inculcated into the infant's sense of self. Equally compelling is the recent evidence indicating that a spectrum of affective disorders may be genetically transmitted, so that even if the infant were removed from his or her biological caregiver and raised in an optimal environment, he or she would still harbor an innate vulnerability to the subsequent development of an affective disorder. In essence, then, the specter of parental depression infuses infant maturation and exerts an invidious effect with respect to each of the developmental hallmarks that have been discussed.

In addition to this distressing portrait, recent evidence suggests that both the incidence of maternal depression and the subtle variations this disorder can assume may be more widespread than previously suspected. Such conditions as postpartum depression—which can affect an infant during the earliest months of life—and premenstrual syndrome—which surfaces on a regular, cyclical basis—may pose threats to infant development that have previously been overlooked.

Maternal depression may represent such an overwhelming risk to newborns and young children perhaps because it intrudes on and disrupts the processes whereby the infant exercises his or her discriminatory capacities and perceptions of contingency. If these processes are tampered with, the infant may be prevented from engaging in the form of regulation necessary for eventually developing an unimpaired sense of self. In fact, exposure to either persistent or intermittent maternal depression may provoke dysregulation of infant behavioral response.

Finally, it is within the arena of maternal depression, that the analog of learned helplessness depression is most productively applied. Maternal depression is likely to expose the infant to noncontingency responses and to inadequate maternal response to infant behavior. As such, the infant will eventually perceive the environment as a domain in which expected principles of cause and effect do not operate. This environment, then, is uncontrollable and the realization of uncontrollability is likely to evoke feelings of helplessness. Since the helplessness has, from the infant's perception, no attributable source, he or she may come to attribute failed outcomes either to his or her own deficits or to attribute dashed expectations to a hostile universe in which he or she is a vulnerable pawn of arbitrary forces. In either case, learned helplessness, with its concomitant symptomatology, may ensue. These themes are explored in depth in this chapter.

At any arbitrary point in time, between 10 and 20 percent of the adult population in the United States suffers from depressive symptomatology, according to a review of the epidemiological literature conducted by Boyd and Weissman (1981). As many as one quarter of all women will experience a nonbipolar depressive episode during some period in their lifespan (Boyd & Weissman, 1981). By any standard, these figures qualify depression as a significant mental health problem. But the statistics are even more disturbing, in light of the well-documented fact that depression tends to "cluster" in families.

Estimates of the incidence of depression in the offspring of depressed parents range from 14 percent (Kashani, Burk, & Reid, 1985) to almost 50 percent (McKnew, Cytryn, Efron, Gershon, & Bunney, 1979) of the children of depressed parents. According to a recent survey of the literature by Weissman and Boyd (1985), depression in one member of a family magnifies the risk for other family members by a factor of two or three. Thus, by virtue of their parents' disorder, a significant portion of the child population faces a heightened risk of succumbing to depression. Moreover, the period during which the child is at risk may extend over a longer stretch of time than has generally been considered. Although major affective disorder has typically been construed as a self-limiting illness, with episodes enduring for 6 to 18 months (Beck, Sethin, & Tuthill, 1963), some evidence suggests that a sizable minority of cases do not remit completely for many years. In a sample of 120 patients treated for major depressive episode, whose disorder began between the ages of 30 and 60, 39 percent continued to present DSM-III symptoms for an entire year. Symptoms in one subject lasted into the fourth year, and then remitted only partially (Ceroni, Neri, & Pezzoli, 1984).

For many years documentation of a familial clustering phenomenon in other mental illnesses, principally schizophrenia, overshadowed interest in the effects of parental depression on children. In recent years, however, researchers have increasingly concerned themselves with the high rates of depression seemingly spawned by a family history of affective disorders and/or depression. Research into the relationship between parental and child depression actually began over half a century ago. As early as 1921, Kraepelin reported evidence of "psychic degeneration" in 52 percent of a group of 44 children of manic-depressive patients. Over the ensuing decades, many researchers have confirmed the comparatively high incidence of depression among relatives of depressed individuals. Investigations have documented the correlation between parental and offspring psychopathology from two orientations. Studies using clinically depressed children as probands have found a high incidence of depression in their parents (McKnew & Cytryn, 1973; Philips, 1979; Poznanski & Zrull, 1970; Strober, 1984). Conversely, research on clinically depressed parents has detected an unusually high incidence of depression among their children and first-degree relatives (Brumbeck et al., 1977; Gamer et al., 1977; Klein et al., 1985; Price et al., 1984; Weissman et al., 1984).

Although studies of the relationship between parental and childhood depression have been plagued by inconsistencies and methodological problems such as small sample sizes, inadequate control groups, and absence of uniform diagnostic criteria, most research indicates that parental depression does, in fact, increase the risk that a child will develop depression. Recognition of this phenomenon has prompted investigators to focus more broadly on this child population at risk, in an effort to pinpoint not only clinically significant cases of depression, but also the precursors and correlates of such psychopathology. Indeed, researchers have demonstrated that irrespective of the children's clinical diagnosis, offspring of depressed parents differ significantly on a number of cognitive and emotional measures from children of nondepressed parents. Weintraub, Winters, and Neale (1986), for example, have found that teachers and peers of the offspring of affectively ill parents view them as less competent on a number of dimensions than they see the children of parents without mental illness. Moreover, although the evidence is far from definitive, several important studies reveal significant differences between children of depressed parents and children of parents with no psychopathology (Cohler, Grunebaum, Weiss, Gamer, & Gaueest, 1977; Kauffman, Grunebaum, Cohler, & Gamer, 1979). For example, Weintraub et al. (1986) discerned differences between the offspring of affectively ill and normal parents and detected a remarkable similarity between the former and the children of parents with other psychiatric disorders. Most recently, researchers have begun to uncover important behavioral differences among children of different types of depressives (Radke-Yarrow et al., 1985; Zahn-Waxler et al., 1984a). This finding is not without controversy, as exemplified by the research of Kashani, Burk, and Reid (1985). Their investigations confirmed significant differences in symptomatology between control children and 50 offspring of patients with major affective disorder but failed to establish comparable distinctions between children of parents with different subtypes of affective disorder.

Studies describing differences between children of depressed parents and children of nondepressed parents—either clinically normal parents or parents with other types of psychopathology—have provided important clues about the mechanisms by which depression in one generation can either genetically transmit or environmentally induce depression in the next generation. The difference between these two processes is highly pertinent. Genetic transmission implies a direct replication of the original, parental facsimile of psychopathology. Environmentally induced depression, on the other hand, suggests a process by which intermediate variables interact to culminate in depression. Etiologic theories have been formulated based on

both types of mechanisms. Numerous studies have shown that depression
—at least bipolar depression—may be conveyed to children through genetic
transmission (Gershon, Bunney, Leckman, Eerdewesh, & DeBauche, 1976;
Mahmood et al., 1983; Mendlewicz & Rainer, 1977). Certain environmental
explanations also imply a mechanism which may incorporate a transmission
component. For example, theories of mirroring and imitation, as well as
Stern's model of affect attunement (1984), assume a more or less direct
replication of parental experiences of depression.

Other explanations of childhood depression posit a more circuitous route
whereby the offspring of depressed parents may develop a depressive
predisposition, if not depression per se. These theories focus on the impact
of parental depression on critical developmental functions such as
attachment formation, affect regulation, and cognitive functioning—each
of which plays a seminal role in the etiology of childhood depression.
Research has, for example, implicated parental emotional dysregulation
(Zahn-Waxler et al., 1984) as leading to a child's experience of
noncontingency, a prerequisite of learned helplessness depression, and
impaired parental functioning as resulting in lack of involvement with or
even meaningful contact with the child.

Identifying the causal mechanism in an episode of parental depression
can be problematic because depression is often precipitated by multivariate
factors. Other parental pathology, such as anxiety disorders, alcoholism, or
abuse and neglect, often accompanies such depression. Some of these
disorders, whether or not they occur in tandem with full-fledged
depression, also have well-documented links to depression (Weissman,
Gershon, et al., 1984a). In fact, the literature has frequently cited abuse and
neglect as major causes of infant and childhood depression. Clearly,
however, parental depression accompanied by abuse or other psychopathology will compound the risk to the child. In reality, it is often difficult to
segregate these many forms of psychopathology impinging on the child, but
for practical purposes it is useful to make the attempt. Therefore, this
chapter will focus exclusively on the role of parental depression in the
etiology of childhood depression.

Since depression is both episodic and heterogeneous in manifestation, the
disorder can present with varied symptomatology and in different degrees
of severity among children at risk. This phenomenon was underscored by
the investigations of Weintraub, Winters, and Neale (1986), who noted that
no singular behavioral pattern adequately encompassed all of the children
of affectively ill parents. As a consequence, this discussion does not remain
limited to the development of depression per se in the infants and children
of depressed caregivers. Rather, the commentary extends to the full
spectrum of depressive symptomatology, as well as to both the precursors
and correlates of depression.

Investigations focusing on the symptomatology rather than the syndrome level of depression provide insight into the continuous or discontinuous nature of affective illness. They are especially important given the lack of consensus about whether infant and childhood depression constitutes a similar or fundamentally distinct disorder from adult depression. Thus even those investigators who deny that affective disorders can be reliably diagnosed with existing operational criteria prior to the age of 5 years recognize that certain early symptoms may represent developmentally determined precursors of adult affective illness (Cytryn, McKnew, Zahn-Waxler, & Gershon, 1986).

This chapter is divided into three sections. Initially, discussion concentrates on the epidemiological literature identifying and measuring the at-risk population for depression passed from parent to offspring. Next the cognitive and emotional development of these at-risk children is probed to ascertain how the impact of parental depression may thwart normal developmental processes. A portrait of the developmental status of these children will then permit presentation and evaluation of several alternative hypotheses explaining how depression in parents is often replicated by depression among their offspring. Accordingly, this portion of the chapter will describe the behavioral characteristics, including rates of psychopathology as well as depressive symptomatology, encountered among the children of depressed parents. The final portion of the chapter will present several explanatory paradigms, including both genetic and environmental theories, which posit mechanisms whereby parental depression can create depression in offspring. Ultimately, this chapter seeks to offer explanations for the particularly high incidence of depression and depressive symptomatology within this child population.

EPIDEMIOLOGY OF DEPRESSION

Although researchers have for over half a century suspected that affective disorders cluster in families, only within the last ten years have they accumulated sufficiently reliable data to support this claim. Indeed, researchers have confronted, and continue to confront, an array of investigative difficulties that, while not the primary concern of this chapter, are important to understand when evaluating the epidemiological evidence. First, a definitional problem arises, since these investigations are attempting to measure a secondary risk—a risk derived from another risk. The size of the infant and child population at risk for depression by virtue of parental affective disorder is a function of two main risk factors: the risk that parents will develop the disorder and the degree of risk that parental depression imposes on the child.

The definitional complexities with which researchers have grappled in attempting to explain the apparent clustering of depression within families cannot be ignored. Disagreement over which phenomena constitute depression has made it difficult to delimit the parental population whose children face increased risk for depression. Definitional problems have surfaced in debates on such issues as the existence of depressive spectrum disease and the intergenerational passage of psychopathologies (e.g., substance abuse and anxiety disorders) that often accompany depression. Evidence increasingly demands that researchers concern themselves with differentiating populations with different types of affective disorder— bipolar and nonbipolar—as well as with subclassifications of major depression. Nevertheless, a climate of controversy still surrounds these nosological questions. Moreover, dispute remains about whether some of the well-accepted subclassifications of affective disorder represent discrete clinical entities (Trad, 1986).

The currently prevailing view (Leonhard, 1957) is that affective disorders may be divided into two broad categories as determined by the presence or absence of mania. This view supplanted Kraepelin's (1921) conception that a single morbid process was responsible for both bipolar and unipolar depression. Indeed, Kraepelin's view has regained credibility as an outgrowth of investigations discerning similarity in the symptomatology exhibited by the offspring of bipolar and unipolar depressives (Kashani, Burk, & Reid, 1985) and research on genetic transmission mechanisms of depression (Baron, Klotz, Mendlewicz, & Rainer, 1981). For example, research on multiple-threshold transmission mechanisms raises the possibility that the two disorders—bipolar and unipolar depression—are more reliably seen as a single morbid process on a single genetic-environmental continuum in which bipolar disorder is the more deviant (Baron, Klotz, Mendlewicz, & Rainer, 1981).

Greater specificity in defining the parent population clearly dictates greater specificity in evaluating the degree of risk to children. Implicit in the effort to differentiate disorders within the parent population is the assumption that the risk to relatives of one type of disorder may not equal the risk presented by another. As we shall see, when an assessment of the degree of risk is isolated, investigators have found substantial support for this assumption.

Methodological problems have also arisen with respect to data collection and interpretation in parental depression studies. Formerly, epidemiologists were pessimistic about the prospects of achieving a level of subject interviewing and diagnostic uniformity that would facilitate consistency among the numerous studies assessing the magnitude of affective disorders both in this country and worldwide. Reviews of the epidemiological literature yielded widely varying estimates on rates of affective disorder, reinforcing this grim outlook (Boyd & Weissman, 1981). Recently, however, improved diagnostic techniques have promised to add confidence to major community studies on affective disorders. The refinement of diagnostic criteria for identifying psychiatric disorders, coupled with structured interview techniques for eliciting the behavioral information needed to detect disordered symptoms has provided encouraging, although by no means uniform, results. More systematic use of instruments such as the Research Diagnostic Criteria (RDC) and DSM-III for classification, and structured interviews, such as the Renard Diagnostic Interview (Helzer et al., 1981) and the Schedule for Affective Disorders and Schizophrenia (SADS) (Weissman and Myers, 1978) have only begun to provide the quality of data needed to embrace the full spectrum of risk factors associated with parental depression.

Inconsistencies have arisen as a result of differing diagnostic techniques, as well as the use of different epidemiological measures to estimate risk in sample populations. Detailed analysis of the adequacy of various measures is beyond the scope of this chapter. Nevertheless, several general definitions are helpful in interpreting the data, although the reader is cautioned that specific studies may have applied variations of these epidemiological measures of risk.

1. *Point prevalence* refers to the percentage of the population that, at a given point in time, manifests the disorder under study.
2. *Period prevalence* measures the proportion of the entire population that has the disorder at the commencement period or is developing the disorder over a specified period of time.
3. *Incidence* documents the rate at which new cases of the disorder develop in the risk population during a designated interval, usually a year.
4. Lifetime risk is the proportion of a population that may develop a particular disorder if those individuals lived to a specified age. *Lifetime risk* is often—albeit imprecisely—used interchangeably with "morbid risk," "disease expectancy," and "lifetime prevalence."

Analysis of the epidemiology data on the impact of parental depression properly begins with a discussion of available evidence on the prevalence of parental depression, since the child population in which we are interested is a derivative of this group. Although newer research reports on the full range of affective disorders, much of the older research distinguishes only bipolar and nonbipolar depressives. This section will provide data on each of these major groups of depressives, breaking them into further subgroups to the extent such data are available.

Nonbipolar Depression

Contained within this category are individuals in several diagnostic subgroups, belying the multiplicity of classification schemes that have been used during the last half century. The category of nonbipolar depression encompasses patients with postpartum depression, as well as patients in several other diagnostic classifications of depression, such as melancholic, involutional, reactive, and endogenous. Greater standardization with the advent of DSM-III and RDC has helped to minimize the imprecision in defining the exact contours of this seemingly broad group. In general, however, the category should be interpreted as including depressed individuals *without* mania—irrespective of accompanying disorder, time of onset, or severity of depression.

Because of the comparatively recent attempts to employ standard diagnostic categories, prevalence rates still vary for nonbipolar depression. In one of the initial efforts to apply the RDC to the study of affective disorders, Weissman and Myers (1978) selected a single adult from each of 1095 randomly selected households. Of these adults, 938 agreed to an interview in 1967 and 720 consented to another in 1975-1976. Using the SADS and RDC in the 1975-1976 study, the researchers calculated a 4.3 percent point prevalence for major depression and a 2.5 percent rate for minor depression, yielding a combined rate of 6.8 percent for both major and minor depression combined. (These figures include both definite and probable cases.) Lifetime prevalence rates, also including both probable and definite cases, were 20 percent for major depression and 9.2 percent for minor depression, as calculated by Weissman and Myers. The researchers also observed that the overwhelming majority (86 percent) of depressions were primary, with alcoholism as the most frequent preceding disorder for the remaining secondary depressions.

Boyd and Weissman's (1981) review of the literature on affective disorders includes other community surveys based on SADS, RDC, DSM-III, and comparable interview and classification methods used outside the United States. Even with stringent use of these instruments, research yields discrepant findings. Such differences notwithstanding, the authors concluded that the new research tools have narrowed the discrepancies found in older studies. Among the 16 studies reviewed, the majority of which were performed in industrialized nations, the point prevalence of depression ranged from 1.1 percent to 10.8 percent of the population. Murphy, Sobol, and Neff (1984) found a similar incidence of depression that was replicated over almost a 20-year period in two cross-sectional surveys centered in Stirling County, Canada. In 1952, these researchers calculated a 5.3 percent point prevalence for severe and moderate depression combined, and a rate of 5.6 percent for 1970. These figures coincide with others reported in the literature. The point prevalence for severe depression changed only slightly (from 1.4 to 1.5 percent) in 1970, while the rate of moderate depression escalated only slightly (from 3.9 to 4.1 percent), as well, during this period.

Point prevalence for women often exceeded that reported for men in the studies reviewed by Boyd and Weissman (1981). These studies on nonbipolar depression detected a point prevalence of 1.8 to 3.2 cases per hundred for men and 2.0 to 9.8 cases per hundred for women. While most of the period prevalance studies reviewed by Boyd and Weissman were based on treatment records rather than on the new community survey methods, the two studies using community interviews found period prevalence of nonbipolar depression among women ranging from 8.4 to 14.8 percent. These studies did not measure period prevalence for men or for men and women combined.

Less reliable data are available for the *incidences* of nonbipolar depression since most studies are based on case registries, which tend to underestimate true risk because only a fraction of depressives ever receive treatment. The only study utilizing new diagnostic methods reports an annual incidence of 7800 per 100,000. Boyd and Weissman (1981) caution that this figure needs further substantiation.

The lifetime risk studies reviewed by Boyd and Weissman (1981) posed greater interpretive difficulties, since the six studies evaluated did not employ the same measurement of risk. Some relied on lifetime prevalance, while others employed disease expectancy. However, as the authors observe, the two investigations using SADS, RDC, and a similar lifetime risk measurement achieved notably similar results. (In contrast, however, the two period prevalance studies, both using the same diagnostic criteria, did not achieve the same degree of consistency.) One study performed on six communities showed an 8.3 percent lifetime risk for men and a 20.3 percent risk for women, while the other study, performed in one community, revealed a 12.3 percent lifetime risk for men and a 25.8 percent risk for women.

Some of the most ambitious recent research, performed under the Epidemiological Catchment Area (ECA) program in collaboration with the National Institute of Mental Health (NIMH), detects a magnitude of risk for major depression similar to that reported in the studies described above (Meyers et al., 1984). Researchers examined many kinds of psychiatric disorders among more than 9000 adults in three communities, Baltimore, St. Louis, and New Haven—the latter the subject of an earlier study. Myers et al. found comparable 6-month period prevalence for major depression among the three communities. Baltimore had a 6-month period prevalence of 2.2 percent, while St. Louis and New Haven showed slightly higher levels of 3.2 percent and 3.5 percent respectively. Notably, rates of individual affective disorders except bereavement and dysthymia, declined with age. The highest levels of major depression and dysthymia were found among women in the 25–44 age group. Incidence of depression among women in this group exceeded that of men in the same age group by a factor of nearly 3; dysthymia incidence among women was nearly double that of men in a similar age group.

Measures of lifetime prevalence (Robins, Helzer, & Weissman, 1984) diverged somewhat more among the sites, but still remained in basic concurrence. Once again, New Haven showed the highest lifetime prevalence (6.7 percent), compared with St. Louis (5.5 percent) and Baltimore (3.7 percent). Rates for lifetime diagnosis of dysthymia were approximately the same. While concordant among themselves, these lifetime prevalence rates fall significantly below most other rates reported in the literature. In further confirmation of the apparent greater susceptibility of women to affective disorders, the analysis revealed that rates for both depression and dysthymia were significantly higher for women than for men in all three communities.

Premenstrual Dysphoric Changes. Recent investigations into the high degree of overlap between major depressive disorder and premenstrual dysphoric changes suggest that women with premenstrual aberrations may represent a significant, previously overlooked, population at risk to transmit depression to their offspring. Mood and behavioral disturbances occurring prior to the onset of menstruation have long been recognized. Only lately, however, have the correlations between these changes and major depressive disorder been documented sufficiently, such that the offspring of women with premenstrual syndrome may be considered at risk for depression. Halbreich and Endicott (1985) reported that 84 percent of those who met the criteria of depressive symptomatology, as measured with the Premenstrual Assessment Form, also met the criteria for lifetime RDC diagnosis of major depressive disorder. The researchers characterized the correlation as high but variable, indicating that prospective studies are needed to ascertain how reliably premenstrual changes predict or coincide with major depressive disorder.

From the few studies conducted on premenstrual irregularities, it appears that this disorder more closely resembles unipolar than bipolar depression (Dejons, Rubinow, Roy-Byrne, Hoban, & Grover, 1985). Halbreich and Endicott (1985) caution against attempting to define a single premenstrual syndrome but comment that the changes observed in their research do not replicate the classic picture of endogenous depression. Symptoms—such as overeating, anxiety, hostility, and hypersomnia—that are typical of other depressive subtypes appear more pronounced among women with diagnosed premenstrual syndrome.

Postpartum Depression. Dramatic mood alterations and depressive symptomatology that do not meet DSM-III's chronicity requirements for affective disorders may, nonetheless, interfere sufficiently in an individual's life to present risk for depression in offspring. Although women with particular types of postpartum depression may be excluded from depressed populations when DSM-III chronicity standards are adhered to, the timing—both onset and periodicity—of their altered mood states and their varying degrees of short-lived incapacity suggest that these women may represent an important omission from the overall depressed population from which the child population at risk is derived. Thus it is important to ascertain the full prevalence and impact of postpartum conditions.

By far, the epidemiology of postpartum depression is better understood than the nature of unipolar depression. Postpartum psychosis is generally thought to be rare, according to a review of the literature performed by Stern & Kruckman (1983), occurring in perhaps 1 of 1000 live births. Moderate depression (depressive neurosis) occurs far more often, possibly as frequently as one in five births (Stern & Kruckman, 1983). Most studies reviewed by these researchers documented that as few as half, and as many as four fifths of postpartum women suffer from mild, transitory affective disturbance. If, as researchers such as Klaus and Kennel (1976) have suggested, there is a period of "bonding" occurring immediately after birth that is critical for subsequent attachment formation, the potential for diminished responsivity as a result of postpartum depression qualifies this disorder, however brief, as a legitimate threat to the mother-infant relationship. A mother whose postpartum depression impedes her capacity to provide the infant with early contingency experiences, may thus be depriving the infant of the environmental responsivity requisite for the development of self-regulation (Trad, 1986).

In a discussion of postpartum depression, Kennerley and Gath (1985) reported that puerperal depression of a mild to moderate intensity is far more common than postpartum psychosis. According to these researchers, the incidence of peurperal depression is approximately in the range of 10 to 20 percent of births. Onset generally begins 2 weeks after delivery, with the disorder remitting a few months. Often, such manifestations as tiredness, irritability and anxiety (occasionally phobic) are more pronounced than depressed mood. While it is uncertain whether peurperum depression occurs in greater frequency in those women with a previous history of psychiatric depression, there is some preliminary data indicating that depression following birth carries an increased risk for future psychiatric disorder.

Depressed Mood in Fathers. Recent data suggests that a series of phenomena previously believed to be associated primarily with mothers following birth, may also be manifested by fathers. Until now, the scant literature on psychological difficulties in new fathers discussed severe reactions (Cavenar & Butts, 1977). However, data generated by Zaslow, Pederson, Cain, Suwalsky, and Kramer (1985) indicates that such phenomena as mild to moderate after birth depression or "blue" periods may be relatively prevalent in fathers.

In the Zaslow et al. study, a sample of 37 middle-class families with first born infants was investigated when the infant was 4 months old. The findings disclosed that 62 percent of fathers reported feeling "blue" at some time after the birth. In contrast, when the mothers were interviewed, 89 percent commented that they had undergone a "blue" period.

In families where the father reported mild depression lasting for more than 8 days, interactive behavior with the infant differed from behavior manifested by fathers who had not reported depression. For example, blue fathers engaged in fewer vocalizations with their infants, touched the infants less frequently, and displayed diminished proximity to the infant. In addition, those fathers who experienced depression identified other problems associated with the birth, and specifically commented on changes in the spousal relationship and in an increased need for support. Such fathers often attributed their "blues" to the spousal relationship.

Commenting on the results of the investigation, the researchers hypothesized that greater direct involvement of fathers with infants is associated with a more positive subjective psychological state, with a better spousal relationship, and with more spousal communication concerning the infant. For the purposes of this discussion, paternal depression is significant in that the father represents yet another significant figure with which the infant interacts from the first months of life onwards.

Measures of Bipolar Depression

Bipolar disorders are much less frequent than unipolar depressions and the epidemiological data pertaining to this psychopathology are more scarce. A number of inconsistencies arising from different classification criteria present questions about the reliability of the data obtained prior to the use of RDC. In the first community-wide application of this diagnostic tool, Weissman and Myers (1978) found a lifetime prevalence of 0.6 percent for bipolar I (major depression with mania) and a comparable rate for bipolar II (major depression with hypomania). Lifetime prevalences calculated by Robins et al. (1984) for the years 1980-1981 corresponded with this earlier figure. Among the three sites studied, New Haven, Baltimore, and St. Louis, the research team found lifetime prevalences of 1.1 percent, 0.6 percent and 1.1 percent respectively for bipolar disorder. These findings result in a lifetime prevalence of only about one tenth of that found for major depressive episodes. Notably, the 6-month prevalence rates closely parallel the lifetime prevalence (Myers et al., 1984).

Seasonal Affective Disorder. Only very recently have investigators begun to recognize the significance of what may be a mild variant of bipolar disorder (Rosenthal, Sack, & Gillin, 1984) known as seasonal affective disorder (SAD). As the diagnostic label implies, individuals suffering from SAD exhibit depressive symptomatology that fluctuates rhythmically with the seasons. Whether this disorder is, in fact, a variant on bipolar disorder, as has been suggested by Rosenthal and colleagues, or whether it is equally prevalent among unipolar depressives is still unclear. Because of the seasonal nature of the disorder it has been difficult to determine the precise population actually afflicted with SAD. As a result, many of those who suffer from SAD may not be accounted for adequately in large-scale epidemiological calculations of affective disorders. The difficulty in identifying SAD is further compounded by a lack of consensus on the precise pattern of symptomatology—that is, when periods of mania are evident and when they are replaced by periods of depression (Frangos, Athanassenas, Tsitourides, Psilolingnos, et al., 1980; Rosenthal, Sack, Gillin, Lewy, Goodwin, Davenport, & Mueller, 1984).

Nevertheless, several characteristics of patients diagnosed with SAD suggest that the offspring of this population represent a significant—albeit inadequately measured—risk group for depression. For example, a family history of major affective disorder is common among patients with SAD. Over two thirds of those with SAD had a first-degree relative with major affective disorder, although a family history of SAD itself is far less common. Legitimate cause for concern is raised by the preponderance of women, particularly those of childbearing age, among this population. Well over three quarters (86 percent) of the SAD population studied by Rosenthal, Sack, Gillin, Lewy et al. (1984) were women. Moreover, the mean age of SAD onset was 27 years.

IMPACT OF PARENTAL DEPRESSION ON CHILDREN

Ann was first brought to the clinic at 6 months of age. During the visit, Ann responded to both her mother and the physician, and during testing she functioned more effectively when her mother was nearby. This phenomenon suggested that an attachment had been formed. Decreased activity and delay in motor development were visible, but not severe. Ann was unable to maintain her trunk erect when placed in a sitting position, and she was less interested in toys than were other children of her age. Although her capacity for discrimination of acoustic stimuli, as well as objects in her visual environment, was good, she reacted to the sound of a bell and to some other noises by closing her eyes, as though attempting to shut out these stimuli. At this examination, her mother reported that Ann took long daytime naps.

When Ann was next seen, at 7 months, 3 weeks, a dramatic decline in all aspects of development was observed. Indeed, the examiners described the infant as being outwardly depressed. Language was the most severely retarded function and averaged 6 weeks below age level. Ann neither imitated sounds nor responded to her name. Gross motor achievement was more retarded than before and muscle tone was described as poor for the first time. Indeed, Ann displayed more vigor in getting rid of objects than in obtaining them. In addition, she displayed an apparent preference for stimulation of low intensity, as well as a tendency toward withdrawal. The infant seemed to find more pleasure in contact with toys than in social contact.

Also evident at this visit was the markedly disturbed relationship between Ann and her mother. For example, Ann cried repeatedly when her mother approached but could be comforted by the pediatrician. The infant also demonstrated more overt signs of affective pleasure at contact with the pediatrician, as opposed to the affect she demonstrated with her mother.

Significantly, Ann's mother was extremely depressed at this time. Interviews revealed that she was dissatisfied, lonely, bored, and angry at her husband. It was suspected that this negative affect had been conveyed to Ann during the mother-infant interaction. Ann's mother commented that although she felt guilty about her feelings for her daughter, she seemed unable to modify her behavior. In addition, Ann's mother noted that the infant had screaming spells of approximately 10 minutes duration which seemed to coincide with her own depressed moods.

Ann's heightened attention to acoustic and visual stimuli, her increased anxiety, and particularly her distress at the approach of her mother suggested to the examiners that Ann now responded to familiar stimuli in the external world with fear. This response was paralleled by a relative decrease in libidinal attachment behaviors, as reflected by the infant's tenuous ties to human objects, her relative incapacity to play, and her low investment in toys. The emotional tie between mother and infant was characterized as weak, and Ann fit the classic description of a miserable and depressed infant. Her cry was a loud shriek of distress and she had lost weight. In general, then, Ann had ceased to thrive, both physically and psychologically.

From the available evidence, Ann's temperamental characteristics fall between the "slow-to-warm-up" and "difficult" categories of the NYLS typologies (Thomas, Chess, Hertzig, Birch, and Korn, 1963). She displayed evidence of low activity, withdrawal, poor motor control and negative mood. She was also reported to prefer stimulation of low intensity, suggesting a diminished threshold of response. As the information available spans such a short amount of time, it is not possible to make any judgments on the development of these characteristics—that is, how much these behaviors are influenced by genetic factors contributing to Ann's depression or how much they have been environmentally induced.

At 7 months, 3 weeks, Ann showed signs of avoidant attachment. For instance, she resisted the approach of her mother, preferring the pediatrician, and did not exhibit pleasure during free play. We may infer that the infant had not received consistent or sufficient contact with her mother, and possibly that the quality of the contact she experienced was unpleasant (Provence, 1983).

A growing volume of literature has recently documented rather conclusively that when one member of a family, such as Ann's mother, is depressed, other members of the family—in this instance, Ann—are also likely to exhibit disordered behavior, presumably as a result of parental depression. This coincident behavior may include merely disordered symptoms as well as overt psychopathology. In this section we are concerned with the full spectrum of aberrant effects, in order to identify not only existing cases of childhood depression, but behaviors which appear likely to evolve in the direction of full-fledged psychopathology.

Rates of Depression Among Children with Depressed Parents

Much of the literature addresses the phenomenon of offspring psychopathology rather broadly, using first-degree relatives of probands to assess the risk that depression in one family member will be reflected in depressed conditions in other family members. Only very recently have researchers gathered data focusing exclusively on depression in the children of depressed parents (Weissman et al., 1984; Kashani, Burk, & Reid, 1985).

Weissman et al. (1984) compared the offspring of probands with major or minor depression (but not bipolar disorder) with a sample of children whose parents had no psychiatric illness. They found that depression in parents conferred a three times greater risk of some DSM-III diagnosis—although not necessarily depression—on the child. Major depression was the most common diagnosis encountered in the children of depressives, approximately 13 percent of whom received such a diagnosis. None of the control children had the symptomatology of major depression. Other diagnoses that often overlap with depression in children, such as attention deficit and separation anxiety disorders, also accounted for a substantial portion of diagnosed children of depressed parents. Fully 10 percent of the children of depressives had each of these disorders. Although the researchers acknowledged the preliminary nature of these findings—since they were based on family histories rather than on direct interviews with the children—they viewed their findings as supportive of the often disputed existence of depression in prepubescents.

Cytryn, McKnew, Bartko, Lamour, and Hamovitt (1982), unlike Weissman et al., used direct interviews to sustain the hypothesis that offspring of depressed parents face a heightened susceptibility to developing depression than offspring of well parents. They found more than twice as much depressive symptomatology among children (5 to 15 years old) of depressed parents than among children of parents without psychiatric impairment. On the basis of DSM-III criteria, more than two thirds of the index families had one or more depressed children, compared with less than one fourth of the controls. Moreover, of the nine proband families with depressed children, one third had children with major depressive disorder. In sharp contrast, the control group included only one child with this disorder. In both groups, the remaining children with an affective disorder had dysthymic disorder. Additionally, children in two proband families and one control family received diagnoses of overanxious disorder.

Kashani, Burk, and Reid (1985) used children as the probands to demonstrate the strong correlation between parental and childhood depression. In evaluating 50 children whose parents suffered from either a nonbipolar or bipolar disorder, the researchers observed that 14 percent received a DSM-III diagnosis of depression, and that depression represented the most frequent disorder among parents with affective disorders. This study matches the findings of Weissman et al. (1984) and offers the additional evidence of direct child interviews, which Weissman et al. lacked.

McKnew et al. (1979) also used direct interviewing techniques in their study of 30 children (14 boys and 16 girls ages 5 to 15 years). The researchers conducted two separate interviews at 4-month intervals using the Weinberg criteria (Weinberg et al., 1973). The researchers noted that nine of the children whose parents had either bipolar or unipolar disorders were diagnosed as depressed at both interviews, while almost half the children were depressed at one interview. However, McKnew et al. published their findings before the articulation of DSM-III criteria for childhood depression. Therefore, differences in diagnostic instruments employed by McKnew et al. and Kashani's team may explain some of the discrepancy between the statistical incidence of psychopathology emerging from these two studies.

Several studies have focused exclusively on the transmission aspects of depression in the children of bipolar parents. Decina, Kestenbaum, Farber, Kron, Gargan, Sackeim, and Fieve (1983) examined 31 children (ages 7 to 14) of bipolar parents. These researchers found dramatically higher rates of psychopathology among such children than among a sample of controls. While over half of the 31 index children received some psychiatric diagnosis based on DSM-III and RDC, only one of the 18 controls was assessed as having a psychiatric impairment. Moreover, half of the psychiatrically impaired children of bipolar probands received a diagnosis of major or minor depressive disorder. In their examination of children 6 to 18 years old of bipolar parents, Kuyler et al. (1980) also found a high level—although less than that noted by Decina et al. (1983)—of psychopathology. Of these 49 children, 4 were diagnosed with an affective disorder, while 18 were considered to have undiagnosed psychopathology.

With certain types of cyclical affective disorders it may be difficult to establish a relationship between psychopathology in the parent and disorder in a relative. Often the symptomatology manifests in atypical form. For example, in Halbreich and Endicott's (1985) research on premenstrual disorders, they found that well over half of the female relatives (41) of inpatients (35) in their sample had previously experienced major depressive disorder and that only seven of the relatives had never been mentally ill. Moreover, of those who had had major depressive disorder, half also met the criteria for full depression. Thus premenstrual abnormalities may be one indicator of depression that has passed from one generation to the next.

These studies fill an important gap that has long existed in research on the transmission of affective disorders. Several significant gaps still exist, however. For example, scant research exists on the prevalence of depression among infants and very young children of depressed parents. To some degree, this may reflect the difficulty in diagnosing depression among this young population. At best, investigators have been forced to identify aberrant individual manifestations—in such areas as attachment behavior or attention span—that may signal depression. One recent study of young infants, however, attempted to measure depression by observing whether infants of clinically normal mothers behaved in a disorganized and distressed way when their mothers were instructed to simulate depressed affect (Field, 1984a). It was found that infants of mothers who had confirmed postpartum depression showed continuity of behavior during this simulation, while many of the infants of mothers who feigned depression responded with active protest to their mothers' seemingly depressed behavior. This finding suggested to Field that children of depressed mothers may have already integrated their caregiver's depressed behavior, thereby displaying no apparent change when their mothers simulated depression. Field's study represents an important initial step in compiling a literature on depression, rather than depressive symptoms or depressive precursors, among the very young offspring of depressed parents. Diagnostic difficulties notwithstanding, more research is clearly needed in this area (Trad, 1986).

Diagnostic Specificity

Many of the offspring studies reviewed thus far were designed primarily to test general theories about the genetic transmission of depression. Often these investigations make no effort to ascertain whether there is any specificity to the disorder produced in children. That is, the studies test a comprehensive group consisting of many types of depressives against controls, or they test children of parents with a particular disorder against a control group. But there is a dearth of research analyzing the ability of one type of affective disorder—for example, bipolar disease—to reproduce itself or to induce other types of affective illness such as unipolar depression. Failure to incorporate these analyses may obscure potential heterogeneity in the mechanisms by which different types of depression produce depression in offspring. Although the Collaborative Family Study of Depression— undertaken jointly by Yale University and NIMH—used a sample of all first-degree relatives of probands and did not limit itself to children of depressed parents, its findings indicate that there is, indeed, some diagnostic specificity to the transmission of risk (Weissman, Gershon et al., 1984). The study found that bipolar disorder created additional risk of both major depression and bipolar disorder. By contrast, unipolar disorders apparently produce elevated levels of unipolar disorder among first-degree relatives, but did not produce bipolar disorders.

Several researchers have found even greater specificity in regard to the transmission of affective disorders. Price, Nelson, Charney, and Quinlan (1984) and Perris (1966) observed that unipolar depression in the proband correlated more with unipolar than bipolar depression in family members, and that bipolar correlated with bipolar. Moreover, according to Price et al., unipolar depression confers a heightened risk to family members. Price et al. project a risk of 16.5 percent for family members of unipolar depressives and 9.2 percent for relatives of those with bipolar disorder—figures coinciding with those in the literature.

The findings of Kashani, Burk, and Reid (1985), as well as some investigations into genetic transmission mechanisms, tend to refute the notion of diagnostic specificity. In a sample of 50 children (ages 7 to 17 years) of parents with affective illness, Kashani and colleagues did not find parental diagnosis to be a differentiating variable in describing the children's symptomatology. One of the few adoption studies tracing affective disorders between generations found that biological parents of bipolar subjects actually had higher levels of unipolar, rather than bipolar disorder (Mendlewicz & Rainer, 1977). Multiple-threshold theories of genetic transmission also suggest one underlying morbid process which may affect an offspring in degree rather than in kind (Baron, Klotz, Mendlewicz, & Rainer, 1981).

One of the few studies focusing exclusively on the offspring, rather than first-degree relatives, of bipolar patients provides some limited confirmation of a distinctive pattern for the transmission of bipolar disorder. Klein, Depue, and Slater (1985) examined two groups of young women (ages 15 to 21) who were the offspring of patients with bipolar disorder and nonaffective psychiatric disorders. Diagnostic interviews based on the SADS were conducted by interviewers blind to the parental psychiatric status, and diagnoses were made using RDC. The bipolar offspring demonstrated higher rates of affective disorder than the comparison group. Moreover, 24 percent of the bipolar offspring, and none of the other group, received a diagnosis of cyclothymia.

Depressive Spectrum Disease

These studies raise important questions about the discrete nature of certain types of affective illness and, by extension, about the boundaries of the parental population from which the child risk population is drawn.

These studies also raise broader questions about the discrete nature of depression in relation to other psychopathology. Such issues have been framed in the debate about the existence of what has been referred to as depressive spectrum disease, first described by Winokur et al. (1971). When Winokur et al. demonstrated that depression in some probands tended to produce not only depression per se, but also alcoholism and sociopathy, in effect they redefined the population at risk for depression. If, as the depressive spectrum concept proposes, depression can transmit other types of psychopathology—that is, if depression lies within a spectrum of disorders, each of which may reflect a different expression of a single common underlying pathology, and each of which may be capable of transmitting other disorders in the spectrum—then the population at risk for depression may be substantially broader than would appear when employing a limited definition of affective disorder.

Even when a spectrum approach is adopted, the breadth of the spectrum is still a matter of contention. Winokur et al. (1971) applied the concept very narrowly, examining the relationship between depression on the one hand and alcoholism and sociopathy on the other. Other investigators have examined different conceptualizations that may encompass other psychopathology such as anxiety disorders (Weissman et al., 1984) and conduct disorders/antisocial personality disorders (Merikangas et al., 1985). If, as seems evident, depression in one generation tends to pass to the next, then from an epidemiological vantage point, establishing the validity of the depressive spectrum construct is essential for delimiting the parental population at risk for transmitting depression to offspring. Does this population, for example, include alcoholics? What other variants of psychopathology might fruitfully be viewed as a differing manifestation of depression, thereby increasing the risk for overt depression?

Answers to these questions are by no means definitive. However, the evidence of an intergenerational relationship between depression and other disorders seems best for three types of disorder—alcoholism, anxiety disorders, and conduct disorders/antisocial personality. Tentative though the findings may be, they merit careful examination given the general prevalence of these disorders in the community and thus, by inference, the potentially substantial numbers of children who remain unaccounted for in estimates of those at risk for depression. Bedi and Halikas (1985), for example, describe alcoholism as the country's third most serious health problem, behind cardiovascular disease and cancer. According to estimates from three community surveys conducted as part of the program, alcoholism is roughly as prevalent as affective disorders, with about 5 percent of those surveyed developing the disorder during a 6-month period (Myers et al., 1984), and between 10 and 20 percent of Americans developing it at some point during their lives (Robins et al., 1984). Roughly 10 percent of those studied experienced panic or phobic disorders during the 6-month period encompassed by the Myers et al. study, and 9 to 25 percent had suffered such disorders at some point during their lives. Conduct disorders/antisocial personality are far less prevalent, with about 1 percent of the population receiving such a diagnosis during a 6-month period, and 2 to 3 percent receiving such a diagnosis over the course of their lives.

   The Impact of Single Versus Multiple Disorders.   A rigid conceptualization of depressive spectrum disease would suggest that offspring of parents with any of these diagnoses should be considered at risk for depression. Much of the literature on psychopathology in the offspring of parents with a single primary diagnosis—that is, in the absense of a secondary condition—reports levels of disorder that do not significantly exceed those of children of nondisordered parents. The evidence varies, though, depending on the disorder. With respect to alcoholism and affective disorder, opinion is still very much divided. Schuckit's (1986) review of the literature on the genetic and clinical implications of alcoholism and affective disorder examined the relationship between this psychopathology from two perspectives to determine whether alcoholism produced affective disorder and whether affective disorder tended to produce alcoholism. On both counts the researcher found little basis for concluding that a genetic relationship existed between alcoholism and affective disorder. The relationship was examined from two perspectives—assessment of the level of alcoholism among the affectively ill and assessment of the rate of affective disorders among alcoholics.

   In contrast to Winokur, Cadoret, Dorzab, and Baker's (1971) findings with respect to depressive spectrum disease, Weissman et al.'s (1984c) family study of psychiatric disorders among first-degree relatives of those with varying degrees of affective disorders found no significant differences in the rate of alcoholism among the offspring of the affectively ill, the offspring of those without affective illness, and the general population. Similarly, Merikangas et al. (1985) observed in a sample drawn from those in treatment at Yale's Depression Research Unit and other facilities of the Department of Psychiatry, that depression without alcoholism did not transmit alcoholism. Even when both parents were depressed, the level of alcoholism among offspring did not rise. Nor was the converse demonstrated: The level of affective disorder did not increase significantly when both parents were alcoholics. Not unless alcoholism accompanied depression did the investigators detect a significant increase in the level of depression among the children of the affectively ill. Indeed, the secondary alcoholism in such parents conferred a three times greater risk of alcoholism than observed among the children of parents with depression only. This finding suggests that the presence of alcoholism, not affective disorder, was responsible for the elevation in alcoholism among children of parents with both disorders, and supports the notion of distinct transmission mechanisms for affective disorders and alcoholism. As Schuckit (1986) notes, however, the evidence is somewhat less conclusive with respect to the ability of alcoholism to elevate the risk for affective disorder in offspring.

Evidence from the other perspective—the degree of depression among the offspring of alcoholics, as opposed to the degree of alcoholism among offspring of depressives—contradicts the findings of Weissman et al. (1984) and Merikangas et al. (1985). Steinhausen, Gobel, and Nestler (1984) discerned a clear elevation in psychiatric risk among the children of alcoholics compared to children of nonalcoholic parents. According to the preliminary findings of this study, the child's psychiatric diagnosis varied depending on whether the mother and/or father were alcoholics. Maternal alcoholism, whether alone or accompanied by paternal alcoholism, tended to produce emotional disorders, while paternal alcoholism alone often resulted in conduct disorder.

The investigations of Moos and Billings (1982) also support part of Winokur et al.'s (1971) conceptualization of an interfamilial relationship between alcoholism and affective disorders. In a study of the children of relapsed and recovered alcoholics, Moos and Billings found significantly more depression and anxiety among the former than among both the latter and matched controls. More than half of the children of relapsed alcoholics had two or more emotional problems (depression, anxiety, nightmares, indigestion, or headaches) as reported by their mothers. In contrast, less than a quarter of the children of controls and less than 15 percent of the children of recovered alcoholics experienced such psychopathology. Twice as many of the children of relapsed alcoholics, as compared to controls, were reported to suffer from depression ("feeling sad or blue"). Other possibly depressive symptomatology, such as sleeping problems (nightmares) and eating problems (indigestion) also appeared significantly more prominently among the children of relapsed alcoholics. Interestingly, on two of the three measures most closely related to depression (reports of depression and indigestion) the children of recovered alcoholics were the least symptomatic of the three groups. The authors noted, however, that it is still not clear how long the children of recovered alcoholics will remain symptom-free. They speculated that the effects of alcoholism may create long-term underlying vulnerability that stressors later in life can aggravate. Only longitudinal investigation of these children will elucidate the long-range implications of parental alcoholism on children.

In some cases there may be a teratogenic basis for the psychological impairment caused by parental depression and its correlates. Research on the impact of maternal alcoholism has associated a number of physical, emotional, and intellectual deficits with high levels of consumption during pregnancy (Streissguth, 1983). Many of the characteristics of fetal alcohol syndrome (FAS)—including degrees of mental retardation, susceptibility to illness, hyperactivity, inattentiveness, impulsiveness, as well as eating and sleeping difficulties (Streissguth, 1983)—may reveal incipient signs of depressive symptomatology. Even more significantly, as in the discussions of the impact of illness and handicapping conditions on children, the symptomatology of FAS may have a number of indirect repercussions that increase the risk for depression in the child. Illness, lack of attention, and hyperactivity, for example, may make an infant or child temperamentally difficult and may interfere with successful parent-child interactions. Mental retardation may cause a variety of strains in such interactions. Furthermore, illness or mental retardation stemming from FAS may necessitate hospitalization. These themes are treated in greater depth in other chapters. For now, it is significant simply to recognize the multiplicity of risk factors—prenatal, perinatal, biological, and environmental—that set the children of alcoholic mothers at risk for depression. Moreover, it is important to recognize, as Steinhausen, Gobel, and Nestler (1984) have noted, that while some of the symptomatology of FAS may abate over time, there are enduring consequences. These investigators showed that while certain indicators or emotional and intellectual functioning revealed improvement in 30 FAS children evaluated at 36 months, hyperactivity persisted. To the extent that this symptom interferes with a child's social interactions, the impact of FAS should be conceived of as seriously damaging.

The evidence on the ability of anxiety disorder to transmit affective disorders, or vice versa, is somewhat more conclusive than research pertaining to alcoholism and affective disorders. The study by Weissman et al. (1984) seems to support Schuckit's (1986) belief in discrete diagnostic entities with little genetic overlap. In studying how depression and anxiety, both separately and in combination, affect children, these investigators observed that depression alone did not convey significantly higher risk for anxiety disorder in children. Nor did agoraphobia or panic disorders correlate with an increase in affective disorders among first-degree relatives evaluated in a family study of agoraphobia (Crowe, Noyes, Pauls, & Slymen, 1983). Crowe and colleagues (1983) observed a familial component to panic disorders, similar to that discerned in affective disorders and alcoholism, but they found a specificity to the transmission of these disorders. First-degree relatives of probands with panic disorder had almost a 25 percent chance of developing the disorder in their lifetime, in contrast to a 5 percent chance if the proband had no panic disorder. Although the investigators acknowledged that the inclusion of some controls with familial disorders, such as depression and alcoholism (but without panic disorder), may have distorted the comparison of the prevalence of such disorders among relatives of index and control families, they observed that the presence of panic disorder in the proband did not confer significantly greater risk for any other type of psychopathology, including major depression, alcoholism, or other anxiety disorders. If these disorders genuinely lie within one spectrum, depression by itself would have been expected to lead to higher levels of anxiety in children, and vice versa.

Despite the lack of correlation between anxiety disorders and primary affective disorders, Crowe and colleagues (1983) detected a significant rise in the level of secondary depression among proband relatives who had developed anxiety disorder. More than twice as many of the latter, as compared to controls in the sample studied by Crowe's research team, experienced secondary depression.

The Impact of Multiple Disorders.   From the evidence reviewed thus far it does not appear that a single disorder within any of the different conceptualizations of the depressive spectrum—however widely it is conceived—increases the risk for depression among offspring. Thus offspring of neither the total population of alcoholics nor those with anxiety disorders can be considered at a significantly higher risk for depression than the offspring of nondisordered parents. Nevertheless, it is possible that the occurrence of these disorders in conjunction with each other leads to an exacerbated risk of depression.

Some of the clearest evidence in support of this hypothesis is revealed in the clustering of anxiety disorders with affective disorders. The investigations of Weissman et al. (1984) found, for example, that certain anxiety disorders (panic disorder and agoraphobia) accompanying parental depression resulted in greater risk for depression than depression without anxiety disorder. While none of the children of nonpsychiatrically ill parents and only 11 percent of those with depression alone received a DSM-III diagnosis of major depression, approximately one quarter of each group whose parents had agoraphobia or panic disorder accompanying depression were also depressed. The authors interpreted this finding as confirmation of a partially shared diathesis for certain cases of major depression and panic disorders. This result contrasted with their observation noted earlier that major depression alone (i.e., without anxiety disorder) did not produce anxiety disorder in children.

Data gathered in this study also point to an increased level of potentially depressive symptomatology in the children of parents with depression and anxiety, although this level is not necessarily indicative of full depressive disorder. This implication is apparent in increased levels of separation anxiety, which may be suggestive of underlying depression. Depression alone did not appear to result in any separation anxiety among children with depressed parents. Separation anxiety was, however, documented in more than 10 percent of the offspring of depressive agoraphobics and in over 33 percent of the children whose parents had depression and panic disorder. The resemblance between separation anxiety and depression in children has been reported by Bernstein and Garfinkel (1986) in an assessment of depressive symptomatology among school phobic children. Their study, one of the first to report on the overlap between anxious and depressive symptomatology in school phobics, used a combination of structured interview, self-report, and clinical rating scales and found that over two thirds of the chronic school refusers met DSM-III criteria for affective disorder—most for major depressive episode. Depressed children showed significantly more anxiety symptoms than nondepressed children. Moreover, higher levels of anxiety correlated with more pronounced depressive symptoms. School refusers with high anxiety had significantly more depressed feelings, sleep disturbances, depressed affect, weeping, anhedonia, suicidal ideation, hypoactivity, social problems, guilt, and low self-esteem than those with low anxiety. The breadth of the overlap led Bernstein and Garfinkel to conclude that severe anxiety may be indistinguishable from depression. Depressed children, however, elaborated on this relationship in describing their symptomatology, while anxious children often failed to report depressive symptoms.

The increased risk for childhood psychopathology related to parental multiple diagnoses is evident from the significantly higher levels of multiple diagnoses in the offspring of psychopathologic parents. Only 3 percent of the offspring of parents with depression alone had two or more diagnoses, while more than a quarter of the children of depressive agoraphobics received two or more diagnoses (Weissman et al., 1984). Depression accompanied by panic conferred the greatest risk on the child, with almost one third of the offspring of such parents receiving two or more diagnoses.

A similar degree of familial risk appears to arise from the combination of depression and panic disorder (Leckman et al., 1983). First-degree relatives of probands with major depression accompanied by either panic disorder or general anxiety disorder had twice as much major depression and twice as much alcoholism as relatives of probands with major depression alone. In contrast to Weissman et al. (1984), however, the increase in major depression in Leckman et al.'s study was associated only with the combination of major depression and panic/general anxiety disorder. Leckman et al. did not detect significant differences in the rates of depression among relatives of probands with major depression and agoraphobia. Notably, the levels of major depression and alcoholism in relatives of probands were roughly comparable for each type or combination of proband diagnosis, suggesting some possible link between the combination of proband anxiety and depression on the one hand, and the relative's combination of alcoholism and depression on the other.

Leckman et al. (1983) concluded from their investigation that panic disorders and major depression may have a common diathesis, but that such a hypothesis must be tested prospectively. The investigators also implied that the observed link between major depression in relatives and the combination of panic and major depression in probands may not necessarily be limited to combinations of affective disorders and other disorders. They noted that most studies of the impact of a single disorder on relatives employ diagnostic grouping schemes and sample selection criteria—such as exclusion of those with overlapping diagnoses—that may obscure some correlations.

Examination of the temporal relationship between panic disorders and depression further confirms the notion of a common underlying process and hence of familial risk if both disorders are present. Breier, Charney, and Heninger (1984) investigated time of onset of major depression episodes in relation to panic and agoraphobic disorders, determining that depression usually precedes panic and that a history of depression tends to aggravate the severity of the panic when it occurs. These observations, coupled with the finding that over 70 percent of the depressions were endogenous, led the researchers to refute the notion of depression as the experience of demoralizaton related to incapacitating panic in favor of a spectrum conceptualization.

Merikangas et al. (1985), who ruled out a link between primary depression and alcoholism, have raised the possibility that there may be some specificity to the transmission of a combination of disorders. They found that offspring of parents with primary affective disorder and secondary alcoholism had a five times greater risk of conduct disorder/antisocial personality than did offspring of those with depression alone. Given the observed overlap between depression and conduct disorders in prepubertal populations (Puig-Antich, 1982), this study may indeed confirm the hypothesis that a constellation of affective and other disorders in a parent may markedly increase the risk for depression in the child. Indeed, Merikangas et al. concluded that despite the small absolute number of children with conduct disorders in their study, their findings tend to support Puig-Antich's claim that conduct disorders may appear as precursors of either alcoholism or affective disorder. Puig-Antich found that one third of the boys they studied who could be designated as depressed according to RDC criteria, also fit DSM-III criteria for conduct disorder.

Perhaps, therefore, a substantial portion of those receiving a diagnosis of conduct disorder (14.3 percent of the 6 to 17 year old offspring of probands with depression and alcoholism) in the study of Merikangas et al. (1985) were actually depressed. Their findings may be particularly significant given the added risk for conduct disorder associated with each additional alcoholic parent. For example, when neither affectively ill parent received a diagnosis of alcoholism only 2.8 percent of the offspring were classified as conduct disordered/antisocial personality. One parental diagnosis of secondary alcoholism raised the rate of conduct disorder/antisocial personality to almost 10 percent of the offspring, and when both parents were diagnosed as alcoholic roughly one third of the offspring met the criteria for conduct disorder/antisocial personality.

How conduct disorders relate to depression, both at the time they are diagnosed and in their long-term prognosis, is not yet clear. If conduct disorders are viewed as nonspecific behavioral pathology or as precursors of depression, then, as Merikangas et al. (1985) note, it is unlikely that they will persist or increase into adulthood. While the rate of major depression among the offspring of those with depression and alcoholism remained roughly equal in the two age groups (6 to 17 years and 18 or more years), the rate of antisocial personality in the older age group was double that of the younger. Confirmation of the hypothesis that those with conduct disorders went on to develop antisocial personality rather than depression would require longitudinal tracking of the younger group.

The apparent ability of clustered disorders to increase the incidence of depression and depressive-like phenomena in offspring significantly above the level produced by parental depression alone raises the issue of how frequently multiple disorders or overlapping symptomatology aggregate in a single individual and within families. Many studies indicate a significant degree of coincidence between alcoholism and anxiety disorders on the one hand and depression on the other. One of the strongest relationships observed is that between anxiety disorders and depression. Breier, Charney, and Heninger (1984) studied 60 patients with agoraphobia and panic disorder and found that over two thirds had experienced an episode of major depression, most often endogenous. Almost half of the cases of depression were primary.

Leckman et al. (1983) took another perspective on the overlap between depression and anxiety disorders. They estimated that well over half of those with major depression displayed sufficient anxiety symptoms to meet DSM-III criteria for agoraphobia, panic disorder, or generalized anxiety disorder. In the overwhelming majority of cases, the investigators found that the anxiety symptoms were associated with depressive episodes. Based on these two studies, it seems reasonable to assume that a large subset of parents with anxiety disorders will also exhibit depressive symptomatology. Offspring of these parents should, therefore, be considered at risk for depression.

A somewhat smaller, but nonetheless significant, degree of overlap has been documented between alcoholism and depression. Schuckit's (1986) review of the literature estimated that between 25 and 66 percent of alcoholics suffer sufficient depressive symptomatology to interfere in their daily lives and that severe depression associated with alcoholism occurs in between 30 to 40 percent of alcoholics. Weissman and Myers (1978) reported that almost three quarters of alcoholics have another psychiatric diagnosis at some point in their lives. Most of these diagnoses involved depression. Over 40 percent of alcoholics had previously experienced a major depression at some point in their lives, 15 percent had suffered from a minor depression, 6 percent had had bipolar disorder, and slightly less than 20 percent had received an earlier diagnosis of depressive personality.

Comparable figures were reported by Bedi and Halikas (1985). When they evaluated 421 new admissions to an alcohol treatment facility, these researchers found that one third of the alcoholics had been diagnosed with an affective disorder at some point in their life. In their sample the combination of alcoholism and depression appeared prominently among women 20 to 30 years old, 60 percent of whom displayed both disorders simultaneously.

Significant as this overlap may be, the clinical course of such a depression may differ from primary depression and thus may affect children differently. Some evidence suggests that the depressions accompanying alcoholism, although severe, may remit spontaneously with sobriety. Schuckit (1986) concluded that although intense depression is very common in conjunction with heavy drinking, it is almost always a secondary depression that rarely follows the clinical course of primary depression. This view was confirmed by Dackis, Gold, Pottash, and Sweeney (1986), who found that within 2 weeks of abstinence, 80 percent of alcoholics with major depression were no longer depressed. Thus it seems that the risk to the child is a function of the chronicity of the alcoholism. In a related vein, Jacob, Dunn, and Leonard (1983) have observed that the pattern of drinking, rather than drinking per se, determined the impact of alcoholism on the family. Although the high proportion of alcoholics who also experience depression might imply that definition of the child population at risk for depression would be understated if restricted to the children of parents with depression alone, it might also be overstated if broadened to include children of all alcoholics who have received a lifetime diagnosis of depression.

Firm conclusions about the risk for depression stemming from any of the disorders thought to overlap significantly with affective disorders are not yet possible given the current state of research. Most research has focused on clinically significant cases of depression. For the most part, studies have failed to penetrate below the syndrome level to the level of symptomatology in the children they evaluate. Researchers know very little about how concurrent parental disorders within the depressive spectrum affect a child's temperamental predisposition or the attachment behaviors established between parent and child. Nor is there much evidence on how such disorders influence the child's representational capacities. More definitive conclusions will require careful, longitudinal study of the symptomatology of children whose parents have disorders thought to lie within the various conceptualizations of a depressive spectrum. Most current research has taken a snapshot of these children at a single point in time. Only by tracing the patterns of symptomatology temporally will researchers be able to discern how these disorders relate to one another and to gauge the full ramifications of these disorders for the population at risk.

Depressive Symptomatology

The evidence presented thus far clearly demonstrates a high level of full-fledged clinical depression among the children and relatives of parents who are depressed. Not surprisingly, the literature describes an even higher level of depressive symptomatology and subclinical impairment. Among 12 studies compiled using depressive symptom scales, the point prevalence of depressive symptoms ranged between 9 and 20 percent of the population (Boyd & Weissman, 1981). The presence of such symptoms may reveal early signs of depression or depressive predisposition.

The literature abounds with descriptions of both cognitive and emotional deficits in children whose parents are depressed. While none of these symptoms alone constitutes depression, considered as components of a syndrome they form part of a clinical picture that, at the very least, predisposes a child to depression. Weintraub, Winters, and Neale (1986), who found little evidence of depression that had reached significant clinical proportions, described distinctively different behavior patterns, defying a single description, among the offspring of depressed parents. The following section will describe a number of the characteristics identified by these investigators and by others. (See Table 7).

Temperament. Although temperament is generally viewed as a set of inherent genetically determined characteristics, many current researchers (Buss & Plomin, 1975; Goldsmith & Campos, 1982; Rothbart & Derryberry, 1981, 1982; Thomas & Chess, 1984) feel that these characteristics are mediated by the environment. As an infant's parents are perhaps the most salient feature of its environment, parental depression can be assumed both to be affected by, and in turn to have a strong effect on, the infant's temperament. For a parent whose functioning is already impaired by depressive disorder, coping with a temperamentally difficult child (as defined by Thomas & Chess' typology) may present overwhelming difficulties. By contrast, a child of low-intensity reactions and low activity—a portrait fitting the "slow-to-warm-up" temperament typology—would present fewer difficulties and might receive more positive affect from the parent. This smoother interaction could improve the quality of the child's attachment to the mother.

Temperament is one of the most basic indices for attempting to differentiate children of depressed and nondepressed parents. Indeed, some research suggests a correlation between parental depression, temperament, and child behavior problems at a young age. The dynamics between these factors are still unclear, although a mutually exacerbating relationship between infant temperament and maternal depression is likely. A review of the literature on postpartum depression conducted by Kraus and Redman (1986) cited potential temperamental "mismatch" as a partial

Table 7. Behavioral Features of Offspring of Maternally Depressed Compared with DSM-III Criteria

Maternal Depressed Features	DSM-III Criteria for Major Depression (1980, pp. 213-214)	DSM-III Criteria for Dysthymic Disorder (1980, pp. 222-223)
Dysphoric mood (1,2,3,4,5,6,7,8,9,10)	Dysphoric mood	Dysphoric mood
Sleep disturbances, (1,9)	Sleep disturbances	Sleep disturbances
Eating disturbances (1,2,3)	Eating disturbances	
Psychomotor agitation/retardation (1,8)	Psychomotor agitation/retardation	Psychomotor agitation/retardation
Loss of interest/pleasure in usual activities (1,4,7,9)	Loss of interest/pleasure	Loss of interest/pleasure
Decreased attention/concentration (1,2,5,7,8,9)	Cognitive disturbances	Decreased attention/concentration
Social withdrawal (1,2,4,7,8,10)		Social withdrawal
Irritability/excessive anger/aggression (1,3,4,5,6,7,8,10)		Irritability/excessive anger
Inability to respond with pleasure (4,5,10)		Inability to respond with pleasure
Tearfulness/excessive crying (3,9,10)		Tearfulness/excessive crying
Hypochondria (6,9)		Hypochondria
Suicidal ideation or behavior (9)		Suicidal ideation or behavior

Sources:
1. Anthony (1983);
2. Bemesderfer & Cohler (1983);
3. Fergusson et al. (1984);
4. Gaensbauer et al. (1978);
5. Grunebaum et al. (1978);
6. Mahler (1966);
7. Weintraub et al. (1975);
8. Weissman et al. (1972);
9. Welner et al. (1977);
10. Zahn-Waxler et al. (1984a,b).

cause of maternal depression. At the same time, preexisting maternal depression appears to contribute to temperamental difficultness and behavior problems. A longitudinal study measuring these variables at four intervals until the child was 42 months old showed that maternal depression coupled with certain temperamental profiles at 4 months of age related to behavior problems at 42 months (Wolkind & De Salis, 1982). The fact that correlations for maternal depression and child behavior problems were significant only if the child had a "difficult" or "easy" temperament at 4 months old—and not if the child was "slow to warm up"—may suggest mediation by ambivalent mother-child interaction (see Table 8).

Attachment.   Differences in attachment behavior also differentiate the children of depressed parents. For example, in a sample of 2- and 3-year-olds, Radke-Yarrow et al. (1985) found more than twice as many children of parents with major depression had insecure attachments compared with children with clinically normal parents or parents with mild depression. Gaensbauer et al. (1984) found similarly disturbed attachment behavior among even younger offspring of depressed parents. This team compared a control group against seven male infants at 12, 15, and 18 months of age. Each proband had one bipolar parent—four mothers and three fathers. Although in the first evaluation none of the probands, and one control behaved negatively toward the mother, an increasing number of probands displayed such negativism by the third evaluation at 18 months. By then, three probands and no controls were seen as negative.

This progressive pattern was reflected in the infants' Ainsworth classifications. Among probands, more than half (four) received a classification of "insecure" attachment at 15 months and almost all (six) were so classified by 18 months. Half as many of the controls received such Ainsworth classifications at 18 months, making the differences in attachment at 18 months significant between probands and controls.

Given the disordered nature of the attachment behavior of the offspring of the depressed, it is not surprising that such infants frequently fail to seek the kind of support that other infants typically seek from their caregiver. Zahn-Waxler, Cummings, McKnew, and Radke-Yarrow (1984) have observed that when confronted with the distress of another, the infants of bipolar families were significantly less likely to use their caregiver as a source of direction and reassurance. Difficulties in prosocial functioning also extended to relationships with peers in this study, with children of bipolar parents showing significantly less altruism to their peers. Thus the portrait painted is one of extreme difficulty in regulating the emotions arising from interactions with both adults and peers.

Despite this evidence and the plausibility of a link between episodic parental impairments and insecure attachment, Naslund, Persson-Blennow, McNeil, Kaij, and Malmquist-Larsson (1984) introduced contradictory

Table 8. *Dimensions of Temperament Compared with Offspring of Maternally Depressed*

Maternal Depressed Profile	Thomas, Chess, Birch, Hertzig and Korn (1963)	Buss and Plomin (1975)	Rothbart (1981)
Dysphoric mood (1,2,3,4,5,6,7,8,9,10)	Adaptability Approach/withdrawal Mood	Emotionality Impulsivity	Smiling and laughter Fear Distress to limitations
Sleep disturbances (1,9)	Rhythmicity	Activity	Activity level Duration of orienting
Eating disturbances (1,2,3)	Rhythmicity	Sociability	Smiling and laughter Fear
Decreased attention/concentration (1,2,5,7,8,9)	Activity level Attention span/persistence	Emotionality Sociability	Duration of orienting Smiling and laughter
Social withdrawal (1,2,4,7,8,10)	Approach/withdrawal Mood	Emotionality Sociability Emotionality Sociability	Smiling and laughter Distress to limitations Soothability
Loss of interest/pleasure in usual activities (1,4,7,9)	Approach/withdrawal Mood Attention span/persistence	Emotionality Sociability	Smiling and laughter Soothability
Irritability/Excessive anger/ aggression (1,3,4,5,6,7,8,10)	Intensity Adaptability Mood	Activity	Activity level
Inability to respond with pleasure (4,5,10)	Intensity Mood	Emotionality Sociability	Smiling and laughter Distress to limitations
Psychomotor agitation/ retardation (1,8)	Activity level Approach/withdrawal Intensity Attention span/persistence	Sociability	Fear Duration of orienting
Tearfulness/excessive crying (3,9,10)	Intensity Mood	Sociability Impulsivity	Smiling and laughter Duration of orienting
Avoidant/anxiously attached (1,4,6)	Approach/withdrawal		
Communication problems (2,5,7,10)	Approach/withdrawal Intensity		
Hypochondria (6,9)			
Suicidal ideation or behavior (9)			

Sources:
1. Anthony (1983);
2. Bemesderfer & Cohler (1983);
3. Fergusson et al (1984);
4. Gaensbauer et al (1984);
5. Grunebaum et al (1978);
6. Mahler (1966);
7. Weintraub et al (1975);
8. Weissman et al (1972);
9. Welner et al (1977);
10. Zahn-Waxler et al (1984 a.b.).

evidence using a modified version of the Strange Situation Procedure. Their data show that "anxious" attachment among 1-year-old children of cycloid and affective psychotics was either equal to or less frequent than anxious attachment among a matched control group. More than three quarters of children with cycloid or affective psychotic parents had secure attachments—a level which the authors note exceeds the percentage (66 percent) of securely attached infants that Ainsworth (1971, 1973) found in her samples. Notably, the only infants demonstrating significantly higher levels of anxious attachment than their controls were those with schizophrenic parents. Even when the researchers reassigned certain subjects to different classification groups using RDC guidelines, they found that more than half of the offspring of schizophrenics showed anxious attachment compared with only about 10 percent of the children of affectives. Compelling as their observations may appear, Naslund et al.'s findings remain in the minority.

In the context of attachment studies, some investigators have also examined other aspects of children's interactional development. Observation of the infants' emotional regulation also revealed discernible differences between offspring of depressed and normal children according to Gaensbauer et al. (1984). Overall, the infants of depressed parents showed dampened affect and less flexible responses. Maladaptive affective patterns progressed, in a similar manner to affiliative behavior, over the course of the experiment. At 12 months, fear and sadness among the probands distinguished them from the controls during the lower-stress periods (i.e. free play and reunion with the mother). Fear and sadness among controls was not only less pervasive in an absolute sense, but diminished quickly on reunion with the mother. By 15 months, in situations where probands would have been expected to show a high level of fear during separation, they instead displayed less fear than controls, suggesting a dampening of affect. Probands also showed greater stress than controls in both low-stress free play with the mother and during higher-stress testing at 18 months.

Evidence of emotional dysregulation in the context of parent–child interactions may surface even in early infancy, as the research of Field et al. (1985) discloses. Analysis of face-to-face interactions of the 3- to 5-month-old infants of postpartum depressed and nondepressed mothers revealed that those with depressed mothers had a less optimal state, characterized by frequent drowsiness. They also relaxed less, exhibited fewer contented expressions, and fussed more than infants of mothers who did not experience postpartum depression. Depressed mothers also described their infants' moods as being more labile. Again, however, the investigators underscored the uncertainty surrounding the direction of the causal relationship between infant and maternal behavior. They questioned whether the mothers' observed lack of contingent behavior was provoked by their own depression or by the lability of their infants' emotions.

Burland (1986) taps the infants' internal experiences well, writing that:

In observations of mother-infant pairs of this kind, one sees little in the way of a social smile and no specific smiling response. Eye contact between the two is fleeting at best, if not altogether absent. There is little 'dialogue'; the mutual cueing, the sensitivity to each other's rhythms is strikingly absent. In severe instances it is as though the mother does not exist for the infant, who remains promiscuous in his equal responsiveness to anyone who offers to meet his immediate needs. . . . The babies show litle joy, and little evidence of an early structuralization polarity based on pleasure versus unpleasure; . . . they are either apathetic and vacant, or in distress. . . . There is little evidence that internal images are being elaborated; that is, others are not related to in a recognizably differentiated manner, and self-stimulation lacks the consistent pattern that would speak of some degree of organization of internal experiences. (p. 327)

Self-Representation. Interactions with the external world of objects serve as the medium through which infants and children define themselves as separate and unique beings. The process begins early in infancy, with the mother's ministrations helping infants form a sense of the continuity. Responsive caregiving and the development of neurologic structures facilitate the development of memory traces containing sequences of events and responses, most notably the sequence of hunger, satiation, and bliss. With the additional recognition and anticipation that these memory traces help to build, infants assume a more active participation in their interactions with caregivers and begin to construct the sense of personal agency that is critical for a stable self-concept (Burland, 1986). Interactions with the caregiver sharpen perceptual abilities and further help young infants demarcate themselves from objects in their environment. By the middle of the first year infants will shift from coenesthetic to diacritic responsiveness. Throughout the next 2 years of life, caregivers serve as a fulcrum, enabling infants to explore their environment and elaborate their internal images of objects and themselves. The inner resources marshalled through their explorations during the first year and a half of life help infants negotiate successfully through the rapprochement crisis and continue on the route to object constancy and, ultimately, self-constancy (Trad, 1986).

The self is thus sculpted, both directly and indirectly, from the mother-infant relationship. To the extent that infants are deprived of this relationship, self-development can be expected to suffer. Evidence of such deficits among the offspring of the depressed is based largely on clinical observation rather than empirical study. Burland (1986), who has studied many children suffering from the kind of maternal deprivation not uncommon among the offspring of the depressed, has cited failure to achieve self/object differentiation and constancy as one of the four salient characteristics of these children. According to Burland's observations, "hatching"—the process by which infants emerge from what the researcher refers to as the autistic shell and adapt to the impingements of the environment—may be delayed or absent. Thus these infants may encounter difficulty in consolidating their physical—much less their psychological—separateness. Such infants often fail to develop fully elaborated and stable internal images of others and themselves. As a result, Burland has found that many children who have suffered maternal deprivation falter in the face of the rapprochement crisis, the first major test of their ability to surmount the fears associated with the awareness of their separateness. Their inability to resolve the ambivalence of the rapprochement crisis may prolong, if not entrench, the naturally occurring (and, under normal circumstances, naturally disappearing) depression often observed during this developmental period.

Aggression. Not surprisingly, the constellation of emotional deficits frequently encountered among the offspring of depressed parents often leads to a variety of maladaptive interpersonal interactions, including conduct disturbances and aggression (Decina et al., 1983; Weissman et al., 1984; Welner, Welner, McCravy, & Leonard, 1977). The clinical observations of Burland (1986) confirm the prominence of aggression in the constellation of symptomatology presented by maternally deprived children who seem incapable of neutralizing the phallic aggressiveness that Burland describes as a compensation for a depressive core. Writing of the children he has observed, Burland says

> *Almost all activities are destructive. . . . It is a chilling experience being in a playroom with several of these mother-infant pairs: there is no joy whatsoever; play activity is markedly destructive, the toys and furniture broken and scattered; the only verbalizations are angry, with people screaming past one another, ignoring what others say. It is a Pinteresque scene. (p. 327)*

The prevalence of aggression and a host of related behaviors among the offspring of the depressed has been demonstrated empirically in two investigations by Zahn-Waxler et al. (1984a, b). The first study focused exclusively on the children of bipolar parents. These children, studied longitudinally at the ages 1 year and between 2 and 2.5, were measured for aggression, altruism, social interactions, and emotional expressiveness. Aggression appeared to dominate these children's behavior when compared with that of a control group. Their aggression was both more persistent and more intense than that of the offspring of nondepressed parents. Moreover, aggression was directed both at the unfamiliar adult in the testing situation and at their peers. At the same time, however, these children typically adopted a passive role when they were the object of aggression. Separation from their mothers, in particular, appeared likely to provoke aggressive responses in these children.

In their second study, Zahn-Waxler et al. (1984b) expanded on their original work and uncovered important variations not only between children of normal and bipolar parents, but also in the conduct profiles of children whose parents have different affective disorders. They found that, in fact, of the three groups of children under study—control, bipolar, and unipolar offspring—bipolar offspring were the most likely to be aggressive toward the experimenter. Children of unipolar depressed mothers were less likely, even than control children, to show aggression toward peers.

Other Emotional Symptoms.   Higher levels of anxiety, whether in the form of separation anxiety or various phobias, have been rigorously documented among children of the affectively ill (Weissman et al., 1984). According to Weissman et al.'s data, although depression alone does not confer greater risk for anxiety in children, depression accompanied by agoraphobia or panic produced especially high levels of separation anxiety in offspring. For example, more than one third of the children of parents with depression and panic disorder developed separation anxiety. None of the children of normal parents displayed separation anxiety in the reseachers' best-estimate of DSM-III diagnoses. Over 10 percent of children with depressive and agoraphobic parents received diagnoses of separation anxiety and/or social phobia.

Inordinate preoccupation with pain in others also seems to typify children of depressed parents, as Zahn-Waxler et al. (1984a) observed. While control children often turned away from others in distress, conflict appeared to engage the sensitivities of children with depressed parents. Despite their seeming absorption in others' distress, the offspring of depressed parents exhibited less altruistic behavior than might be anticipated by Hoffman's (1977, 1982b) model of empathic development. Possibly the degree of distress experienced by these children disables this response function. The offspring of the bipolar parents were not only unable to find a constructive outlet for their distress while in the midst of a stressful situation, but—notwithstanding their heightened upset in stressful testing situations—they found greater difficulty than controls in returning to a pleasurable state after the cause for distress disappeared. The rigid, inflexible responses that the offspring of the depressed develop may inhibit them from developing adaptive strategies for coping with aversive circumstances. As the authors note, emotional dysregulation of the type displayed by such children may thus predispose them to a learned-helpless form of behavior characteristic of depression.

There may be important differences in the ways parental subtypes of depression affect offspring's emotional regulation. Children of unipolar parents impressed the researchers as somewhat more controlled in their expression of upset than did the offspring of other parents, particularly the bipolar probands, whom the researchers characterized as emotionally dysregulated.

Cognitive Deficits. Deficits in many facets of emotional development clearly mark the children of the affectively disordered. However, these deficits do not exhaust the list of repercussions of parental depression. Investigators have commonly observed cognitive deficits, especially attention deficits among the children of depressed parents. In the Gaensbauer et al. (1984) study, 18-month–olds evaluated with the Strange Situation maintained less interest in toys during periods of frustration and on reunion with the mother. Cohler et al. (1977) demonstrated that such children (ages 5 to 6 years) showed greater intellectual impairment and inability to attend to a task than children of schizophrenic or well mothers. Although they found no significant differences in attention between children of schizophrenic and depressive psychotics, Gamer et al. (1977) revealed that the children of the psychiatrically impaired group as a whole performed more poorly on measures of attention than children of well mothers. Weissman et al. (1984) found that over 10 percent of the children (ages 6 to 17 years) of parents with major depression had attention deficit disorders. These deficits revealed themselves particularly strongly when complex and difficult tasks were involved. Decina et al. (1983) also commented on such deficits among children of bipolar parents. Notably, the attention deficits observed by Decina et al. occurred among the children not diagnosed as clinically impaired.

Summary. Overall, Kauffman et al. (1979) has characterized the offspring population of depressed mothers as generally less competent in many spheres of functioning. Ranking children on social functioning in relation to children of mothers with other types of mental illness, they found that five of the six least competent had mothers who were depressed. In summarizing the clinical data on those proband children in their study who had not received a formal psychiatric diagnosis, Decina et al. (1983) described them as characterized by

> *extroversion with expansiveness leading to grandiosity; excitability; exhibitionism; need for constant attention and admiration; need for constant reassurance; separation anxiety; and disturbances in interpersonal functioning with overdependency, lack of empathy, and egocentrism. (p. 549)*

RISK FACTORS FOR DEPRESSION

Embedded with many of the aggregate measures for prevalence of depression among the children of depressed parents lie important trends revealing a differential impact of this phenomenon on specific types of families. Not every depressed parent passes this depression on to his or her child. Measurement of risk factors permits understanding of why one child at risk develops the disorder and another does not. However, it is perplexing to speak of risk factors without simultaneously offering explanations for how depression in one generation seems to produce high levels of depression in the next. Accordingly, this section will present a brief review of the epidemiological evidence on specific risk factors.

The derivative nature of the risk presented to the child—that is, the risk that a parent will develop depression and the risk that the depression will filter down to the child—often makes it confusing to isolate only those risk factors that heighten offspring risk. Clearly factors that increase risk to parents enlarge the risk to which children are exposed. However, not all risk factors for parental depression translate into risk for the child. The literature tends to obscure this important distinction. Weissman et al. (1984), however, have applied great rigor to the process of identifying specifically those factors pertaining to a parent's illness that present risk to offspring. These researchers identified four factors found to contribute to significantly greater incidences of major depression or other DSM-III diagnosis in the child of a depressed parent: (1) early onset of the parent's depression, (2) increased numbers of first-degree relatives with depression, (3) increased number of relatives with other psychopathology, and (4) marital instability or death of a spouse.

These observations have gained additional support in the literature. In another family study, focusing on first-degree relatives rather than exclusively on children of depressed probands, Weissman and another group of colleagues (Weissman, Wickramaratne, et al., 1984) found increased risk associated with early onset depression. They observed that the risk of major depression in relatives of those whose depression began before age 20, was greater than three times that of control relatives. If the depression began after the age of 40, however, the risk to relatives dropped more than 50 percent. Kuyler, Rosenthal, Igel, Dunner, and Fieve (1980) also showed that divorce predicted higher levels of psychopathology in the children of bipolar parents.

Interestingly, the severity of a parent's psychopathology does not appear to increase the risk of depression among children. Although they caution about drawing firm conclusions from their relatively small sample of bipolar offspring, Kuyler et al. (1980) did not detect significant differences among more severe cases (defined as Bipolar I) of bipolar disorder. A lack of correlation between severity of parental illness and development of depression in relatives has also been observed for unipolar depression. Price et al. (1984), who used melancholia as an index of severity, determined that the morbidity risk for unipolar depression among relatives of nonmelancholic individuals exceeded the risk of morbidity for relatives of melancholics.

It is not yet known whether different types of depressive disorders present variant degrees of risk—for the same disorder or for other disorders—within the general contours described by researchers such as Weissman et al.

Epidemiologic research to date falls short in its treatment of risk factors specifically associated with different subtypes of parental affective illness. As indicated, there appears to be a certain amount of diagnostic specificity in the passage of types of depression between generations, implying different risk factors for different depressive disorders. Indeed, Leckman et al. (1984) reported in a family study that different degrees of risk were associated with different subtypes of nonbipolar depression among first-degree relatives of probands with major depression. Unfortunately, while epidemiologic research on adults has developed an ample literature on different risk factors for bipolar and unipolar disorders, little research is available specifically on children—perhaps because of the comparative rarity of bipolar disorder in all but the oldest members of this age group. Thus most epidemiological studies attempting to identify risk factors in children either ignore the specific depressive diagnosis of the parent or examine only children of parents with a particular disorder.

Developmentally oriented research on the risks arising from parental depression is also hampered by the lack of comparative data on the prevalence of depression and depressive symptomatology among high-risk children in different age groups. Continued controversy about the existence of prepubertal depression may be largely responsible for this lack of data. The absence of such information, however, makes it difficult to determine whether children of different ages and at different developmental levels face variant degrees of risk from their parent's disorder.

EXPLANATORY MODELS

Measures of depression, depressive symptomatology, and other deficits provide convincing support for a strong relationship between parental depression and depression in offspring. But one major piece of this puzzle still remains unsolved: Specifically, how are depression and depressive-like phenomena conveyed from one generation to the next?

The high degree of family clustering in depression makes it tempting to attribute the phenomenon's apparent transmission to genetic factors. However, families share not only genes, but common environments as well. Most research suggests that a dynamic combination of genetic and environmental factors coalesces in cases of children of depressed parents who themselves display signs of depression. This section will outline the evidence in favor of both genetic and environmental theories.

Genetic Theories of Depression

Morbidity risk estimates for depression—which, as we have seen, are higher for children of depressed parents than for children of other parents—do not, by themselves, verify that a genetic factor operates. Far too frequently, research has relied on such specious reasoning either explicitly or implicitly. Proving genetic hypotheses requires the identification of an experimental mechanism to control for genetic similarities and differences. Studies of twins and adopted children traditionally have been employed for this purpose. When researchers detect a higher concordance between the rates of disorder among monozygotic (MZ) than among dizygotic (DZ) twins, they typically interpret this finding as evidence of genetic contribution for a particular disorder. (A higher MZ concordance for one disorder over another, when DZ concordance is comparable, implies greater genetic involvement in that disorder.) Similarly, researchers often stress genetic explanations when it is determined that the biological parents of adopted children with disorders display greater rates of disorder than adoptive parents.

Twin and adoptive studies of affective disorders are still too few, and the literature is far richer for bipolar disorders than for unipolar depression. A recent adoption study—a technique particularly effective in isolating genetic from environmental influences—by Cadoret, O'Gorman, Heywood, and Troughton (1985) failed to demonstrate a significant genetic contribution to affective disorders and suggested that environmental factors occurring prior to adulthood have a more significant impact on the risk for depression. To the extent that genetics are a factor in transmitting affective disorders, their role appears to be greater in bipolar, than in unipolar, depression.

Results of a study performed by Conners, Himmelhock, Goyette, Ulrich, and Neil (1979)—although not a twin or adoption study—demonstrate a stronger genetic influence for bipolar than for unipolar disorder. A recent review of the literature conducted by Mahmood et al. (1983) also confirms the widely held view that genetic factors exercise a stronger role in transmission of bipolar disorder than unipolar depression. Indeed the limited evidence on genetics in bipolar disorder reveals a significant genetic influence. Gershon et al. (1976) established a concordance rate of almost five times higher for bipolar disorder among MZ twins than among DZ twins. Both the MZ twins had bipolar disorder in almost 70 percent of the 91 pairs studied. By contrast, less than 15 percent of the 226 pairs of DZ twins studied had bipolar disorders. With reference to the specific transmission mechanism, Fieve, Mendlewicz, and Fleiss (1973) suggest a relationship between bipolar disorder and the Xg blood group marker a genetic marker—located on the X chromosome.

One of the few adoption studies investigating bipolar disorder among the biological and adoptive parents of adoptees showed a significant genetic contribution to bipolar disorder (Mendlewicz & Rainer, 1977). The study, performed in Belgium because of the availability of adoption registers, found higher levels of bipolar disorder in biological parents of adoptees than in their adoptive parents. While only one of the adoptive parents of 29 bipolar adoptees was diagnosed as bipolar, four of the biological parents received such a diagnosis. Notably, however, biological parents of the bipolar probands showed even higher levels of unipolar disorder than of bipolar disorder—suggesting a nondiagnostic specific genetic factor. Biological parents of bipolar adoptees still showed higher levels of psychopathology (albeit unipolar disorder) than adoptive parents, only half as many of whom had a diagnosed case of unipolar depression. These findings would be consistent with the multiple-threshold hypothesis in which bipolar and unipolar disorders are thought to exist on a single continuum of severity in the degree of risk they present (Baron, Klotz, Mendlewicz, & Rainer, 1981).

A shortage of twin and adoption data for probands with unipolar depression makes an assessment of the genetic influence in this disorder tentative at best. The two studies reviewed in Mahmood et al.'s (1983) survey of genetic studies in affective and anxiety disorders, (Allen, 1976; Bertelsen et al., 1977), both show higher concordance among MZ than DZ unipolar depressives, suggesting a genetic contribution to unipolar disorder. Nonetheless, these studies show that genetic factors do not seem to weigh as heavily in unipolar disorder as in bipolar. While DZ twins in Bertelsen et al. showed similar concordance rates, concordance for MZ bipolars was half as much as for MZ unipolars. Allen's (1976) review of nine twin studies in affective illness arrived at comparable results. When he calculated concordance rates of all twins in the studies, he showed comparable DZ concordance for unipolar and bipolar disorder, but almost twice the rate of MZ concordance for bipolar than for unipolar MZ twins. Notably, the levels of concordance for DZ twins (14 percent for bipolar and 11 percent for unipolar disorder) roughly match those of Bertelsen et al. (17 percent for bipolar and 19 percent for unipolar), as do the concordance levels for MZ twins (72 percent for bipolar disorder and 40 percent for unipolar in Allen's review versus 74 percent and 43 percent for Bertelsen et al.'s bipolar and unipolar MZ twins).

Temperament studies offer further insights into the modes whereby depression may be influenced genetically. A number of researchers conceive of temperament as based on heritable characteristics (Allport, 1937; Buss & Plomin, 1975; Rothbart & Derryberry, 1982; Thomas & Chess, 1980). As outlined earlier, an infant may be at risk by virtue of being temperamentally predisposed to depressive disorders when in an environment that includes parental depression. Although temperament, viewed in this light, may introduce a genetic risk factor if it is accompanied by a depressive environment, this is not equivalent to saying that the infant is predisposed to depression with respect to temperament alone (Trad, 1986).

Environmental Theories

Depressive disorders, although widespread, often remain untreated. Even when they are treated, hospitalization is infrequent. Individuals with depressive disorders typically remain with their families, thus exposing offspring to changes of mood, emotional dysregulation, and potential impairments in parenting. Given the continued interaction between a child and his or her depressed parent, it is not surprising that research has taken a great interest in how parent-child relations may lead to depression in the child.

Two hypotheses, each with variations on a basic model, have attempted to examine childhood depression as a function of the parent-child interaction. One general theory suggests that parental depression passes directly to the child through mechanisms such as mirroring and empathy. The other theory implicates impaired parental functioning over any specific parental diagnosis. This latter theory posits a less direct chain of causality in which parental incompetence leads to developmental deficits in the child, and these deficits in turn produce depression. This section will explore each of these basic models.

Mirroring. The sharing or communication of affect between parent and child may provide an important medium through which young children, even infants, can experience depression. Although experimental research has documented this process in a number of ways, relatively little research has dealt exclusively with the transmission of depressed affect to children. One study that observed the sharing of affect between young infants and their mothers suggested that depression among some infants may reflect a mirroring of their depressed mothers' behaviors (Field, 1984a). By comparing the interactions of dyads with depressed and nondepressed mothers, the researcher found that changes in a mother's behavior elicited changes in the infant's behavior, while continuity in maternal behavior predicted continuity in the infant. Field observed three mother-child interactions. During the first and third interaction mothers were instructed to act spontaneously. In the second interactive sequence, however, mothers were told to act depressed by gazing directly and without expression at the infant, speaking in a monotone and minimizing body movement. Those infants with nondepressed mothers reacted with greater protest to the change in maternal behavior, while infants of depressed mothers showed remarkable continuity—perhaps because they had grown accustomed to their mother's depressed affect. Field suggests that the different response of the infants may indicate mirroring, that is, behavior reflecting the infant's internalization of its mother's passive, depressed interactional style. Since the mirroring theory relies only on the ability of the infant to imitate its parent, its strength lies in its ability to predict depression even in early infancy.

Mirroring may also occur in cognitive rather than affective style as a recent study on school-age children's attributional style suggests (Seligman, Peterson, Kaslow, Tanenbaum, Alloy, & Abramson, 1984). This study, one of the first to apply the learned helplessness model of depression to school-age children, sought to determine whether children's attributional styles corresponded to the debilitated style that learned helplessness theorists have found among adults. In addition, by comparing the attributional style and depressive symptomatology of parents and children, the study attempted to assess whether children learn their attributional style from their parents. Findings revealed that the children's explanations for bad events correlated significantly with those of their mothers and that the children's depressive symptoms also correlated significantly with those of their mothers. These findings led the authors to suggest that depressed mothers may transmit a depressive cognitive style to their children.

The Role of Empathy. Mirroring implies similarities in the behaviors of parent and child. But transmission of depression may not actually require faithful duplication of the parent's depressed interactional style. Instead, transmission may occur through a process sometimes described as empathic contagion whereby parent and child share psychic states, although not necessarily similar behaviors. Theories such as secondary intersubjectivity (Trevarthen & Hubley, 1978) and affect attunement (Stern, 1984) describe a general process by which the parent's affect informs the infant of the parent's affective state and manipulates the affect of the infant. These theories can be applied to an understanding of the transmission of depression between parent and child (Trad, 1986).

Although secondary intersubjectivity applies largely to the realm of motivation, and affect attunement refers to affects and emotions, they share an underlying mechanism that may be responsible for transmitting depression. Trevarthen and Hubley (1978) describe secondary intersubjectivity, the first signs of which can be discerned at about 9 months, as "a deliberately sought sharing of experiences about events and things for the first time" (p. 184). Beginning at this time, the infant's intentions, as reflected in movement and communication, reveal a new orientation toward others. Infants begin to discover not only that they have a mental self as well as a physical self, but also that others have mental selves distinct from their own. Indeed, at this developmental stage infants realize that the two mental selves can be interfaced. This cognitive realization forms the basis of empathy which, in turn, serves as a channel through which depression may travel from parent to child.

Hoffman (1984) posits that empathic distress can precede recognition of others as distinct entities. He writes:

> *Infants can probably experience empathic distress through one or more of the simpler arousal modes (e.g., conditioning, mimicry) long before they acquire a sense of others as distinct physical entities. Through much of the first year, . . . witnessing someone in distress probably results in a global empathic response. . . Since the infants cannot yet differentiate themselves from the other, they must . . . be unclear as to who is experiencing any distress that they witness and they may at times behave as though what is happening to the other is happening to them. (pp. 111-112)*

This notion of empathic distress offers an alternative explanation for the results in Field's (1984a) study. For the very young, there may be no shield against the experience of another's distressed emotional state. Throughout the early years of a child's life, empathy becomes more differentiated and more mature, eventually including a sympathetic as well as an empathic component.

Although as yet little research supports the application of these theories to the intergenerational transmission of depression, studies in children revealing high levels of preoccupation with others' pain (Zahn-Waxler et al., 1984b) can be viewed as partial support for this theory.

Impaired Parenting.   With processes such as empathic contagion, we might expect most of the children of depressed parents to become depressed. In fact, most do not. This does not diminish the potentially harmful impact of parental depression. Rather, it suggests that in the future, predictive models should focus on the early impact of parent-child interaction as it affects the broader indices of child competence—cognitive and emotional—influencing the longer-term development of depression. Models implicating parental impairment generally, rather than a specific diagnosis, take this approach. Such studies focus on the impact of parental depression on the child's ability to experience certain emotions and perceptions thought to be essential for establishing a sense of mastery and competence in its environment. According to this theory, unresponsive, detached, or helpless parenting, which is the likely product of depression (Bromet & Cornely, 1984; Crook, Raskin, & Eliot, 1981; Davenport, Zahn-Waxler, Adland, & Mayfield, 1984; Susman, Trickett, Ianotti, Hollenbeck, & Zahn-Waxler, 1985; Weissman, Paykel, and Klerman, 1972), deprive children of the building blocks of mastery, thereby rendering them more likely to develop depression whether in childhood or subsequently.

Three avenues of investigation—the impact of depression on attention, emotional regulation, and attachment formation—have figured prominently into this model because of their links to early development of mastery (Fisher, Harder, & Kokes, 1980; Gamer et al., 1977; Kauffman et al., 1979; Zahn-Waxler et al., 1984). Although these investigations focus on different measures, they all point to diminished competence in the offspring of depressed parents—despite potentially higher levels of innate competence, such as IQ (Fisher et al., 1980). Unable to elicit predictable responses from their parents, to persist in the face of distress, and to seek parental support under such circumstances, these children may slowly acquire a helpless response to the demands of development. Indeed, as Kashani et al. (1985) note, the high level of anxiety found among these children, may reflect their inability to exercise control over threats in their environment. Weintraub, Winters, and Neale (1986) have implicated diminished social and cognitive competence as a cause, rather than a product, of depression.

Emde and Sorce's concept of "maternal referencing" (1983) provides a useful theoretical framework in which to understand how parental depression can set the stage for childhood depression. They described the process as "the infant's developing capacity to make use of the mother's emotional signals to guide exploration and learning." According to the authors, infants use facial patterns for regulating their own behavior and emotions. Dampened maternal affect or lack of emotional availability as a result of depression can therefore deprive a child of important regulatory devices. For example, a child trying to express happiness to its mother, but reading sadness in her expressions, can become confused about his or her own internal state and ability to communicate that state. Since the child expects the mother to greet smiles with positive affects, a saddened affect would violate this expectancy and cause the child to experience a lack of control. Zahn-Waxler et al. (1984a) write of unpredictability and emotional dysregulation experienced by children of both unipolar and bipolar depressives. Depressed mothers, who have been described as helpless in child care, irritable, uninvolved, and unaffectionate (Weissman, Paykel, & Klerman, 1972), can thus foster noncontingency in their infants, making it difficult for their offspring to draw on their own resources in responding to developmental tasks such as attachment formation. Withdrawal and perhaps isolation—the potential upshot of an inability to form secure attachments—can thus augment the original sense of helplessness. Indeed, as we have seen, children of depressed parents exhibit significantly greater than normal levels of insecure attachments.

It is tempting, but unfair, to focus entirely on parental impairment in functioning as the precipitant of a chain of events that threaten an infant's ability to build mastery and establish secure attachments—in short, to bolster the self against the possible development of depression. An infant's temperament may also exert a strong influence on the parent-child interaction. A difficult temperament may elicit a depressive response from a competent parent seeking but failing to relieve a difficult infant's seeming distress. Incompetence in the parent can only aggravate this situation. Inability to offer comfort to a fussy child may further reinforce a preexisting parental sense of futility.

Table 9. Offspring of Depressed Mothers Compared with Three Risk Populations

Abuse/Neglect	Hospitalization	Handicapped
Offspring of depressed parents are more likely to be maltreated (5,9,11,12,13,16)	Hospitalized child is at greater risk with an emotionally disturbed parent (15)	Parents of handicapped children are more likely to be depressed (4,6,7)
Both maltreating parent and maltreated child are likely depressed (2)	Depressed mothers have better chance of recovery if not separated from infants (8)	Parents of handicapped children show more depressive symptoms, but not more MDD (3)
Parent degree of psychopathology affects perception of child difficulty (10)		Parents of handicapped children experience heightened stress (1)
Brain-damaged parents are more likely to maltreat their children (14)		
Depressed mothers show a "dampening" of behavior, with greater risk of neglect; and they continue to have difficulty with child after recovery (17,18)		

Sources:
1. Bernheimer, Young, & Winton (1983);
2. Bible & French (1979);
3. Breslau & Davis (1985);
4. Burden (1980);
5. Conger et al. (1981);
6. Cummings (1976);
7. Cummings, Bayley, & Rie (1966);
8. Douglas (1956);
9. Ebeling & Hill (1975);
10. Estroff et al. (1984);
11. Galdston (1965);
12. Johnson & Morse (1968);
13. Kaplan et al. (1983);
14. Lezak (1978);
15. Mason (1965):
16. Steele & Pollack (1968);
17. Weissman et al. (1972);
18. Weissman & Paykel (1974).

Whatever the causes, many studies have found attention deficits, insecure attachment, and overall lack of competence in mastering challenges from the environment among the children of depressed parents. What is notable, however, is the remarkable similarity these children have to the children of parents with other types of mental illness. This finding seems to support the view that parental impairment generally, rather than a specific type of impairment, can heighten a child's risk for depression. Indeed, Gamer et al. (1977) found no differences between diagnostic groups on measures of attention, but did find distinctions between high-risk and control children.

This view finds further support in the studies that show a higher risk to children whose parents had early onset of depression (Weissman et al., 1984). If parental depression coincides with the critical developmental period when the infant first begins to establish mastery over his or her environment, it may threaten the child's development. In this context, postpartum depression may present an especially serious risk to the child. Unfortunately, epidemiological data on the risk factors to children do not yet provide much information on the sources of depression among the group of parents whose comparatively early onset of disorder may correlate with higher risk to their children. (See Table 9, which provides a comparison with the other three populations at risk.)

CONCLUSION

Parental psychopathology represents the quintessential risk factor for infant and childhood depression. Not only has evidence demonstrated that depressed caregivers can induce psychopathology in their offspring by emitting particular behaviors and functioning in a distinctive manner in the environment, but recent data also reveal that depression may be transmitted to children by genetic mechanisms. The chapter has explored several previously omitted examples of maternal depression, including premenstrual dysphoric change, postpartum depression, and seasonal affective disorder, and advocates that therapists acquaint parents with the affects such psychopathology can have on offspring, particularly young infants.

CHAPTER SEVEN

Abuse and Neglect as Risk Factors for Infant and Childhood Depression

As a population at risk for developing depression, infants and children who have been abused and/or neglected are in a particularly poignant situation. In these children, the precise emblems of psychopathology—either in the form of physical injuries and scars or organic wasting—are painfully evident. Unlike a handicapping condition or a hospitalization experience, virtually no single factor can be found in a case of abuse and/or neglect. Within such a population, the therapist can only hope that the incident was too fleeting to leave an indelible mark or that the infant had sufficiently developed resources to bolster him or her against the onslaught of such treatment.

Tracing the etiology of depression in an infant or child who has been a victim of abuse/neglect is not difficult. First, such behavior can interfere with the exhibition of what would be normal temperamental displays in another situation. Abuse from a primary caregiver will also warp the dyadic interaction between parent and child, generating an attachment which is characteristically either avoidant or resistant. Finally, this behavior will have an inevitable effect on the infant's incipient sense of self, resulting most likely in a deficit of self-esteem (Trad, 1986).

The model of learned helplessness depression should be discussed in this context. Infants and children confront extreme examples of noncontingency each time they undergo an episode of abuse/neglect. As with the population of offspring of depressed caregivers, these infants and children face a confusing dilemma: Are they responsible for the abuse or is the abuse/neglect merely one facet of an incomprehensible universe? Perceptions of this type are likely to be incorporated into the self-concept and are virtually identical to the self-esteem deficits described in cases of full-fledged learned helplessness depression.

Approximately 25 percent of American families are at risk for abuse. Many factors, which are explored in depth in this chapter, contribute to this alarmingly high potential for domestic violence. When this potential materializes into overt abuse or neglect, virtually every aspect of the child's early development is affected. Abuse and neglect leave indelible imprints on the child's temperament and sense of object relations, as well as on the child's empathic development and capacity for self-representation. The physical repercussions, dramatic as they may be, may not betray the extent of psychological damage caused by abuse and neglect. According to some studies, abuse and neglect are the primary causes—with the exception of loss or separation from a mother figure—of childhood depression (Blumberg, 1981; Garbarino, 1977; Wolfe, 1985). Therefore any discussion of infant and childhood depression would be incomplete without a thorough examination of abuse and neglect.

This chapter is devoted to such an analysis. Before investigating the varied causes of abuse/neglect, however, a working definition of both phenomena, coupled with an assessment of the scope and severity of abuse, will be proposed. The chapter will then review the depressive symptomatology that has been observed in abused /neglected children. This review will serve as a basis for theories about the mechanisms whereby maltreatment of children often culminates in depression or depressive-like phenomena. Finally, the chapter will present four different explanatory models—the sociological model, the psychiatric model, the transactional model, and the ecological model—and isolate factors that, by creating risk for maltreatment, also enhance the risk for depression.

One cautionary note is necessary. Understanding abuse and neglect, and their relationship to depression, presents the researcher with one of the most perplexing cause–effect analyses in psychiatric epidemiology. Clearly many of the effects of abuse, such as childhood violence and attachment insecurity, perpetuate it as well. Isolating first causes is virtually impossible. When evaluating the various explanatory models presented, it is imperative to remember that the distinction between cause and effect may not be clearcut; much of the emotional and intellectual fallout of abuse may in fact trigger further episodes. Keeping this dynamic quality in mind will provide a better understanding of one of the most pernicious effects of abuse: its ability to transfer psychopathological behavior from one generation to the next.

DEFINITIONS OF CHILD ABUSE AND NEGLECT

Among the varieties of violent experiences to which humankind can be subjected, child abuse is unique. It is intimate, personal, familial, and infused with emotions that are highly ambivalent (Galdston, 1981). As the study of child abuse has evolved, theorists have advanced several definitions of the phenomenon. Kempe, Silverman, and Steele (1962), in a classic definition, coined the phrase "battered-child syndrome" to characterize the situation of young children who have suffered serious physical abuse, most often from a parent or foster parent. Social workers and health care professionals such as pediatricians, orthopedists, and radiologists often describe abuse as "unrecognized trauma." Whatever the label, working definitions of abuse and neglect provide the criteria for documenting the incidence of the phenomenon.

Several definitions stress the physical result of maltreatment. These definitions, which focus solely on objectively discernible conditions, make the task of documenting abuse more straightforward than most other definitions. Parke and Collmer (1975), for example, suggested that abuse be defined as "behavior that results in injury of another individual." Kaplan et al. (1983) offer a similar definition, stipulating only that the child must be under 12 years of age and that the abuse must be inflicted by an adult caregiver. A further variation on result-oriented definitions requires that the infliction of physical injury be repeated, occurring "within the context of a pathological parent–child and family relationship" (Green, 1983).

Other definitions add the element of intention. In an early attempt to define child abuse, Parke and Collmer (1975) labeled a child as abused if he or she "receives nonaccidental physical injury (or injuries) as a result of acts (or omissions) on the part of his parents or guardians that violate the community standards concerning the treatment of children" (p. 513). Gelles and Straus (1979) also pinpoint intent, calling this violence "an act carried out with the intention of physically hurting another person." One working definition of abuse would then incorporate both isolated and repeated, as well as both minor and fatal, nonaccidental injuries to a child.

Sexual abuse presents a slightly different definitional problem, since it does not necessarily require the infliction of physical injury or emotional stress. Any sexual activity between an adult and a child, whether it is assaultive and produces injury or trauma or nonassaultive and causes little physical injury or apparent emotional stress, falls into the category of sexual abuse.

Gelles and Straus' (1979) definition raises another significant, yet problematic definitional issue—the issue of threats that may not actually culminate in violence. Such threats represent one form of emotional abuse. Threats of abuse or annihilation, whether or not they result in violence, are difficult to define and hence more difficult to document. Nonetheless, a meaningful definition of abuse must incorporate the element of threat since such threats, which can serve to intimidate or terrorize, may have consequences as devastating to the young child as actual assault (Aber & Zigler, 1981).

Emotional abuse assumes other forms as well, although they are difficult to describe precisely and, hence, to document. Emotional neglect, running the gamut from ignoring to blatantly rejecting a child, is one such form. Failure to provide a nurturing environment in which the child can thrive and develop to full potential is another. Not all neglect is as hard to define and document as emotional neglect. Moreover, child neglect has its physical correlates as well. This type of neglect occurs when the caregiver of a person under 18 years old deprives the child of food, shelter, clothing, education, or medical care.

THE SCOPE OF CHILD ABUSE AND NEGLECT

Although researchers have assiduously documented a variety of public health phenomena, until recently they have largely ignored child abuse and neglect. More than 20 years have elapsed since Kempe et al. (1962), in their pioneering study, coined the phrase "battered-child syndrome." But only in the past few years have government agencies begun to compile reliable statistics on the magnitude and severity of child abuse.

Although abuse and neglect statistics vary, most researchers concur that child maltreatment in the general population is pervasive and increasing. It is estimated that between 750,000 and one million cases of abuse are reported each year. In a statistical review compiled by the National Center on Child Abuse, Newberger, Newberger, and Hampton (1983) estimated that 711,000 cases of abuse had occurred in the United States in 1979. The U.S. Department of Health and Human Services offered a somewhat higher figure 1 year later, reporting that just over .5 percent (.57 percent) of the child population was victimized by abuse, translating into about 800,000 children. Three years later, in 1983, the American Humane Association estimated that almost 1.5 million American children had been abused that year (American Humane Association, 1985).

Alarmingly, and perhaps revealingly, abuse commonly victimizes the very young. The earliest studies of abuse found it most frequent among children between 3 months and 3.5 years old (Galdston, 1965; Kempe et al., 1962). Hampton and Newberger (1985) substantiate these earlier studies in an analysis of data drawn from the National Study of the Incidence and Severity of Child Abuse and Neglect. They report that 55 percent of their sample of abused children were less than 5 years old. A review of the 1984 U.S. Census data also indicates that the average age of maltreated children has declined in the last decade from 7.8 to 7.1 years old (American Humane Association, 1985).

Abuse is not only more pervasive than generally recognized, but its incidence may also be on the rise. Newberger et al. (1983) report that child abuse multiplied tenfold between 1969 and 1979, while the Humane Association notes that the number of reported cases increased 121 percent between 1976 and 1983 (American Humane Association, 1985). Whether these figures represent a bona fide increase in abuse or merely an increase in reported cases is still uncertain. Abuse has commanded greater public attention in recent years and this has no doubt fueled a greater willingness to report abuse, thus creating possible distortions in comparative abuse rates over time. Complicating matters further, definitions of abuse and neglect have also changed, potentially leading to additional distortions. Many state reporting agencies, from which data have been collected, have altered their reporting units from abused children to family units where abuse has occurred or from family units to number of abused children. For this reason, the Humane Association (1985) cautions against misconstruing growth figures. Nonetheless, even a small percentage increase in the surface figures signifies a rapidly expanding medical and social problem that warrants more precise documentation.

These statistics on the actual incidence of abuse are startling, and yet the potential for abuse appears even higher. After reviewing surveys on potentially harmful child-rearing attitudes and experiences characteristic of abusers, as well as reports in which adults were asked whether they thought they could injure a child, Garbarino (1977) concluded that fully one quarter of American families are "abuse-prone." This translates into roughly 40 million children at risk for abuse.

THE IMPACT OF CHILD ABUSE AND NEGLECT

The impact of abuse or neglect is felt in many ways in homes where maltreatment has occurred. Abuse can affect virtually every facet of a child's physical and psychological life, from basic physical growth through cognitive and motor development, emergence of temperament and attachments, regulation of affects, and development of self-esteem and coping. When abuse and neglect necessitate hospitalization or separation from abusive parents, the prospects of deleterious pyschological consequences escalate even more. This is particularly true among very young children whose vulnerability to depression from hospitalization is disproportionately high. Thus the group of children most at risk for serious forms of physical maltreatment is also most at risk for a depressive outcome as a consequence of the required treatment of their physical condition.

Death and serious injury are not uncommon results of abuse and neglect. The most conservative statistics of mortality resulting from abuse come from the National Center on Child Abuse and Neglect, which estimated that in 1978, between 2000 and 4000 deaths resulted from abuse. Nongovernment research suggests a more pronounced mortality rate, as well as a higher rate of serious injury. Schmitt and Kempe (1975), for example, concluded that of children who have been physically abused and returned to their parents without intervention, 5 percent are eventually killed and 35 percent suffer serious injury. These figures roughly corroborate Kempe et al.'s (1962) findings on the seriousness of known cases of abuse. In their nationwide survey of hospitals treating abuse victims, Kempe et al. reported that over one quarter (85 cases) of the 302 cases reported suffered brain damage and over 10 percent (33 children) died. Hampton and Newberger (1985) found that 34 percent of the injuries sustained from abuse were serious, while less than .5 percent were fatal. The most recent figures released by the Humane Association (1985) are much lower, however. This organization estimated that only 3.2 percent of abused children experienced major physical injury in 1983, while approximately one quarter sustained either minor physical injuries (18.5 percent) or "unspecified physical injuries" (5.2 percent; American Humane Association, 1985). Most cases (58.4 percent) of reported maltreatment in 1983 arose from the deprivation of necessities (American Humane Association, 1985). The difficulty of diagnosing many types of internal physical injury—particularly anatomical cartilaginous tissue disruptions that do not present in gross distortions—suggests that many instances of significant abuse remain undetected and that many seemingly minor injuries may be more severe than initially suspected.

Whatever the definitive breakdown of the severity of abuse may be, however, cases of severe maltreatment appear to be concentrated among the youngest children (American Humane Association, 1985). Almost two thirds of the reported cases of major or major with minor physical injury were sustained by the 0- to 5-year age group, and almost half of the cases of deprivation of necessities occurred in this group. Additionally, cases of multiple forms of maltreatment are reported more frequently in this age group than in the 6- to 11-year or 12- to 17-year age groups. In contrast, sexual maltreatment appears to occur predominantly among older children, with less than one quarter of known cases occurring among children under 5 years (American Humane Association, 1985).

Abused children receive treatment for their physical injuries more often than for the psychological damage wrought by abuse and neglect. Studies of any type of psychopathology (not just depression) among the abused/ neglected are hampered by the difficulty of answering two questions. First, how many cases of abuse actually receive psychiatric treatment? Second, by implication, how much of a risk factor for serious psychopathology is abuse/neglect? Estimates based on numbers of children in treatment probably understate the prevalence of serious psychopathology. Since many cases of abuse occur in children under 3 years of age, most will not receive psychiatric care. Moreover, the inadequacy of hospital referral procedures means that many of those who should receive psychiatric care for abuse escape the attention of mental-health professionals. In fact, hospital referral committees refer only a small percentage of identified abuse cases to psychologists or psychiatrists.

Kaplan and Zitrin (1983b) studied child abuse assessment procedures in the New York metropolitan area and found that a majority (58 percent) of hospitals referred less than one quarter of known abuse cases to psychiatrists for evaluation. Only about 14 percent referred more than half of the cases for psychiatric evaluation. Thus it is difficult to assess with any confidence how often abuse and neglect lead to serious psychopathology.

Setting aside the shortcomings of the referral process for a moment, and focusing on children already identified by psychiatric treatment facilities, it is clear that a history of abuse is a prominent characteristic of those referred for assessment or treatment. In what may be the first study of its kind on this population, Monane, Leitcher, and Lewis (1984) found that well over one third (42 percent) of the 166 youngsters aged 3 to 17 years admitted to the psychiatric service of a major urban hospital had been abused. Tarter, Hegedus, Winsten, and Alterman (1984), in a study of older children (delinquents with a mean age 15.7 years who had been referred for assessment to a psychiatric facility) found that over one quarter (27 percent) had been abused.

Although it is clear from the literature that a history of abuse and neglect are common among the psychiatrically impaired, few studies have been devoted exclusively to affective disorders in this population. Blumberg (1981) has asserted that abuse and neglect are among the most significant causes of childhood depression, and Bible and French (1979) also discerned significant signs of depression among abused children. Given that the systematic attempt to document infant depression originated in neglected populations (Spitz, 1945), it is somewhat perplexing that the availability of standard diagnostic criteria and sophisticated methodologies have not, in the last 40 years, truly advanced knowledge of the incidence of affective disorders among this population. In part, this may reflect reluctance to become mired in the continued debate about the nature of childhood depression—a debate to which Bible and French (1979) may be alluding with their observation that among the abused, impulsiveness and aggression often mask depression. The investigations by Tarter et al. (1984) are a good example of the shortage of detailed data on affective disorders among the abused. Although these researchers found no significant difference in the level of affective disorders among abused and nonabused delinquents, their study made no effort to probe affective disorders in depth or to account for the polymorphous nature of affective disorders. A caveat issued by the authors hints at the latter problem. They suggested that the expected prevalence of conduct disorders within the population they studied may have overreaching implications for other disorders. Recent investigations on the overlap between conduct disorders and depressive disorders (Puig-Antich, 1984) raise the probability that this speculation is correct.

If the literature on depression as a syndrome among the abused and neglected is rather sparse, it is far richer on specific correlates of depression—for example, depressed affect, disturbed object relations, and eating disorders. The isolated depressive symptoms that have been well documented may not reach clinical significance during childhood, but are nonetheless important since they are precursors of a more severe psychopathology later in life. A review of the literature suggests that maltreated children develop a progressive pattern of symptomatology, much of which may be classified as depressive. (See Table 10).

Table 10. A Spectrum of Depressive Correlates among Abused Children

Years	Response
0–1	Susceptibility to illness and accident increased illness hospitalism
1–5	Combination of withdrawal and aggression unpredictable behavior insecure attachment failure to explore the environment failure to interact with objects and others depression
Greater than 5 years	delinquency school difficulties failure to form stable relationships isolation immaturity violence/abuse

A case study may provide a useful composite of some of these symptoms as they surface in early infancy and should serve as a landscape for a more detailed discussion of the most significant depressive correlates of abuse.

A Case Study in Abuse/Neglect

Gaensbauer (1980) described Jenny, a prototypical case of child abuse and intervention. She was the product of a normal pregnancy and was cared for by both parents—a mother who actively nurtured her and a father who was affectionate but harbored a severe temper. At 2 weeks of age, Jenny presented with a fractured arm. During a well-baby clinic check-up 1 month later, pediatricians noted a small bruise. By the age of 3 months the injuries she sustained grew progressively worse, with a nondepressed skull fracture accompanying a second broken arm. At that time, Jenny was hospitalized for 5 days. She was visually hypervigilant, had a tendency to squirm when held by strangers, and was somewhat fussy. Otherwise, she showed no signs of recent physical abuse.

Jenny was placed in a home in which the foster mother provided minimal physical care, leaving Jenny unattended in her crib for long periods. Jenny's mother visited her three times during the 3 weeks of foster care following hospitalization. The first visit demonstrated that there was a positive relationship between them, as witnessed by a "beaming" response consisting of excitement and smiling. By the next visit 1 week later, Jenny had grown more subdued, according to her mother.

The third encounter was in the laboratory playroom where a 1-hour evaluation took place. Observers noted Jenny's lack of attention, her seeming inability to hold her head erect, and her negative greeting of her mother, and characterized Jenny as emotionally depressed. They noted signs of apathy and disinterest in toys and other objects around her. Jenny was unsmiling and easily upset by overstimulation. When she was placed in a different home with a warm, sensitive foster mother, the sad face observed in the playroom dissipated within a few days and was transformed into smiles and vocalized expressions in response to the new foster mother.

In Jenny's case, measures, such as hospitalization and removal to a foster home, taken to protect the infant from further physical abuse, appear to have contributed as much to her apparent depression as the abuse itself. Prior to her hospitalization, Jenny was described as a happy and engaging infant who interacted well with her mother and others. Jenny appears to have undergone the classic response to maternal loss, whether in the form of brief or permanent separations, described by Spitz and Wolf (1946) and Robertson and Bowlby (1952), and often viewed as the central precipitant of depression in the very young. Indeed, Jenny may have been responding to three specific losses—abrupt weaning, separation from her mother, and neglect by her foster mother—which combined to leave the infant with what

Gaensbauer (1980) terms the loss of the mothering function. During her mother's first visit to Jenny in a foster home, the infant still responded positively, but as time passed Jenny became more subdued. The description of her behavior during her mother's third visit, while Jenny was still living with her neglecting foster mother, is typical of the "despair" phase of an infant's response to separation (Bowlby, 1969; Robertson & Bowlby, 1952). Neglect at the hands of her first foster mother deprived Jenny of sufficient interaction to form any substantial attachment in her mother's absence. The description of Jenny's second foster mother as "warm" and "sensitive" is substantiated by the description of Jenny's positive affect in response to her.

Jenny's case illustrates not only the common depressive symptoms resulting from abuse, but also hints at how some of these symptoms may perpetuate further abuse. Although the information concerning Jenny is too limited to yield definitive statements about the etiology of her abuse, there are clues that help elucidate the nature of the abusive or neglectful caregiver behavior. From the standpoint of temperament, we know little about Jenny beyond the characterization of her as fussy and irritable. It is possible that she was a temperamentally "difficult" infant (Thomas et al., 1963; Thomas, Chess, & Birch, 1968). By description, she was high in activity (tendency to squirm) and intense in reaction, and she had a negative mood–characteristics that, in the Thomas and Chess typology, would classify her as a difficult infant. Jenny also grew progressively unresponsive to people and objects in her environment. These qualities may have provoked frustration in her caregivers, who may have felt deprived of the gratification generally derived from a calm and engaging baby. Their frustration may have surfaced in different ways. Her father apparently abused her physically and her first foster mother, overtaxed with other foster children, neglected her.

Nonorganic Failure to Thrive

Disturbances of bodily function, especially eating and sleeping disturbances, often serve as the earliest indicators of adult depression. Increased illness may be a form of protest, the first stage of a child's response to maternal neglect or separation as delineated by Bowlby (1958, 1960). In infants and children, eating disturbances, which can also betoken underlying depression, may manifest as a failure to grow physically. Charting an infant's or child's physical growth may, in fact, be one of the most reliable means of detecting incipient or existing depression in the very young. Indeed, failure to thrive physically was one of the most prominent signs of depression in the depressed infants Spitz (1945) first described.

Nonorganic failure to thrive (NOFT) includes any significant growth retardation that cannot be attributed to organic causes, such as congenital heart disease, Central Nervous System (CNS) abnormalities, malabsorption, and various congenital defects. The standards most commonly used for measuring growth retardation are the Boston and Harvard Growth Standards. A child can be diagnosed for NOFT if his or her height and weight fall below the third percentile for his or her chronological weight (Politt & Eichler, 1976).

The causal relationship between abuse and NOFT is still unclear. One theory holds that abuse and neglect predict NOFT, illness, and developmental delays, while another hypothesis advocates the opposite view, namely that the strain of having ill children elevates the likelihood of abuse (Hunter, Kilstrom, Kraybill, & Loda, 1978; Klein & Stern, 1971). A recent study by Sherrod, O'Connor, and Vietze (1984) arrived at surprising conclusions when attempting to clarify this relationship. The study found that a high incidence of illness and NOFT shortly after birth, tended to decline with time. This finding appears to refute the hypothesis that abuse causes ill health.

Kavanagh (1982), in contrast, makes the strongest claim for the theory that abuse leads to illness, in a review of the impact of emotional abuse on the physical and psychological state of the child. She concludes that with the marked exception of NOFT, researchers have not reliably linked abuse/neglect with any objective abnormal physical or psychological syndrome.

Data collected by Greenberg (1970) support this claim. The researcher found a significant correlation between neglectful and punitive maternal characteristics and infant feeding problems, including significant lags in weight gain among 42 infants under 2.5 years old. Although the study contained methodological flaws, it established a strong connection between certain maternal behavioral profiles and NOFT. Subsequent studies, many of them retrospective, also detected a relationship between a mother's abusive characteristics and NOFT. Evans, Reinhart, and Succip (1972) found that some mothers of NOFT infants were overtly hostile and angry with their infants, and Pollitt, Eichler, and Chon (1975) observed that mothers of such infants were less affectionate and more likely to employ physical punishment than were control mothers from the same socioeconomic background. This relationship has been further substantiated by Money (1977).

Klaus and Kennel (1976) suggest that a high incidence of neglect and abuse may correlate with mother–infant separation at birth. They found both NOFT and child abuse more common among children who had been separated from their mothers shortly after birth, than among children whose mothers had nurtured them from birth. The researchers argued that there was a critical period immediately following birth when it was vital for mothers and children to interact in order to form a secure attachment. Klein and Stern (1971), who posited that low birth weight may lead to battering, also suggested that separation after birth may be a factor in abuse.

Developmental Delays

Some of the clearest evidence on the impact of child maltreatment relates to developmental delays. Researchers have detected developmental deficits in virtually every facet of abused children's functioning (Elmer & Gregg, 1967; Green, 1978a; Kempe & Kempe, 1978; Martin & Beezley, 1977; Morse, Sahler, & Freidman, 1970; Newberger & Cook, 1983; Sandgrund et al., 1974; Spinetta & Rigler, 1972; Steele, 1976). The development of motor skills is especially vulnerable to the effects of abuse. Children maltreated for exercising such age-appropriate motor skills as walking, reaching and "getting into things" will often stop practicing these skills. Speech and language disorders, particularly delayed speech development and problems in articulation and expression once verbal facility has been attained (Green, 1983), have commonly been observed in follow-up studies of abused children (Elmer & Gregg, 1967; Kempe & Kempe, 1978; Martin & Beezley, 1977). Physically abused delinquents, for example, frequently display cognitive defects in tasks involving language capacity (Tarter et al., 1984).

Dietrich, Starr, and Weisfeld (1983) examined 53 mother–infant dyads and established a relationship between maltreatment and developmental status. They also were able to delineate correlations between severity of maltreatment and developmental impact. The research team divided the infants into five groups: (1) those combining nonaccidental trauma with failure to thrive; (2) those with nonaccidental trauma without growth problems, but with iron deficiency anemia; (3) those suffering only from nonaccidental trauma; (4) those with general weight and diagnosis indicating caregiver neglect; and (5) controls. When they applied the indices of the Bayley Mental and Motor Scores to the infants, they found significantly lower scores among infants combining nonaccidental trauma and failure to thrive. Notably this group was the only one of the four abused/neglect groups to present developmental delays. Such evidence substantiates the continuum of impact reflected in severity of maltreatment.

While statistics reveal that many abused/neglected children sustain physical injury and fail to progress in many facets of development, only a small fraction may actually receive injuries serious enough to warrant hospitalization (American Humane Association, 1985). Nonetheless, the age range of highest risk for abuse/neglect—from 6 months to 4 years—is the same period during which children are most prone to the adverse effects of hospitalization (Schaffer & Callender, 1959), particularly depression. In fact, the first descriptions of childhood depression emerged from the institutional context (Spitz & Wolf, 1946; Bowlby, 1944). The abused child is more likely to suffer the ill effects of hospitalization because of a host of factors (most of which correlate with abuse), including insecure attachment, lack of parental support due to either parental anxiety or guilt, increased parental stress, disturbed parents, and fear of abandonment (Douglas,

1975; Jessner, Blom, & Waldfogel, 1952; Kashani et al., 1981; Mason, 1965; Solnit, 1960).

Moreover, the abused child returning home faces a greater risk of further abuse/neglect with its deleterious effects, since childhood hospitalization only exacerbates many of the conditions which can cause additional abuse, such as behavioral difficulties (Ferguson, 1979; Prugh, 1983), depression (Ferguson, 1979; Pilowsky, Bassett, Begg, & Thomas, 1982; Reichelderfer & Rockland, 1963; Spitz & Wolf, 1946), insecure attachment and developmental deficits (Bowlby, 1944), angry, aggressive reactions (Bowlby, 1951; Ferguson, 1979; Langford, 1961), impaired ability to form relationships (Bowlby, 1944, 1951), stress in the home (Prugh et al., 1953). Thus the synergism of these two phenomena—the original abuse/neglect and hospitalization—increases the prospects that these children will suffer not only further abuse, but also developmental retardation, depression, and future psychopathology.

Hospitalization need not, however, result in only harmful effects. The experience can provide an opportunity to identify abuse/neglect and to intervene (Howells, 1963). To do this, hospitals must establish adequate predictive screens that include criteria for recognizing abuse/neglect in hospitalized children under 5 years of age. Medical personnel should strive to recognize abused and neglected children immediately on hospitalization and to identify those likely to be adversely affected by hospitalization.

The cases of two children, presented by Freedman and Brown (1968), graphically illustrate the range of physical deficits and developmental delays arising from abuse and neglect, as well as the positive role hospitals can play in intervention. These children, raised by a psychotic mother, were virtually isolated from all normal human contact. On the recommendation of an investigating social worker, the two were hospitalized. Both ranked below the third percentile in physical development; the girl measured 42.5 inches and weighed 30 pounds at age 6; and the boy stood 37 inches tall and weighed 23 pounds at 4 years. Since the girl had been fed exclusively from a bottle, she could not feed herself. Neither could she speak meaningfully except for a few words and sentences repeated in echolalic fashion. At admission, she was also totally incontinent. When released from the hospital after 8 weeks, she had gained continence and could call some objects by name. A year and a half in foster care brought her to the developmental age of a 4-year-old, despite a chronological age of 8.

Her brother presented a similar portrait of physical and developmental deficiencies. He, too, was incontinent and, with the exception of a few occasional screams, spoke only in grunts. According to the nurses, the boy smeared feces gleefully. Eight weeks of hospital therapy improved his locomotion and taught him to hold a cup, but could not change his chronic headbanging and rocking. Notably, his return to the family setting undermined the basic advances made during hospitalization.

Temperament and Affective Expression

Several qualities studied by temperament researchers coincide with the depressive symptomatology encountered among the abused and neglected. Temperament researchers have concerned themselves with differences in the responsivity of individuals to their environment. Several investigators have observed significant differences in the level of affective response displayed by abused and neglected children. For example, Gaensbauer and Sands (1979) compared 48 abused or neglected infants (aged 6 to 36 months) to normal controls in a structured playroom situation, and described the abused as less expressive than nonabused children. Others have similarly characterized the affect of abused children. Lamb, Gaensbauer, Malkin, and Schultz (1985) referred to the affective expression of maltreated children as generally more muted. Weissman and Paykel (1974) spoke of a "dampening" of behavior and affect.

In further investigations of the facial expressions of abused children, Gaensbauer (1982) confirmed earlier findings. A sample of 12 abused infants between 12 and 19 months compared to 60 normal infants of the same ages, revealed less pleasure, less interaction, less exploration, and a lower overall affective repertoire than found in normal infants (Gaensbauer, 1982). Abused children in a Structured Playroom Paradigm tended to play with fewer objects, and to do so in a stereotypical and repetitive manner (Gaensbauer, 1982). In a later study, Gaensbauer and Hiatt (1984b) compared a severely abused infant (3 months and 25 days old) with 9 abused infants under 27 weeks of age (average age 16.4 weeks) and 9 controls matched for age (within 1 week). All infants were exposed to a series of standardized stimulus conditions based on the Maximally Discriminative Facial Movement Scoring System (MAX). When the severely abused infant was scored, observers noted expressions of sadness and fear in the presence of her mother during the initial free-play period, as well as during and after male stranger approaches. She did not express fear at female stranger approaches, perhaps because her father was her abuser. With both males and females she also frequently expressed anger during holding, pick-ups, and testing periods. In general, she slumped and showed psychomotor retardation. Moreover, when male strangers approached she averted her gaze, withdrew, and displayed signs of what in older infants would be labeled "stranger distress." By contrast, the control infants were predominantly happy. They smiled and expressed interest frequently during the testing.

When lack of affect transforms into an emotional display the child's affect appears distorted and markedly ambivalent, perhaps reflecting unresolved emotional conflicts. Abused children often express sadness, distress, anger, and depression (Gaensbauer & Sands, 1979). Irritability and chronic crying, which may encompass some of the qualities measured by Thomas and Chess' (1977, 1984) temperament dimensions of adaptability and quality of mood, are common among abused and neglected children (Milowe & Lourie, 1964;

Gaensbauer & Sands, 1979; Gaensbauer, 1982; Gaensbauer & Hiatt, 1984). Such irritability may represent the child's protest, in the sense described by Bowlby (1958, 1960), against the perception of separation that results from neglect.

Although such characteristics as muted expressions, irritability, and negative mood have been correlated with abuse and neglect, the direction of the causal relationship—as in the relationship between abuse/neglect and NOFT—is still not clear. On the one hand, much of the literature treats temperament as a possible incipient of abuse. Milowe and Lourie (1964), for example, have linked abuse to infant irritability and chronic crying. This view of the role of temperament also confirms the prevailing belief that most abuse occurs to the very young. Since temperament is conceived of as part of the infant's constitutional endowment, it can trigger responses, perhaps abuse, shortly after birth. There is no developmental achievement required before temperament can affect the environment. This view carries great appeal for investigators who are concerned with formulating cause-effect etiologies. However, this view may not reflect the findings of some current research, which perceives temperament as more plastic, at least as much a product of the environment as of birth. According to this latter approach, temperament operates bidirectionally: it is as much a product of abuse as a primary cause. Crittenden (1985a), for example, has shown that temperament—manifested in such behaviors as uncooperativeness—responds favorably to improvements in the caregiving environment, and that infant behavior, purported to cause maltreatment, does not result from a constitutional trait, but rather, is a product of the environment. In her study investigating abusive mother-infant interactions and the impact of intervention on this dysfunctional behavior, she found that infant passivity or difficult tendencies among maltreated infants depended largely on features of the dyadic exchange and was not inherently different from temperamental displays among normal children.

This view of temperament in the context of abuse finds support in the general concept of temperament advanced by Rothbart and Derryberry (1982), who argue that the dimensions of temperament have certain innate components but change in response to interactions with the environment. These researchers believe that individual differences in the degree, time of onset, and delay of affective response to stimuli are present from birth. Such differences affect the infant's interactions with both the material and social world by evoking a "style" of behavior. The infant's active response to outside stimuli comprises his or her "self-regulatory" system. As the child develops, the quality of his or her reactions to the environment will affect the nature of his or her developing self-regulatory capacities. Thus, Rothbart and Derryberry (1982) hold that the innate elements of temperament are shaped by the physical and social environment, giving temperament a plastic and fluid quality. (See Table 11).

Table 11. Dimensions of Temperament Compared to Abused/Neglected Child Profile

Abused/Neglected Profile	Thomas, Chess, Hertzig, and Korn (1963)	Buss and Plomin (1975)	Rothbart (1981)
Dysphoric mood (1,2)	Adaptability	Emotionality	Smiling & laughter
low or flattened affect (5)	Approach/withdrawal	Impulsivity	Fear
less warmth (7)	Mood		Distress to limitations Soothability
Sleep disturbances (2)	Rhythmicity		
Less compliant/difficult (1,2,4,6,7,8)	Approach/withdrawal Intensity Adaptability Attention span/persistence Mood	Emotionality Sociability Impulsivity	Distress to limitations Soothability Duration of orienting Duration of orienting
Avoidant (1,2,4,5,6,7)	Approach/withdrawal	Sociability	Fear Duration of orienting
Aggression (3,4,6)	Approach/withdrawal Intensity	Sociability Impulsivity	Distress to (3,4,6) Activity level
Communication problems (5,6,7)	Approach/withdrawal Intensity	Emotionality Sociability	Smiling & laughter Duration of orienting

1. Bakwin (1971)
2. Blumberg (1981)
3. Bousha & Twentyman (1984)
4. Crittenden (1985a)
5. Gaensbauer et al. (1980)
6. George & Main (1979)
7. Herrenkohl et al. (1984)
8. Wasserman et al. (1983)

Attachment Behavior

Many of the configurations of temperament and affective expression reflect themselves most conspicuously in atypical patterns of interaction among abused families. Numerous studies demonstate lucidly that abuse damages affective expression in the child and ultimately reveals itself in the style of interaction forged between caregiver and child. Characteristically, abusive homes are marked by social isolation and infrequent exchange of information (Bousha & Twentyman, 1984). Patterns of withdrawal and lack of involvement—both on the part of the parent and on the part of the child—typify interactions in which abuse has occurred (Crittenden & Bonvillian, 1984; Gaensbauer & Sands, 1979). Less maternal gazing, more "hovering," and more physical constraint were observed by Robison and Solomon (1979) during interactions with abused toddlers, and confirmed by Lewis and Schaeffer (1981). Among school-aged abused children and their families, Burgess and Conger (1977,1978) reported lower rates of interaction and fewer encounters than found in nonabusive families. George and Main (1979) noted that abused infants approached their caregivers only about half as frequently as did nonabused infants, and that they actually avoided their caregivers three times more often than did the controls. Gaensbauer and Sands (1979) described the 6- to 36-month-old maltreated infants they studied as being more shallow and unpredictable in their affective relationships. Withdrawal marked these children more than any other quality; they failed to respond to attempts by others to elicit smiles or other pleasurable reactions.

These signs of withdrawal are not only important evidence of depression in their own right, but they also have a profound impact on the development of a child's self-concept. Main, Kaplan, and Cassidy (1985), Lewis, Brooks-Gunn, & Jaskir (1985), among others, have suggested a correlation between attachment behavior and the ability to represent the self. Attachment allows the child to use the mother as "a secure base for exploration" (Ainsworth, 1973; Ainsworth, Bell, & Stayton, 1971). Such exploration permits the securely attached child to forge a self-concept based on numerous sources of information from the environment. It is not surprising, therefore, that the insecurity often accompanying the attachment behavior of abused children also damages their self-concept.

The Strange Situation Procedure, developed by Ainsworth and Wittig (1969), has provided a wealth of reliable documentation pertaining to the effects of abuse on the quality of an infant's attachment with the caregiver. Children who have developed an atypical relationship, as demonstrated by the Strange Situation Procedure, can be categorized as "avoidant" or "resistantly" attached, with each type of attachment characterized by specific affect. "Avoidant" children in the Strange Situation show little affect on reunion with the mother after a short separation. Ainsworth and Wittig

(1969) describe the children categorized as "resistantly attached" either as displaying anger and anxiety throughout the Strange Situation Procedure or as demonstrating overall passivity. "Anxiously attached" (avoidant and resistant combined) infants are characterized by various affect difficulties.

It is rare in psychiatric epidemiology to find such conclusive evidence of affective disorder as the prevalence of insecure attachments among abused children provides. Egeland and Sroufe (1981a), for example, found only about half the rate of secure attachment among abused children as among nonabused children. In one prospective study of abuse and attachment, Egeland and Sroufe evaluated 209 infants at 12 months and 194 of them again at 18 months of age. They distinguished between infants who had received inadequate care—either through abuse, neglect, or poor physical care—and those who had received high quality care from their mothers. Not surprisingly, only 38 percent of the inadequately attended infants were classified as securely attached, while 24 percent were anxious-avoidant and 38 percent anxious-resistant. In contrast, three quarters of the infants in the excellent care group were classified as securely attached, with only 16 percent classified as avoidant and 9 percent as resistant. Although the differences diminished somewhat when the infants were measured again at 18 months, nearly twice as many (44 percent as compared with 24 percent) of the poorly attended infants showed insecure attachments.

The impact of maltreatment on attachment appears particularly significant when abuse is perpetrated by an infant's biological mother. In a recent study, Lamb et al. (1985) examined the differences in attachment behavior among infants abused by their biological mothers and infants abused by others. Using a modification of the Strange Situation Paradigm, the authors evaluated 32 maltreated infants between the ages of 8.7 and 31.8 months. They divided these infants into four groups:

1. Those present with their biological mothers (the M-M group)
2. Those living with foster mothers for at least 1 week (the FM-FM group)
3. Those with their natural mothers but currently living with foster mothers (the FM-M group)
4. Those who had been maltreated by a person other than their biological mothers (the "Other" group)

The authors demonstrated that infants abused or neglected by their natural mothers showed a far higher incidence of insecure attachment than those abused by someone other than their biological mothers. While 78 percent of those abused by someone else showed secure attachments, only 19 percent of those neglected and 14 percent of those abused by their biological mothers had secure attachments. Avoidant, rather than resistant attachment behavior, typified the abused children.

Given these observations, it is not surprising that a study undertaken by DeLozier (1982) several years later found abused children unable to form and maintain caregiver relationships. In many instances, such infants and caregivers actually behave in ways that effectively stifle restoration of interaction. George and Main (1979) observed, for example, that abused infants frequently avoided friendly overtures by caregivers and peers. Moreover, there appears to be a continuum of impact, with the most neglected and maltreated infants displaying the most severe interactional problems (Dietrich et al., 1983).

By undermining secure caregiver attachments, abuse not only establishes maladaptive patterns for formation of future attachments, but also may threaten development of mastery. As DeLozier (1982) has observed, mastery is more easily achieved if a child feels he or she has a secure base from which to operate. Ultimately, failure to experience a sense of mastery can contribute to depression.

Self-Representation

The harmful effect of abuse on affective expression and parent-child interaction reverberates through many developmental challenges the infant and young toddler confront after the first year of life. Abuse's deleterious impact on the growing child's ability to represent the self as distinct from the object, as well as on the ability to form a positive self-representation, are perhaps the most devastating consequences of abuse from the standpoint of depression. The capacity to distinguish between the self and the object is particularly important for abused children, since their parents often display depressive symptoms that the child, who has not yet fully separated, may incorporate into his or her own self-concept.

Many theorists have linked early attachment security with various aspects of self-concept later in life. Main, Kaplan, and Cassidy (1985) have argued that attachment-related events fortify internal working models of relationships and that these representational models control a child's access to information about the self. Security of attachment in their study also related to a child's perceived ability to cope with a prospective separation. Investigators have tied attachment security to self-esteem, positive affect, ego control, resiliency, and autonomous functioning (Arend, Gove, & Sroufe, 1979; Matas, Arend, & Sroufe, 1978; Schneider-Rosen & Cicchetti, 1984; Sroufe, 1983; Waters, 1978; Waters, Wippman, & Sroufe, 1979).

Schneider-Rosen and Cicchetti (1984) elaborated on the extent to which abuse may retard development of a child's capacity for self-representation. In this study, they established a significant relationship between maltreatment, attachment, the capacity for visual self-recognition, and the quality of the recognition. The researchers studied 37 infants, 18 of whom had been maltreated and 19 of whom had not. They observed these infants in the

Strange Situation Paradigm to assess the quality of attachment. At the conclusion of the session, the researchers used the standard mirror and rouge paradigm to test infants' capacity for visual self-recognition. During this test the infants were positioned in front of mirrors and spontaneous reactions to their images were observed to determine whether recognition was present. The infants were then distracted from the mirror and the researchers surreptitiously applied a smudge of blue makeup to their noses. If infants touched their noses while looking in the mirror, the researchers concluded that they recognized themselves. The researchers also evaluated the infants' affective responses on self-recognition.

The researchers were not surprised to find a significant relationship between the quality of attachment and the capacity for visual self-recognition. Of those who displayed visual self-recognition, almost three quarters (73%) were securely attached—whether or not they were maltreated—while 27 percent of those capable of self-recognition were insecurely attached. The study demonstrated no direct link between maltreatment and self-recognition, but rather correlated attachment and self-recognition. However, since there is a well-established connection between maltreatment and attachment, by inference, Schneider-Rosen and Cicchetti's (1984) study may suggest a link—albeit indirect and mediated by attachment—between maltreatment and self-recognition. Moreover, when the researchers evaluated the infants' affective responses once they recognized themselves, they found that nonmaltreated infants displayed an overwhelmingly (74%) positive affect, while only 22 percent of the maltreated infants who recognized themselves showed such a reaction. Instead, the affect of most (78%) of the maltreated infants changed from neutral or positive to sober, staring, concentrating, or crying. In contrast, only 26 percent of the nonmaltreated infants who recognized themselves evinced this reaction.

The stress of abuse and neglect may not merely cause delays in attainment of self-representation, but may also trigger regressions to global, nondifferentiated self-other states. Greenspan (1981) has noted that panic and anger can result in attenuation of the capacity for normal object representation, a capacity that is not well established until after the age of 30 months. Such regressions may prevent the abused or neglected child from achieving object constancy. In these cases, the infant faces the depressive potential arising from both object loss and loss of his or her incipient self partially invested in the object. Alternatively, the child may achieve object constancy, but may introject an "aggressive, pain-inflicting object" (Solnit, 1982). This process may instill in the child a sense of his or her own relative powerlessness and dependency on the whims of a vengeful parent. Since infants are slow, even under the most painful circumstances, to relinquish the attachment relationship, they may instead internalize the belief that a normal parent–child or self–other relationship entails dominance, frustration, dependency, and pain. Self-aggression may result from a perception that the abusive parent's violence is not unusual or that the child is deserving of the pain inflicted by the punitive or neglectful constant object.

Self-esteem and sense of mastery—products of secure attachment—may also be threatened by the insecure attachments common among abused and neglected children. An infant's self-esteem is constructed from early experiences using affective expressions to stimulate control over the environment.

Unsuccessful affective exchange, as might occur with a neglectful parent, deprives the infant of the knowledge that his or her actions will be understood by the caregiver, impeding the infant's opportunity to explore and control his or her environment. This, in turn, can deprive the infant of important reinforcement in experiencing a sense of mastery over the environment and can undermine his or her self-esteem. Asynchronous affect expression disrupts the infant's ability to draw the correct boundaries between cause and effect. Without appropriate and consistent responses to affective expression, the child cannot develop an integrated sense of self, since normal inner sensations are not being validated. This process may cause the infant to regard the self as irrelevant or erroneous, and to disregard any subsequent validation attempts. Since the infant must rely on the outside world for cues and guidance, unsuccessful affective exchange diminishes the infant's sense of self-worth and omnipotence. Not surprisingly, Helfer et al. (1976) have noted that maltreated school-age children between the ages of 4 and 7 were plagued by lack of self-esteem.

Without self-esteem and mastery, children adopt a passive style, lack exploratory activity, and exhibit failure to control people and objects within their environment, as Helfer, McKinney, and Kempe (1976) have observed. Indeed, Main (1983) has demonstrated clear differences in exploratory and social behavior; these differences varied according to the security of attachment between parent and child. As might be expected, insecurely attached children were less spontaneously verbal and had more limited vocabularies than securely attached children. They also avoided playing with adults or children and displayed a comparative lack of interest in toys. This finding suggests that insecurely attached children will not practice skills needed to enhance establishment of a strong self-concept.

Curiously, abused, insecure–ambivalent children between the ages of 6 and 12 months are not usually anxious in the absence of their parents or in the presence of strangers, whereas securely attached children often experience these events as threatening conditions. Abusing parents who do not perform the function of regulating their childrens' internal and external environments may hasten the process of defining self-other and self-object boundaries to a furious pace. Frozen watchfulness, characteristic of abused infants, suggests that they are intensely aware of the environment and that they have developed a precocious, albeit limited, distinction between the self and external objects. Abused children, who are prematurely thrust into the inappropriate but necessary situation of distancing themselves from abusing parents, are cast in a role inappropriate for their young age. This precocious development does not encourage the infant to explore the environment with the security of knowing that the parent is available in cases of fright or failure. Instead, it engenders a sense that the child is alone and vulnerable. The child's limited cognitive apparatus must be devoted to surveillance and defense, precluding normal development in a wide range of fields. Preoccupation with self-defense often leads to deficits in verbal skills, social skills, regulation of aggression, and expression of emotion.

The probability that abuse and neglect will impede exploration and breed the sense of helplessness and passivity so often associated with depression is particularly high during the period when the infant is separating from the primary caregiver, usually the mother. During this time, an infant normally experiences vacillations between the enthusiasm for exploration that accompanied the advent of upright locomotion and a natural sense of helplessness and loneliness resulting from the realization of his or her own separateness. Exaggerated separation responses, resembling responses to object loss, are not an uncommon sign of a child's reaction to the diminution of illusory omnipotence and feelings of helplessness. At this pivotal developmental phase, the image of the mother is also markedly ambivalent—split between the good mother, who protects the child, and the bad mother, who can no longer be instantaneously controlled by the child. Mahler refers to this phenomenon as the rapprochement crisis of separation–individuation, and several theorists have contended that a child's susceptibility to depression may be significantly affected by his or her ability to resolve this psychic dilemma (Anthony, 1983; Mahler, 1972; McDevitt, 1975). A mother's response to her infant during this phase is critical for determining whether the natural depressive tendencies of this period subside or persist. Abusive and neglectful mothers, who are unlikely to respond empathically to a child's needs at this time may perpetuate the splitting of the maternal image and cause the child to introject a "bad" maternal representation. The nonpathological helplessness typical of this period may thus yield to pathological helplessness (McDevitt, 1975). Continued ambivalence may cause impairment of the child's self-concept if he or she views the self as inadequate to resolve the ambivalence of this period (Bemesderfer & Cohler, 1983).

Violence

One frequently noted, but in some respects atypical, depressive symptom (as defined by DSM-III) observed among the abused is violence. As abused children experience the accumulated sequelae of their maltreatment, they can easily become violent, if not abusive, themselves. Thus, the ironic and commonly observed impact of abuse is to create a generation of abusers from the ranks of the abused. While not all of those abused become abusers, the literature reports clearly elevated levels of aggression and violent characteristics among the abused.

George and Main (1979) were among the first to document the high incidence of seemingly child-induced violent interactions among the abused. Their research has pointed to childhood violence and aggression, coupled with avoidant attachments, as differentiating abused and non-abused children. Moreover, they offered strong evidence of abusive patterns among abused infants. The researchers studied 20 children from disadvantaged circumstances. Ten had been battered physically and ten were matched controls. They found that those infants whose parents had physically battered them were more likely to hit, kick, or slap than their stressed and disadvantaged, but unbattered, counterparts. In fact, the aggressive children actually assaulted or threatened to assault their caregivers at a frequency four times greater than did the controls. Almost three quarters (70%) of the battered infants, as compared with only 20 percent of the controls, harassed their caregivers in this manner. On average, the researchers noted this behavior almost four times during a 2-hour period. Bousha and Twentyman (1984) detected similar aggression outweighing positive behavior.

In a later assessment of their study, George and Main (1979) further observed that abused children reacted with diffuse anger, fear, or physical abuse when confronted with distress among their normal peers. Nearly all of the abused children, as opposed to only one of the control infants, displayed such a reaction. This atypical lack of empathy closely parallels part of the detachment phenomenon Bowlby (1969) described.

Moreover, the infants who had been abused were four times more likely to avoid friendly approaches from both peers and caregivers. All of the abused children displayed conflicting approach–avoidance gestures in response to the friendly overtures of their peers, while none of the control infants behaved in such a way.

Violence among older abused children is particularly prominent, as the recent study of Monane et al. (1984) reveals. When the researchers compared the histories of abused and nonabused hospitalized psychiatric patients aged 3 to 17 years, they found that 72 percent of the abused patients had themselves exhibited extreme violence, while only 46 percent of the nonabused children behaved violently. Homicidal fantasies were reported in 51 percent of the charts of the abused, compared to 34 percent among the nonabused.

This violence can be interpreted conceptually in a number of ways. Aggressive behavior may be evidence of detachment, the third phase of a child's response to separation, by either neglect or actual separation. The lack of manifested affect characteristic of this stage may facilitate aggression, delinquency, and future abuse. Alternately, violence among the abused may be a learned behavior by which the rejected child emulates the rejecting parent (Monane et al., 1984). The violence noted among the abused is also reminiscent of the studies of Zahn-Waxler et al. (1984b) on the offspring of affectively ill parents. Since many abusive parents are themselves depressed, it is not implausible that the children of abusive parents would behave similarly to the children of depressed parents. Their violence may, like the aggressiveness of the offspring of the depressed, reflect an inability to alleviate the empathic distress they feel for their parents' condition. Thus, while empathic distress under ordinary circumstances would find an outlet in pro-social action (Hoffman, 1977, 1982a), those who have been neglected or abused and who lack a model of empathic response may ventilate their distress in aberrant ways, through lack of feeling, aggression, and violence.

Suicide

Violence suggestive of underlying depression can be expressed outwardly, as observed in the studies just described. Violence can also, however, turn inward, seizing on the self as its object. Indeed, the depression resulting from abuse and neglect can culminate in childhood suicide. Several authors have addressed how abuse and neglect may contribute to children's suicidal behavior (Gould, 1965; Green, 1978b; Husain & Vandiver, 1984; Kosky, 1983; Monane, Leichter, & Lewis, 1984; Morrison & Collier, 1969; Rosenthal & Rosenthal, 1984; Sabbath, 1969).

   The volatile combination of isolation and aggression, common among both abusive and suicidal families, raises the possibility that a depressive mechanism may unite the two phenomena (Crittenden, 1985b; Garfinkle & Golembeck, 1974; Green, 1978b; Paulsen, 1974; Paulson, Stone, & Sposto, 1978; Pfeffer, 1979, 1981a; Tishler & McKenry, 1982). Such families, moreover, show a history of fighting and conflict. Ackerly (1967) found, for example, that family fighting was common to all 21 of the suicidal children, aged 4 to 12 years, that he studied (see also Garfinkle & Golembeck, 1974). Paulson et al. (1978) suggested that the family profile of accident-prone children, who are often suicidal, resembles that of abusive/neglectful families. Alcoholism, which may be considered along the depressive spectrum (Winokur et al., 1971), also appears frequently among both types of families. (See Table 12.)

RISK FACTORS FOR DEPRESSION

A social phenomenon as abhorrent to basic values as child abuse has quite naturally sparked heated debate with respect to its etiology. From this debate four basic models—the sociological model, the psychiatric model, the

Table 12. Behavioral Features of Abuse/Neglect Compared to DSM-III Criteria

Abuse/Neglect Features	DSM-III for MAJOR DEPRESSION (1980, pp. 213-214)	DSM-III for DYSTHYMIC DISORDER (1980, pp. 222-223)
Dysphoric mood (1,2,3,7,9)	Dysphoric mood	Dysphoric mood
Sleep disturbances (2)	Sleep disturbances	Sleep disturbances
Eating disturbances (3)	Eating disturbances	
Less Compliant/difficult (1,2,3,6,8,9,12)		Irritable/excessive anger
Avoidant (1,2,6,7,8,9,11)		Social withdrawal
Aggression (3,4,6,8)		
Communication problems (3,7,8,9)		
Suicidal ideation (10)	Suicidal ideation	Suicidal ideation

1. Bakan (1971)
2. Blumberg (1981)
3. Bible & French (1979)

4. Bousha & Twentyman (1984)
5. Cohen et al. (1966)
6. Crittenden (1985a)

7. Gaensbauer et al. (1980)
8. George & Main (1979)
9. Herrenkohl et al. (1984)

10. Kosky (1983)
11. Lamb et al. (1985)
12. Wasserman et al. (1983)

247

transactional model, and the ecological model—have emerged to explain the "battered-child syndrome." This section will describe each of these models and present evidence for evaluating the contribution each makes to an understanding of the causes of child abuse. Since child abuse is a leading factor in infant and childhood depression, tracing the etiology of abuse will help identify risk factors for a major social problem, as well as for a significant childhood psychiatric problem.

The Sociological Model

Theorists advancing sociological explanations of abuse focus on social values and sociocultural organizations, rather than on the psychosocial characteristics of individuals (parents or children). This model, one of the earliest, originally gained popularity when abuse was still thought to be a problem confined to the lower socioeconomic classes. Its proponents, such as Gil (1968, 1969), who conducted perhaps the most extensive national survey on the relationship between demographic characteristics and abuse, rely on the prevalence of abuse among lower socioeconomic classes to conclude that the environment of these individuals fosters abuse. As the reforming spirit of the 1960s swelled—with its associated attempt to rectify the plight of the poor—a model linking abuse to poverty, unemployment, poor housing, and lack of education naturally won advocates. According to the sociological explanation of abuse, the multiplicity and consistency of socioeconomic stresses placed on abusers heightens their frustration and reduces restraints against aggressive outbursts (Egeland, Cicchetti, & Taraldson, 1976; Galdston, 1965; Gelles, 1973; Gil, 1970; Kaplan et al, 1983; Spinetta & Rigler 1972; Young, 1964; Zahn-Waxler et al., 1984b). Early childhood illness, prematurity, and perinatal complications—all of which are frequent products of the inadequate prenatal care received by the poor—are commonly cited as contributors to abuse (Elmer & Gregg, 1967; Lynch, 1975; Pollock & Steele, 1972). Gil argued that cultural norms among the underprivileged, which show greater acceptance of physical force as a child-rearing device, further enhance the prospects for abuse.

Indeed, researchers have gathered a wealth of descriptive data correlating abuse with stress-inducing social factors. Giovannoni and Becerra (1979) claim that a family's poverty level provides the best indicator for neglect. Sherrod et al. (1984) support this view with findings that 57 percent of the families of the neglected children they studied depended on financial subsidies, whereas about one quarter of the controls relied on such assistance.

Most studies on isolation, for example, note that isolation from community and family support systems typifies families in which maltreatment occurs (Elmer, 1967; Garbarino, 1977; Merrill, 1962). Garbarino (1976), for example, found that the abuse and maltreatment across New

York state related directly to the support systems available to mothers under economic stress. He found that the degree to which mothers are subject to socioeconomic stress without adequate support accounts for a substantial proportion (36%) of the variance in rates of child maltreatment across counties statewide. In contrast, economic conditions in general accounted for only 16 percent of the variance. Based on this study, Garbarino concluded that establishment of support systems to help mothers provide for basic needs and reduce isolation offers a particularly promising way of reducing abuse.

A more recent study by Egeland, Breitenbucher, and Rosenberg (1980) confirms the relationship between abuse and lack of social support structures. This study followed 267 women throughout their first pregnancies, most on welfare, from the last trimester of their pregnancies until their infants reached 1 year of age. The researchers found significant differences in abuse rates between mothers under stress who had friends and family to help them work out crises and high-stress mothers with no such resources.

Other social forces may also affect the rate of child abuse. Light (1973), who reanalyzed Gil's (1968) data, established a link between paternal unemployment and maltreatment, and Herrenkohl, Herrenkohl, Toedtler, and Yanushefski (1984) detected a strong tie between family income and abusive behavior. Klein and Stern (1971) even correlated abuse with low birth weight, perhaps a product of inadequate prenatal care. However, they acknowledge that other factors, such as the mother's own childhood experiences and current social network, influence the potential for abuse.

This research, mostly retrospective, correlating high incidences of abuse with a variety of socioeconomic stress factors, appears compelling and perhaps suits the need to distance ourselves from the ugly reality of abuse. However, evidence increasingly prevents relegating abuse strictly to sociological factors. In fact, most researchers now assert that abuse spans all socioeconomic classes and is far from limited to the economically disadvantaged (Blumberg, 1977). Evidence of widespread abuse outside the economically poor has been used to repudiate the view that socioeconomic stresses place families at risk for abuse.

On its own, this evidence does not entirely discredit the sociological model. After all, it is possible to broaden the definition of socioeconomic stress and identify a number of socioeconomic stress factors—such as job dissatisfaction, isolation, and marital discord—that may spark aggressive outbursts from middle-class individuals. However, in view of the often mentioned fact that the vast majority of those in the lower economic classes do not abuse their children in spite of their vulnerability to socioeconomic stress, the sociological model diminishes in credibility. If it predicts behavior neither within classes nor across classes, it fails to offer sufficient explanation for the eruption of abuse in a particular social context. Indeed, these findings have led many researchers to propose that sociological factors may predispose some individuals to abuse, while other factors, such as individual psychological differences, actually determine whether abuse results (Newberger, 1977; Wolock & Horowitz, 1984). Steele and Pollock (1968) place sociological factors in the proper perspective when they suggest that such factors merely serve to exacerbate personality-rooted factors.

Egeland et al. (1980) imply that the relevant etiologic factors for abuse are not stress and support per se, as much as individuals' differential abilities to take advantage of these supports. Thus, while socioeconomic stress may place certain individuals at risk for abuse, it appears that individual psychosocial characteristics may either precipitate or prevent this behavior. Crittenden (1985b) adheres to this view, suggesting that it is not lack of a social network as much as the quality of social interaction that may predispose a mother to abuse or neglect. Of the abusive and neglectful mothers the researcher studied, most had at least frequent contact with family, if not a broad social network outside of family as well.

Findings such as these, which mandate increasing recognition of individual differences in coping with stress, whatever its source, have justifiably cast disfavor on purely sociological explanations of abuse.

The Psychiatric Model

Explanations linking individual psychosocial profiles to abuse—while comprising a narrower model than the sociological model—appear to possess greater explanatory power. The psychiatric model focuses on particular personality traits and personal experiences of the parent as signals for potential abuse.

An extensive literature has been amassed on the psychosocial characteristics of abusive parents. After reviewing the data, Main and Goldwyn (1984) found that efforts by psychiatrists, psychologists, and others to assemble a single coherent personality profile of abusing parents yields a confusing picture. Most researchers attempting to depict the abusive parent agree that a combination of traits, rather than any single trait, creates a propensity for abuse (Delsordo, 1963; Merrill, 1962; Zalba, 1967).

Researchers disagree on the specific traits that lead to abuse, as well as on how severe a parental disorder must be before it places a family at risk. Nonetheless, they have pinpointed a number of psychological variables falling into four broad categories: (1) personality and psychiatric disorders, (2) early childhood experiences, (3) cognitive impairments and parenting skills, and (4) coping and defense mechanisms.

Personality and Psychiatric Disorders. Studies of abusive parents portray them with varying degrees of disordered traits and psychopathology. Most researchers, however, concur that abusive parents demonstrate particular difficulty controlling aggression (Galdston, 1981; Helfer, McKinney, & Kempe, 1976; Herrenkohl et al., 1983a). Merrill (1962) was one of the first to develop a typology of abusive parents, and his model is still widely used. In reducing a myriad of this population's personality characteristics into three core categories, he proposed chronic hostility and aggression as one category. Other personality traits, many of them strikingly depressive, also appear to factor into the incidence of abuse. Merrill's second category included characteristics such as rigidity, compulsiveness, and unreasonableness. The third category encompassed passivity and dependence. Several researchers cite a lack of empathy (Melnick & Hurley, 1969; Steele, 1983), impulsiveness, hypersensitivity, and quickness to react (Bousha & Twentyman, 1984; Bryant et al., 1963), self-centeredness (Melnick & Hurley, 1969), avoidance of social interaction, fear of authority, feelings of guilt, and low self-esteem (Helfer, McKinney, & Kempe, 1976; Main & Goldwyn, 1984).

Newer evidence suggests that more than mere clusters of traits are involved. Degrees of psychopathology—ranging from personality disorders to bona fide psychosis—characterize many abusive parents. According to Smith and Hanson (1975), approximately 10 percent of parents of abused children have been diagnosed with a definable psychiatric condition. A number of studies have compared abusive and nonabusive parents for various degrees of psychopathology. In one study, abusive parents showed higher levels than control groups when measured on the Psychopathic Deviate and Hypomania Scales (Paulson et al., 1976). When Smith et al. (1973) used the Eysenck Personality Inventory and the General Health Questionnaire to study the fathers of abused children, they found "abnormal personalities" among almost half (46%) and psychopathology among a third. Almost half of the mothers were diagnosed during an interview as neurotic, with symptoms of depression, anxiety, or a combination of the two. These findings conflict with the conclusions of Spinetta and Rigler (1972) who found little in the literature suggesting a high incidence of psychosis among abusing parents.

Although there is no single personality profile for the abusing parent, depression emerges as one of the prominent types of psychopathology contributing to abuse. Merrill's (1962) passive and dependent classification typically revealed a number of traits of depression including moodiness, unresponsiveness, unhappiness, and depressed feelings. Kaplan et al. (1983) conducted a particularly noteworthy study in which they compared mothers of 76 abused children reported to the New York State Department of Social Services with 38 control mothers. They found nearly four times (51% vs. 13%) as much clinical depression among the mothers of abused children, and half as much depression among fathers (24% vs. 16%). When parents were combined, the contrast was still significant: Twice as many of the abusive parents were clinically depressed. Thus, abusive behavior may serve as an outlet for parental depression, facilitating the passage of this behavior from one generation to another.

The correlation between depression and abusiveness appears particularly significant in light of the similarities in child-rearing practices among the mothers of both the abusive and control groups. When Susman et al. (1985) compared the attitudes and practices of several groups (current major depressives, past major depressives, current minor depressives, abusers, and controls) with the Block Child-Rearing Practices Report, they found that mothers with current depression resembled the abuse mothers in 38 percent of the 21 child-rearing factors they evaluated. Interestingly, the two groups resembled each other most closely on factors concerned with affect expression and development of autonomy. Higher rates of alcoholism, drug abuse, antisocial personality, and labile personality also distinguished the abusive parents from the control group in the study.

A higher level of alcoholism may also characterize abusive parents. As yet, the association between parental alcoholism and child abuse is tentative and inferential at best. Demonstration of a causal relationship between alcohol abuse and child abuse would require proof either that the level of abuse is higher among alcoholics than among nonalcoholics or that alcoholism among known child abusers is significantly more common than alcoholism in the general population. Orme and Rimmer's (1981) review of the literature found no reliable evidence of either of these relationships between alcoholism and child abuse and concluded that there is no support for such a relationship.

On the other hand, several investigators have drawn close parallels between the personality profiles and psychiatric histories of alcoholics and child abusers, suggesting that those known to have alcohol problems may have a higher probability of abusing their children than those without alcohol abuse/dependence. Feelings of powerlessness, ineffectiveness, and worthlessness have, from clinical observations, all been ascribed to both populations. On a more objective level, as we shall see, a childhood history of abuse has also been shown to be common among those who abuse their own children. Similarly, a history of child abuse is also common among alcoholics (Hindeman, 1977). In a questionnaire administered to 178 patients in treatment in the United States and Australia for drug or alcoholic addiction, these researchers found that 84 percent reported a history of abuse as a child. Moreover, alcoholics who have been abused as children often display significantly more depressive symptomatology than those who have not been abused, according to Kroll, Stock, and James (1985). Their retrospective chart review (a technique subject to inconsistencies, incomplete information, and interpretive biases) showed that a history of child abuse among the alcoholics they studied resulted in significantly greater levels of aggressive behavior. Notably, the abused alcoholics directed aggression both at others and at themselves. Domestic violence and violence against authority were common, as were serious suicidal attempts. The relative contributions of alcoholism and history of abuse to the alcoholics' violence is unclear from the study, since it failed to include a group of nonalcoholics who were abused as children.

In summary, clusters of personality traits and comparatively high rates of psychopathology—in the forms of depression, alcoholism, labile personality, and antisocial personality—all give rise to a harsh and punitive child-rearing climate, scapegoating, maternal deprivation, and caregiving interruptions. Often this pathological milieu culminates in psychological or physical abuse.

Early Childhood Experiences. The personality profiles—whether pathological or not—that have been associated with abuse emerge, at least in part, from the parent's own childhood experiences. A group of researchers within the psychiatric orientation on abuse has focused on the impact of these early formative experiences of abusing parents. One of the few points on which researchers in this field agree is that individuals who have themselves experienced violence and abuse as children are more likely than those who have not experienced violence during their childhood to become child or spouse abusers (Bakan, 1971; Byrd, 1979; Cicchetti & Rizley, 1981; Curtis, 1963; Flynn, 1975; Fontana, 1973; Gelles, 1973; Green, 1976; Green, Gaines, & Sandgrund, 1974; Justice & Duncan, 1975; Kempe et al., 1962; Main & Goldwyn, 1984; Silver et al., 1969; Spinetta & Rigler, 1972; Steele & Pollock, 1968, 1974).

Of course, a parent need not experience actual physical abuse in childhood to be at risk for abusing his or her own child. Researchers have observed a particularly close relationship between abuse of one's children and rejection—whether in the form of emotional rejection *or* physical rejection—by one's own parents. Often the latter manifests itself in the form of insecure attachments with the parent's own parents. Galdston (1981) noted that a persistent ambivalent attachment between parents and children can motivate violent reactions that may easily find a target among one's own children, frequently entailing outright abuse.

In a study of the social networks of abusive and neglectful mothers, Crittenden (1985b) observed a correlation between a mother's behavior during general social interaction and her behavior toward her child. This suggested to Crittenden that a unified model of relationships—derived from a parent's own early attachment experiences—infuses all of the parent's familial and extrafamilial relationships. A parent lacking a secure and reciprocal model of attachment may carry this model into the relationship with his or her own child. Crittenden describes two different models, one for abusing mothers and one for neglectful mothers. Both are based on the notion that psychological and physical resources for such individuals are scarce. However, the model for the abusive mother tends to incorporate a need for mastery in meeting one's needs, whereas the neglectful mother's internal representation reflects a sense of helplessness and despair. According to this theory, the representational model created by neglect in a parent's own childhood might pose a greater risk for the offspring's depression than the model evolving from abuse.

This explanation, which suggests that the failure to form a secure attachment in childhood may frustrate attempts to form a secure attachment with one's own children, is particularly useful for explaining how abuse and neglect transmit themselves across generations—a characteristic of abuse that few will dispute. Morris and Gould (1963) were the first to describe a role reversal in which parents who were abused themselves actually turn to their children for nurturance and protection—in short, for satisfaction of unmet dependency needs. DeLozier (1982) hypothesizes that mothers who have, because of their own abused history, developed inadequate representations of attachment figures, interpret the normal behavior of their children as rejecting and respond inappropriately with helplessness, self-blame, and anxiety, all of which may find an outlet in anger and violence. A review of the literature by Ricks (1985) concludes that nonoptimal caregiving occurs most often in families where parents themselves suffered deprivation as children. After studying parents of NOFT infants, Leonard et al. (1966) posit that pregnancy, even under the most favorable circumstances, often activates a mother's need for nurturance which must be satisfied for the mother to fulfill her own role as a new mother. However, when this need is not met—because the pregnancy was unwanted, for example, or the marital relationship is not supportive— the mother often "fails to thrive" as a mother. Should the infant fail to thrive for any reason, such a mother may interpret this as a confirmation of her overwhelming sense of inadequacy. Mother and infant thus become locked in a mutually destructive pattern of unmet dependency needs. These forms of introjection, role reversal, and insecure feelings of attachment are directly correlated with childhood depression and suicide (Adam, 1982; Morris & Gould, 1963; Pfeffer et al., 1979, 1980, 1982).

A number of studies have supported Morris and Gould's (1963) inference that a strong tendency exists among mothers who have been rejected or abused by their mothers to reject their own offspring (DeLozier, 1982; Gil, 1969; Leonard et al., 1966; Main & Goldwyn, 1984; Ricks, 1985; Schneider-Rosen & Cicchetti, 1984; Spinetta & Rigler, 1972). In Leonard et al.'s (1966) study, for example, none of the 12 mothers of NOFT infants and children, described her own parenting as continually nurturant. Melnick and Hurley (1969) also found that severely frustrated dependency needs, a lack of empathy and probable history of emotional deprivation distinguished abusive mothers from control mothers.

Although this model helps explain why parents who have experienced rejection or abuse may maltreat their offspring, it does not clarify why parents not subject to abuse/neglect may maltreat their children. Main and Goldwyn (1984) offer one possible explanation. They suggest that rejection can assume subtle, nonphysical forms that can be equally as damaging to the child's affective response as physical rejection. For a child with a temperamentally high need for stimulation, a low degree of contact from the mother may be perceived as rejection.

Cognitive Impairments and Parenting Skills. A third group within the psychiatric school isolates parental cognitive impairments, which range from low levels of intelligence to lack of awareness about children's developing needs.

Researchers are far from agreeing on the role of low intelligence in the etiology of abuse (Cameron, Johnson, & Camps, 1966; Fisher, 1958; Holter & Friedman, 1968; Kempe et al., 1962; Simpson, 1967, 1968). However, more general cognitive differences appear to operate in conjunction with either sociological or emotional factors to unleash abuse. Main and Goldwyn (1984), hypothesize that the significant interaction occurs between cognition and emotion. According to their model, cognitive impairments may act as the mediating mechanisms between a parent's own abuse and abuse of the child. As Main and Goldwyn (1984) recently illustrated, mothers who themselves had been rejected generally exhibit a variety of cognitive deficiencies. When such women were interviewed using the Berkeley Adult Attachment Audit as part of a study assessing the relationship between the representation of a woman's mother as rejecting and her own rejecting behavior, abused mothers failed to recall details about their childhood, systematically distorted and often idealized their rejecting parent, and spoke incoherently in discussing current attachments. Main and Goldwyn concluded that distortions in representation stemming from rejection and/or abuse play a positive role in conveying child abuse from one generation to another. The researchers tentatively posit that repression of these memories—as apparent in the cognitive distortions or omissions— perpetuates a pattern of "identification with the aggressor," activating abuse in the abused.

Cognitive differences in processing signals from infants also appear to factor into an abusive parent's reaction to its child. Evidence of these differences was found by Friedrich, Tyler, and Clark (1985) in a study comparing abusive, neglectful, and control mothers' reactions to an infant's cry. The research team played an audiotape of an infant's cry to the three sets of mothers and had them rate the cry on a number of dimensions. While they detected no significant differences on reasonably objective dimensions—the age of the child, the length of the cry, and the loudness of the cry—the researchers did find significant differences on more qualitative subjective measures, such as the mother's description of the cry. For example, the abusive and neglectful mothers rated the cry as significantly more angry than did the control mothers. Interestingly, the neglectful and abusive mothers diverged on their rating of how irritating and demanding the cry appeared to be—the neglectful mothers rated the cry as most irritating and demanding, while the abusive mothers found it least irritating and demanding among the three groups of mothers. The authors theorize that the differences in these two dimensions may arise through repression on the part of the abusive mothers and exaggeration on the part of the neglectful mothers.

Inadequate parenting skills, stemming from a variety of sources including cognitive deficits, a parent's own deprivation, or an unwanted pregnancy (Bible & French, 1979; Leonard et al., 1966; Smith & Hanson, 1975), also appear to factor into abuse. Newberger and Cook (1983) emphasize that the developmental maturity of the parent's attitude toward the child has significant implications for his or her functioning as a parent. Gregg and Elmer (1969) found sharp distinctions among abusive and nonabusive mothers in their abilities to provide routine daily care and medical care for their children. Misunderstandings of children's needs and behaviors—particularly as they evolve during the course of development—often lead parents to overestimate the capacities of their children and underestimate the impact of their own actions (Newberger & Cook, 1983). Parents may thus react with abuse at the failure of their children to meet their demands and expectations (Galdston, 1965; Steele & Pollock, 1968). For example, Egeland, Breitenbucher, and Rosenberg (1980) observed that abusive mothers had difficulty recognizing the intent behind seemingly violent behavior of their infants and had less understanding of the importance of responding to infant cues in a solidifying relationship. These flaws in awareness extend to the impact of maltreatment and neglect; several authors note that abusive parents lack cognizance of the impact of their abuse on their children (Gilligan, 1977; Smith, Hanson, & Noble, 1973).

Coping Skills. A parent's ability to adapt to the demands of his or her own changing life and the requirements of the child is a function of many variables—some associated with the magnitude of the demands placed on the parent, some with the parent's own internal coping mechanisms, and some with the external resources available. Different individuals placed under the same types and degrees of stress demonstrate different reactions; not all of them will abuse their children. Clearly, then, some internal coping mechanisms, perhaps a function of earlier adaptations, differentiate those who will abuse from those who will not. Egeland, Breitenbrucher, and Rosenberg (1980) detected clear distinctions between the competence of abusive and nonabusive mothers when both groups were under stress. Traits, such as rigidity and dependence, that have been used to characterize abusive parents (Merrill, 1962) will almost certainly impinge on a parent's ability to adapt to stressful situations successfully. Wolfe (1985) posits that the lack of coping skills sparks abuse in parents seeking to gain control in a stressful environment.

The Transactional Model

Children have traditionally been viewed as the victims, rather than the causes of abuse. While no one has suggested that the personality traits and behaviors of children, by themselves, will provoke abuse, some research assigns the child a larger role in the determination of his or her abuse. Children have expectations and perceptions that shape their caregivers' responses to them (Wolfe, 1985). Infant behaviors and temperament impinging on parents' needs, deficiencies, and vulnerabilities produce disruptions in the caregiving environment that ultimately may lead to abuse. The impact of a child on the caregiver is illustrated most poignantly by the sad fact that foster parents will often abuse a child who has been placed in their care after abuse by the child's biological parents (Bible & French, 1979).

The transactional model may be viewed as incorporating both the psychiatric profile of the abuser and the psychiatric profile of the abused. This paradigm explores the mutual influences of these factors, by concentrating on the detailed interactions between family members. It emphasizes the bidirectional nature of the interaction between abusive parent and abused child (Wolfe, 1985). In this model, both child and parent exercise equal influence in shaping their interaction (Bell & Harper, 1977; Gaensbauer & Sands, 1979). According to Schneider-Rosen and Cicchetti (1984), parent-child communication involves the dynamic interaction of the developmental status of the infant, as well as a number of characteristics of the caregiver—temperament, ability to interpret ambiguous signals from the infant, and quality of affective responses. This dynamic perception of the interaction sets the transactional model apart from the more static sociological or psychiatric models and makes it a particularly constructive tool for understanding the intergenerational transmission of abuse. It is particularly useful for explaining a relatively new area of exploration: the child's contribution to his or her own abuse through attachment behavior, affective expression, and violence. Moreover, the model is consistent with Thomas and Chess' (1984) "interactional" view of temperament, which holds that temperament does not serve to initiate behavior in the infant, but does give clues to and initiate behavior in the caregiver.

In fact, a large body of research supports the notion of bidirectionality as the governing force in shaping an infant–caregiver relationship—whether pathological or not. Robison and Solomon (1979) write of a growing awareness that mutually modulating feedback systems, also documented by Brazelton, Koslowski, and Main (1974) and Stern (1974), develop early in life. Such systems can thus be expected to play a prominent role in any child–caregiver exchange.

Since the interaction is a function of both the cognitive and affective characteristics of parents and children, it is necessarily fragile. In environments where abuse has already occurred, changes in a child's temperament, affect expression, and attachment status will inevitably express themselves in further problematic interactions with caregivers. Failure of this interaction can result from what Schneider-Rosen and Cicchetti (1984) call "decreased responsiveness and reciprocal interactions, aberrations in patterns of initiating, maintaining or terminating interaction, and deviations in the capacity to express emotional states" (p. 382). Abuse ranks among the more probable outcomes of such a failure.

Although researchers have demonstrated amply that failed interactions in a variety of forms characterize homes with abuse, they have fared less well in translating these characteristics—insecure attachments, withdrawal, lack of interaction—into causal models detailing precisely how these characteristics trigger abuse. Although any of these characteristics in isolation may correlate highly with abuse, one factor alone does not necessarily cause it. It is a long interpretive leap to suggest, for example, that insecurely attached children somehow elicit abuse. The facts bear out the absurdity of this logic since certainly not every child with difficulties in affect expression or insecure attachment is abused. The task then is to identify the array of parental characteristics that conspire to unleash abuse. This task is not easy (as is apparent by the relative dearth of such descriptions in the literature), since the bidirectional nature of the model implies that failure can come from both parent and child. Moreover, the dynamic element that this model captures suggests that the effects of abuse, such as insecure attachment, withdrawal, and lack of affect, can also be the causes of abuse.

Failed interactions that manifest themselves in confrontations between violent parents and children who in turn have become violent through abuse are easier to explain than interactions in which patterns of avoidance and insecure attachment culminate in abuse. The former may be conceptualized as an instance of violence meeting violence, particularly since recent evidence indicates that abuse occurs often among older children who, through their own abuse, may have formed a strong capacity for violence. Galdston (1981) suggests that children who have been rejected through abuse may provoke interaction from others in order to relieve the burden of their isolation.

With child avoidance, rather than child aggression and violence, the chain of causality is not as obvious. Clearly, only a small fraction of individuals who might be characterized as withdrawn or insecurely attached find themselves part of an abusive parent-child scenario. Some precipitating factor is needed to ignite the outburst. Parental frustration probably plays a major role. One possible explanation builds on DeLozier's hypothesis (1982) that a failed interaction is condemned to further abuse because the maltreated child's conflicting desires—on the one hand, to approach the attachment figure

Table 13. Depressive Behavior in both Adults and Children

Adult Behavior	Abused Child Behavior
Isolation	Failure to explore environment
Immaturity	Developmental delays
Impulsiveness	Increased impulsiveness
Lack of control over aggression	Tendency to act out aggression on caregivers and other children
Unsympathetic to distress in others	Unsympathetic to distress in others
Increased anxiety	Increased anxiety
Unmet dependency needs	Insecure attachment

and, on the other hand, to avoid the source of danger—prevent the child from initiating remedial action in the relationship. Infants unreceptive to their parents' attempts at engagement—rare though they may be (Wasserman, Green, & Allen, 1983)—can certainly breed frustration. Parents who felt insecure in their ability to provide for their children (Newberger, Newberger, & Hampton, 1983) and who turned, as abusive parents are prone to do (Steele & Pollock, 1968), to their children for the kind of reassurance and comfort that only an adult can provide may find such infantile behavior particularly provocative. A child's lack of affect or depression, themselves products of abuse, may have the same incendiary effect, intensifying parental frustrations and undermining their abilities to cope (Trad, 1986).

A further explanation in the transactional framework focuses on a modeling mechanism, whereby children fashion their behavior after their parents. Child–parent interaction provides continual negative reinforcement of the parents' inadequate coping skills, expressed through abuse. Through this modeling, the seeds of abuse are planted by one generation in the next (Herrenkohl et al., 1984; Monane et al., 1984).

Thus, the abusive adult and the abused child share some of the same symptomatology (see Table 13).

While the abused/abuser system is interactional, there is one exception: Because of the child's need for dependence, he or she ususally acts out his or her aggression with persons other than his or her abuser.

The Ecological Model

Although compelling, the transactional model lacks one important variable. While it incorporates bidirectionality between caregiver and child, it does not move beyond events as they occur and are experienced between individuals; that is, it fails to include environmental risk factors. The ecological model provides this important dimension in a bidirectional framework and thereby expands on the strengths of the transactional model. Indeed, this model offers the most comprehensive approach to understanding the etiology and outcome of child abuse.

The ecological model, which can fruitfully be applied to many facets of human development, was originally defined by Bronfenbrenner (1977), who explained that:

> The ecology of human development is the scientific study of progressive, mutual accommodation, throughout the lifespan, between a growing human organism and the changing immediate environments in which it lives, as this process is affected by relations obtaining within and between these immediate settings, as well as the larger social contexts, both formal and informal, in which the settings are embedded. (p. 514)

The model resembles the biological transactional model of Sameroff and Chandler (1975) in its bidirectionality, and it focuses on mutual adaptation of the organism and environment. However it offers a somewhat broader concept of the environmental variables than that delineated by Sameroff and Chandler. According to Bronfenbrenner, individuals operate at three different ecological levels: (1) in the household, which he calls the microsystem, (2) in society at large, or the exosystem, and (3) amid overriding cultural values, or the macrosystem. In Bronfenbrenner's scheme, the macrosystem provides context, information, and meaning which assume concrete form in the complex interpersonal and personal–environmental relations of the microsystem.

This approach is most useful for connecting the interactions of daily life with overarching cultural values. As Belsky (1980) pointed out, this ecological framework provides a useful scheme for integrating the many factors contributing to child abuse, among them the role of the child, family interaction patterns, socioeconomic stress, and cultural values. An ecological interpretation of child abuse would argue that, as a result of their own development, abusing parents enter the immediate family (microsystem) predisposed to abuse. Stress, arising either from the immediate family or from external environmental factors (the exosystem) may activate the abuse if it finds support in cultural values and child-rearing customs (the macrosystem). Another proponent of the ecological approach, Garbarino (1977) offers a similar explanation of abuse. He explains abuse as:

> destructive organism—environment adaptations . . . "permitted" by ideological support for the use of physical force and by naturally occurring and socially engineered support systems that inadequately monitor deviance and fail to encourage effective parenting. (p. 728)

For example, after analyzing data from the New York State Child Protective Service, Garbarino (1976) attributes abuse to socioeconomic stress combined with lack of support systems for mothers and mothers' inability to take advantage of support.

In applying the ecological model to child abuse, Herrenkohl and Herrenkohl (1981) lay greater emphasis on coping skills. They view development as a series of concentric circles with the child-parent interaction at the center. The social and coping skills that the child acquires from his or her parents instill the sense of self-worth and social competence that the child brings to areas of interaction within the family and the wider community. In cases of abuse or neglect, parent-child interaction provides a medium that reinforces the defective coping skills of the parents and transmits them to the child. Modeling of such inadequate coping strategies in an environment that is not supportive and does not encourage development of self-reliance and self-esteem enmeshes the parent-child dyad in a vicious cycle of negative reinforcement that may evolve into child abuse or neglect (see Table 14).

Summary and Future Directions

These models cite a multiplicity of factors contributing to child abuse and neglect. Many researchers have abandoned efforts to isolate any single causal agent (Alvy, 1975; Belsky, 1980; Cicchetti & Rizley, 1981; Green, 1968; Herrenkohl & Herrenkohl, 1981; Parke & Collmer, 1975; Polansky, 1976; Starr et al., 1976). Each of the four models contributes further nuances to the understanding of abuse and thus helps to identify the predictive factors. The parent who suffered from abuse or neglect—or at least from attachment dysfunction in childhood—or who is currently depressed or isolated has a greater predisposition to abuse. However, such a predisposition may remain latent unless activated by some external provocation. This incitement can have numerous sources—socioeconomic stress, a child's illness, or a child's temperament. The psychiatric model focuses too narrowly on the psychosocial characteristics of the abusive parent, while the sociological model overlooks these factors. Predictions of child abuse/neglect require a comprehensive examination of intrafamily dynamics, as well as of family environment dynamics.

Research on the roles played by each of these factors is still plagued by a number of theoretical and methodological problems: small, non-representational samples, lack of adequate control groups, imprecise definitions of the problem, and retrospective analyses. A great deal of attention has been focused on correlates, but not enough on etiologies of abuse, as Cicchetti and Rizley (1981) contend. These researchers correctly urge greater emphasis on prospective longitudinal studies—both to identify

Table 14. *Abuse/Neglect Population Compared with Three Risk Populations*

Maternal Depression	Hospitalization	Handicapped
Offspring of depressed parents are more likely to be maltreated. (1)	Abused/neglected children have more illnesses, especially in first six months. (2)	Handicapped child is more likely to be maltreated. (3)
Both maltreating parent and maltreated child are likely to be depressed. (4)	Birth complications are associated with increased maltreatment. (5)	Parents of handicapped children experience heightened stress. (6)
Parent degree of psychopathology affects perception of child difficulty. (7)		Handicapped child is more likely to be "difficult," which may lead to maltreatment. (8)
Depressed mothers show a "dampening" of behavior, with greater risk of neglect; and they continue to have difficulty with child after recovery. (9)		Handicapped child is more likely to have more disturbing cry. (10)
		Handicapped child is more likely to suffer from poor dyadic relationship and experience less positive attachment behaviors. (11)

1. Conger et al. (1981); Ebeling & Hill (1975); Galdston (1965); Johnson & Morse (1968); Kaplan et al. (1983); Steele & Pollock (1968)
2. Sherrod et al. (1984)
3. Blacher & Meyers (1983); Friedrich & Boriskin (1976); Jaudes & Diamond (1985); Lynch & Roberts (1977); Meyers, Zetlin, & Blacher-Dixon (1981)
4. Bible & French (1979)
5. Elmer & Gregg (1967); Hunter et al. (1978); Klein & Stern (1971)
6. Bernheimer, Young, & Winton (1983)
7. Estroff et al. (1984)
8. Frodi (1981); Steinhausen (1981); Shindi (1983)
9. Weissman et al. (1972); Weissman & Paykel (1974)
10. Ostwald & Peltzman (1974)
11. Blacher (1984); Emde & Brown (1978); Helfer (1975); Stone & Chesney (1978)

more reliably the risk factors and predictive variables and to guide intervention.

We are only beginning to develop the methodologies for accomplishing these objectives. Altemeier, Vietze, and Sherrod (1979) have developed what is, to date, the best tool for identifying factors associated with or predictive of child abuse. When administered to prospective mothers and evaluated against their child's condition at about 1 year old, their questionnaire achieved impressive predictability. Three quarters of the reported abuse and over half of the neglect cases had occurred in the families identified by the study as "high risk." An estimated 43 percent of the NOFT cases belonged to the high-risk group. The original questionnaire and short interview produced impressive results when first administered, but can be refined to provide even greater predictive validity. Future refinements should include measures of aggression, for potentially abusive mothers, and measures of withdrawal/passivity, for potentially neglectful mothers. This tool might also play a valuable role in identifying potentially abusive mothers at a point, probably during their pregnancy, when intervention can be most efficacious. If, as seems likely, patterns of abuse begin with a failure of interaction during the first year of life—with the risk of abuse highest before the child reaches 3.5 years old—early identification and intervention are essential.

CONCLUSION

Abuse and neglect are prominent risk factors for depression and depressive-like phenomena in young populations. This chapter has analyzed four etiologic models of abusive/neglectful behavior displayed by parents toward their children. The psychiatric and transactional models propose that such deviant behavioral manifestations are attributable to intrapsychic disturbance on the part of caregivers or between the members of the infant–caregiver dyad. The sociological and ecological models advance a more macroanalytical approach. These theories suggest that environmental stress factors, such as poverty or lack of social support systems, precipitate instances of abuse and neglect. But regardless of the source, documentation reveals that infant or child abuse/neglect leaves an indelible imprint on the victim, invariably generating a cycle of depression or depressive-like phenomena. Abuse and neglect may serve as such potent risk factors for depression because they represent external examples of noncontingency in a hostile universe to a young child ill-equipped to cope with this treatment. In these cases, intervention is mandatory to ward off the debilitating effects of psycopathology.

CHAPTER EIGHT

Sickness and Hospitalization as Risk Factors for Infant and Childhood Depression

This chapter isolates a distinct category of infants and children who experience a higher incidence of depression and depressive-like phenomena than their healthy counterparts, namely, those with illness or histories of hospitalization. This population has been given special status for a number of reasons. First, since depression has been documented among these infants and children, the paradigm of illness or hospitalization enables a detailed description of the etiologic factors precipitating such disorders in these young populations. Second, infant and childhood depression linked to a bout with illness or an episode of hospitalization is so well encapsulated— onset and duration can be pinpointed fairly precisely. Thus, such depression and depressive-like phenomena may be compared directly with other analogs of depression, such as learned helplessness, to discern similarities among the broad spectrum of affective disorders. Indeed, as the chapter will suggest, infant and childhood depression which first manifests during illness or hospitalization may replicate, in many respects, both the genesis and ultimate aftermath of learned-helplessness depression. Finally, focusing on this population permits us to reevaluate one of the underlying themes of this text—regulation and its converse, dysregulation—in a specifically defined group of infants and children.

Ultimately, illness and hospitalization tax the child's resources in a highly stressful manner, often imposing feelings of loss of control (as a consequence of a body that, for the first time, has gone "haywire"), maternal separation, and an alien environment. These phenomena, which stress the infant and/or child from both the perspective of genetic endowment and environmental influences, must be regulated by the young patient into his or her internal representation in a manner that enables adaptation and optimal response. But if the young child lacks the capacity, resources, or incentive to engage in such regulatory efforts, his or her response may be characterized as "dysregulatory," and as the data will suggest, such a response primes the infant or child for depression, with its inherent ravaging effects.

Depression can occur in any patient with a physical illness. The patient may feel at the mercy of uncontrollable changes occurring in his or her body and is often reduced to a state of helpless dependence on others. Thus, an episode of illness may create a situation which, in many respects, resembles the debilitation encountered by an individual experiencing learned-helplessness depression. However, what may amount to a transient episode of illness in an adult's life can, for infants and children, assume proportions far beyond the significance of the actual physical problem. Moreover, the psychological aftermath of childhood illness may persist in acute form long after the physical problem has been resolved. Hospitalization, which typically entails frustration of attachment bonds by separating the child from loved ones and isolating him or her in a seemingly hostile environment, can further magnify the impact of illness, enhancing the prospects that a confusing and painful experience will result in lasting repercussions.

Anna Freud (1953) wrote that the significance of an early life experience is determined not so much by its value in external reality as by its psychic reality—the realm in which a child's unconscious fantasies and anxieties operate to invest even the most harmless and trivial of events with sinister inner meaning. Illness and hospitalization activate many of these fantasies, causing children to interpret such experiences as confirmation of their most terrifying fears.

Throughout the century, pediatricians have recognized the deleterious physical effects of hospitalization on children. High mortality rates in infant institutions and pediatric facilities—while no doubt attributable in part to the state of medical knowledge—have commonly been cited as evidence of the harmful side effects of child hospitalization. By the middle of this century, researchers began to recognize that the impact of surgical procedures and hospitalization was far from limited to the child's physical condition. With Spitz's (1945) graphic depiction of the impact of long-term institutionalization on British infants during World War II, the medical community first began to appreciate more fully the devastating psychological impact of hospitalization on infants. Since then a number of researchers have clearly demonstrated that the experience of hospitalization can thwart a child's development toward greater adaptiveness and lead to emotional and behavioral problems. (Douglas, 1975; Levy, 1945; Lindemann, 1941; Michaels, 1943; Prugh et al., 1953; Quinton & Rutter, 1976; Robertson, 1953; Robertson & Bowlby, 1952; Schaffer & Callender, 1959). Recognition of this phenomenon even gave rise to the term "hospitalism," which was used by Spitz to describe the weakened and vitiated condition of the body due to long confinement or to the morbid atmosphere frequently encountered in the hospital setting.

Researchers have documented a myriad of affective and cognitive deficits associated with childhood illness and hospitalization. Depression or depressive symptomatology appears in virtually every description of the adverse effects of sickness and hospitalization. Most recently, such psychopathology has been documented among (AIDS) Acquired Immune Deficiency Syndrome victims, a growing number of whom are infants and children (Dilley, Ochtill, Perl, & Volberding, 1985; Holland & Tross, 1985). By the end of 1985, over 200 cases of AIDS in patients under the age of 13 had been reported to the Centers for Disease Control (Church, Allen, & Stiehm, 1985).

Despite the seemingly widespread recognition of the prevalence of depression among sick and hospitalized children, researchers have taken a broadbrush approach to understanding the problem of childhood depression in the context of illness and hospitalization. While a number of researchers have made a commendable effort to add a developmental component to studies focusing on the effects of hospitalization in general—seeking to outline risk factors with differential age-dependent effects—depression has received no such analysis. Instead, perhaps because depression appears at many ages, researchers have tended to assume that children of all ages are equally vulnerable to hospitalization-related depression and that the depression will unfold in a common pattern. This research suggests that risk factors exercise a uniform impact throughout childhood, and by implication, that intervention strategies appropriate for one age are probably appropriate for another.

Such a uniformity of approach ignores the heterogeneity of childhood depression. Children confront illness and hospitalization—and potentially, depression—with differing vulnerabilities and coping mechanisms based on their stage in development and on skills that they have acquired at previous stages of development. For example, Levy (1945) claims that surgery presented the greatest psychological risk to those in the birth to 2-year age group because of what he characterizes as the greater physiologic vulnerability to pain possessed by these infants and young children, their heavy reliance on attachment to the maternal figure, their circumscribed social contacts, and their limited ability to dispel anxiety. The implication of other research (Jessner et al., 1952; Kenny, 1975; Prugh et al., 1953) is that children's unconscious wishes during the Oedipal period—when fears of mutilation and loss of bodily integrity occupy a child's fantasies—may make that period one of enhanced vulnerability to depression. These two viewpoints serve only to illustrate that risk factors for depression present different threats throughout childhood and that children who are ill and/or hospitalized can therefore suffer different types of depressions which may require different forms of intervention. Tracing the etiology of a hospitalization-induced depression, therefore, requires an understanding of both the nature of the hospitalization experience—including interactions with family and medical personnel—as well as the child's developmental status.

Much research to date has suffered from another flaw as well. The experiences of hospitalization and illness have often been lumped together, so that conclusions about hospitalization have been drawn from observations of sickness. While the two experiences overlap in that illness often leads to hospitalization, they retain distinct identities and present unique demands for the child as well. Therefore, each entails a different type and different degree of risk factor predisposing the child to depression. Clearly, since hospitalization presupposes sickness, it poses a greater challenge to a child's development than does sickness alone. Nevertheless, illness by itself threatens some of the growing child's strongest bulwarks against depression. Even in the absence of hospitalization, it can result in depressive symptomatology, if not in full-fledged depression. When evaluating the empirical evidence on the impact of sickness and hospitalization—particularly with respect to developing intervention strategies—we must be cautious about blurring this distinction.

This chapter will begin by reviewing the scope of child hospitalization, to provide a rough estimate of the potential population at risk for depression. Next, discussion will turn to a review of the depressive symptomatology found in sick and hospitalized children. In the course of this discussion, the prominence of DSM-III depressive symptomatology will emerge clearly. However, the discussion will not limit itself to those symptoms detailed in DSM-III. Instead, it will address additional characteristics that also place the child at risk for depression.

The chapter will then focus on the major risk factors and their mode of interaction in triggering depression. Conceptually, these factors can be divided into three groups: (1) those stemming from the nature of the illness, (2) those relating to hospital procedures and practices, and (3) those relating to the child's family and social environment. Operationally, however, all three types of factors interact to determine the ultimate impact of hospitalization. A developmental framework would suggest that an analysis of these risk factors should revolve around the child's psychological resources for coping with the stresses that illness and hospitalization impose. Accordingly, this chapter will review such exogenous risk factors from the vantage point of the developing child's perception of the experience and his or her competence in coping with it.

THE SCOPE OF HOSPITALIZATION

Every infant or child experiences sickness in some degree during childhood. Few confront chronic illness, however. While it is difficult to estimate how many infants and children are chronically ill and thus at risk for depression, hospitalization figures provide some indication of the risk population. Risk is a function of many factors including age at time of hospitalization, length of stay, and type of procedures performed. Simply stated, infants and children hospitalized early, repeatedly, and for long periods of time face the most serious risk for depression. Most developmental research, categorizes the 0–5-year age group as being at high risk. Government statistics reveal that infants and children in this group represent the overwhelming majority of pediatric hospitalizations. According to the U.S. Department of Health and Human Services, in 1983 almost 4 million children under 15 years old were discharged from short-stay, nonfederal hospitals in the United States in 1983. Children under 1 year old accounted for slightly more than a quarter of the discharges, and children under 4 years old comprised well over half of the hospitalized population. Thus, we may conclude that the majority of hospitalized children fall into the population which, from a developmental perspective, exhibits the highest risk for depression.

This risk group is also increasing in relation to other age groups of hospitalized children. Although the total population of hospitalized children has not grown since 1973, the numbers and rates of discharge for infants less than 1 year almost doubled, rising from 15 percent of all children in 1973 to 26 percent in 1983. Moreover, infants less than 1 year also spend more time in the hospital than any other group of children. Earlier admissions and longer stays among the youngest populations combine to expose this group, far beyond any other group of children, to higher risk for depression.

Age at time of admission, length of stay, and purpose of hospitalization represent three significant variables in determining the likelihood of emerging depression. Moreover, surgery may be characterized as a major risk factor, particularly among children under 5 years. Government statistics reveal that the large majority (60 percent) of all hospitalized infants and children will thus be exposed to a procedure possibly disposing them to depression.

THE IMPACT OF ILLNESS AND HOSPITALIZATION ON CHILDREN

Psychotherapist Joyce Robertson (1956) kept a diary outlining the behavior of her 4-year-old daughter, Jean, before, during, and after a tonsillectomy. When Jean learned that she was to undergo an operation, she requested that her mother stay with her in the hospital. Her mother agreed. Jean's behavior became more aggressive after she learned that the operation was to occur. On one occasion, for example, she scratched her younger sister with little provocation. Temper tantrums became common. Soon after the change in behavior, she woke up one night screaming and complained that her mouth hurt. A trip to the dentist the next day found nothing unusual. A few days later, when asked why she had scratched her sister, Jean retorted to her mother, "We didn't talk about the hospital yesterday. That's why."

When the time came to go to the hospital, the child was quiet and tense. She said several times that she did not want to have her tonsils removed and wanted to go home. Yet that evening she had no trouble getting to sleep. The following morning, the day of the tonsillectomy, Jean continued her opposition to the operation. She would not cooperate with the hospital staff, and when given an injection of Atropine in the leg, she began crying bitterly. The operation proceeded without complication. Afterwards, Jean complained of pain, but was otherwise normal and slept well.

The morning after the operation, Jean was active and talkative. She claimed that her throat didn't hurt, but after further questioning by her mother, she admitted that it did hurt. She played with the other children in the hospital, but continued to ask to go home. The following morning, she was still impatient about going home, complained of a sore throat, and resisted attempts to take her temperature. When a doctor came for a final look at her throat before release, she clenched her teeth and cried.

Jean's first day at home was uneventful. On the second day, however, she had several aggressive outbursts, once slapping her mother and saying, "I don't like you because you took me to the hospital." On the fifth day at home, Jean examined and displayed her genitals, laughing and looking at her mother to get her attention. At bedtime, she mentioned that her tonsils had been removed without her knowledge. The following morning she sang a song about "wobbly"—her word for penis. Her mother told her she could be more active when her tonsils were better, to which she responded, "I haven't got tonsils, only a throat." She continued to exhibit her genitals several times that day.

On the twelfth day, Jean began engaging in temper tantrums. She asked many "why" questions for the next 2 days. She also wondered aloud why a nurse had stuck a needle into her leg before the operation. She told her little sister how she had hit the nurse in the leg with a toy. While playing "doctor" with another child, using her doll as the patient, Jean said, "You must hurt her leg and then you make her better."

On the twentieth day home from the hospital, mother and child visited the hospital and the nurse who had taken care of Jean. Jean was relaxed and happy, and even took her little sister on a tour of the hospital. Three weeks after the operation, Jean had apparently worked through her hospital experience.

This case demonstrates only some of the visible impact of sickness and hospitalization on a young child. Indeed, in this instance, the anticipation of the hospitalization, the hospitalization experience itself, and the concomitant surgery all appeared to provoke disruptive and aberrant behavior in a normally well-behaved 4-year-old girl. Although Jean's symptomatology did not coincide with traditional depressive criteria, her overall behavior, which might be alternatively labeled as regressive or aggressive, revealed patterns often known to be precipitates of depressive episodes. In Jean's case, we may speculate that the supportive response provided by the maternal figure served to counteract the disruptive psychological impact of the hospitalization experience and perhaps short-circuited the onset of full-fledged depressive symptomatology.

Nevertheless, a review of the literature demonstrates conclusively that depressive symptoms, and depression itself, figure prominently in the clinical picture of sick and hospitalized children at all ages. Many studies have concluded that hospitalization, particularly in the first 5 years of a child's life, predisposes the child to development of depressive illness or actually causes a depressive episode (Beck et al., 1963; Blumberg, 1977; Pilowsky, Bassett, Begg, & Thomas, 1982; Prugh, 1983; Spitz, 1945).

Two major conclusions emerge from the several major studies assessing the impact of sickness and hospitalization on children. First, most of the DSM-III symptoms for major depressive episode appear among sick and hospitalized children, substantiating the commonly held view that hospitalization can lead to childhood depression. Children studied by these researchers show signs of *eating and sleep disturbances* (Douglas, 1975; Ferguson, 1979; Illingworth & Holt, 1955; Jessner et al., 1952; Kashani et al., 1981; Mrazek, 1984; Pearson, 1941; Prugh et al., 1953; Reichelderfer & Rockland, 1963; Robertson & Robertson, 1971; Schaffer, 1958; Schaffer & Callender, 1959; Vaughan, 1957), *psychomotor retardation or hypoactivity* (Douglas, 1975; Jessner et al., 1952; Kashani et al., 1981; Prugh et al., 1953; Reichelderfer & Rockland, 1963; Robertson & Robertson, 1971; Schaffer, 1958; Schaffer & Callender, 1959; Spitz & Wolf, 1946; Stoddard and O'Connell, 1983; Vaughan, 1957), *apathy* (Ferguson, 1979; Illingworth & Holt, 1955; Jessner et al., 1952; Kashani et al., 1981; Mrazek, 1984; Prugh et al., 1953; Reichelderfer & Rockland, 1963; Robertson & Robertson, 1971; Schaffer, 1958; Schaffer & Callender, 1959), *lethargy* (Ferguson, 1979; Kashani et al., 1981), *self-reproach/guilt* (Kashani et al., 1981), and *suicidal ideation* (Jessner et al., 1952; Kashani et al., 1981).

The second, and perhaps more significant conclusion concerns those symptoms detected by the researchers but not enumerated in DSM-III. Much documented symptomatology falls into this category. Two different, though not necessarily incompatible, theories can explain this finding. On the one hand, these latter symptoms may reflect other pathology accompanying the depression associated with child illness and hospitalization. On the other hand, these unenumerated symptoms may constitute manifestations of depression that change over time and are not adequately depicted by the static DSM-III. As alluded to in other chapters of this book, although DSM-III criteria for childhood depression provide indispensible guidelines for the diagnostician, the symptomatology enumerated may not fully exhaust the range of behaviors suggestive of childhood depression. For this reason, DSM-III should be considered as a supplemental tool to aid the researcher, while other clues to childhood depression extracted from the literature should also be accorded weight.

Indeed, the literature supports the view that children's reactions—whether depressive or not—to illness and hospitalization evolve throughout childhood. In a developmental framework, many of the behaviors described in the literature can be viewed as expressions of depressive phenomena that vary with the emotional and intellectual resources with which children of different ages are equipped to adapt to sickness and hospitalization. While some symptoms of depression arising from illness or hospitalization can appear at a very young age and surface again throughout childhood, other symptoms emerge only in particular developmental contexts. Thus, depression will manifest differently throughout infancy and childhood (Trad, 1986).

DSM-III Depressive Symptomatology

The literature provides ample descriptions of the different depressive symptoms that reveal how infants and children experience illness and hospitalization as they grow older. Most of the symptoms cited in the literature and found as well in DSM-III can appear at virtually any stage of infancy or childhood.

Many researchers have observed that, beginning at a very early age, children react to both illness and hospitalization with sleep and eating disturbances which may represent a response to maternal deprivation (Schaffer, 1958; Schaffer & Callender, 1959; Spitz, 1945). While these symptoms can persist throughout childhood and adolescence, Prugh et al. (1953) demonstrated that they are comparatively more pronounced in children less than 5 years old.

After aberrations in eating and sleeping behavior, a child's temperament often shows the earliest signs of the impact of illness—whether or not the illness culminates in hospitalization. Quinton and Rutter (1976) note that children who suffer from chronic illness and repeated early hospitalization differ from other children in behavior and temperament. Depending on the specific nature of the temperamental reaction, these children manifest a common propensity for, if not an outward display of, depression.

Two key temperamental traits related to depression—irritability/restlessness, which refers to the child's fussing, crying, or overall distress, and negative quality of mood, encompassing the degree of unpleasantness, crying, or unfriendly behavior exhibited by the child—appear repeatedly in the literature on childhood illness and hospitalization. In DSM-III parlance, these symptoms might be labeled "psychomotor agitation" and "retardation." They surface among all age groups, beginning in early infancy (Schaffer & Callender, 1959; Spitz, 1945) and running through adolescence (Illingworth & Holt; 1955; Jessner et al., 1952; Kashani et al., 1981; Mrazek, 1984; Prugh et al., 1953; Robertson & Robertson, 1971; Stoddard & O'Connell, 1983). Schaffer (1958) and Schaffer and Callender (1959) detected such symptoms from 3 weeks through the end of the first year, Reichelderfer and Rockland (1963) in the middle of the second year, and numerous researchers have observed them from ages 2 to 14 (Douglas, 1975; Illingworth & Holt, 1955; Prugh et al., 1953; Vaughan, 1957).

Moreover, specific illnesses appear to prompt specific temperamental responses that may accompany, if not cause, depressive symptomatology. For example, Kim et al. (1980, 1981) found distractability and reactive intensity among epileptics. Mrazek (1984) observed increased irritability among severe asthmatics. (See Table 15).

Hospitalization can create its own set of depressive symptoms, as has been well documented since Spitz (1945) described hospitalism in British institutions during World War II. The impact of hospitalization can be seen

Table 15. Dimensions of Temperament Compared to Profile of Hospitalized Child

Hospitalized Profile	Thomas, Chess, Birch, Hertzig, and Korn (1963)	Buss and Plomin (1975)	Rothbart (1981)
Dysphoric mood (2,3,4,5,6,7,8,9,11)	Adaptability	Emotionality	Smiling and laughter
Withdrawal (2,10)	Approach/withdrawal Mood	Impulsivity	Fear Distress to limitations Soothability
Sleep disturbances (1,2,5,6,7,10,11,12)	Rhythmicity		
Eating disturbances (1,2,5,7,8,9,10,11,12)	Rhythmicity		
Psychomotor agitation/ retardation (1,3,4,5,6,7,8,9,10,11)	Activity level Approach/withdrawal	Activity	Activity level
Loss of interest/ pleasure in activities (5,6,8,9,10)	Approach/withdrawal Distractability Mood	Emotionality Sociability	Smiling and laughter Duration of orienting
Less compliant/difficult (1,2,4,6,7,8)	Approach withdrawal Intensity Adaptability Attention span/persistence Mood	Emotionality Sociability Impulsivity	Distress to limitations Soothability Duration of orienting
Avoidant (5,9,11)	Approach/withdrawal	Sociability	Fear Duration of orienting
Aggression (2,3,4,5,6,7,9,12)	Approach/withdrawal Intensity	Sociability Impulsivity	Activity level Distress to limitations
Anxiety/fear (2,3,4,5,7,9,10,12)	Approach/withdrawal Mood Intensity	Emotionality Sociability	Smiling and laughter Fear Distress to limitations

1. Douglas (1975)
2. Ferguson (1979)
3. Illingworth & Holt (1955)
4. Jessner et al. (1952)
5. Kashani et al. (1981)
6. Mrazek (1984)
7. Prugh et al. (1953)
8. Reichelderfer & Rockland (1963)
9. Robertson & Robertson (1971)
10. Schaffer & Callender (1959)
11. Spitz (1945)
12. Vaughan (1957)

both in isolated symptoms and as a full-fledged depressive syndrome. A study conducted by Kashani et al. (1981) found that 7 percent of the children (mean age, 9.5 years old) admitted to a nonpsychiatric, inpatient pediatric ward were depressed and 38 percent displayed dysphoric mood. Although the depression in these children may have preceded the hospitalization experience, it was only within the hospital environment that the symptomatology became sufficiently overt for a diagnosis of depression to be confirmed. Thus, the implication is that the hospital environment itself, symbolizing an exaggerated form of separation and isolation, may trigger the emergence of underlying depression. The researchers diagnosed depression through parent and child interviews using DSM-III Diagnostic Criteria for Major Depression and the Bellevue Index of Depression (BID).

Among the most vivid DSM-III depressive symptoms in hospitalized infants are changes in affect. A number of studies comment on chronic crying and fretfulness, apparently beginning around the sixth or seventh month (Spitz & Wolf, 1946; Schaffer & Callender, 1959). This forms the first stage of an infant's response to hospitalization, according to Bowlby, Robertson, and Rosenbluth's (1952) classic model. Within this model, Robertson and Bowlby (1952) discerned three distinct stages in the response of infants and children to maternal separation. The first stage, labeled "protest," is characterized by high agitation and attempts to return to the mother. "Despair" represents the benchmark of the second stage, during which weeping and other despondent behaviors are prevalent. Finally, the "detachment" stage brings a general withdrawal from activity and a rejection of attempts by the caretaker to reestablish a relationship. Notably, studies of younger infants do not report such behavior, but rather comment on silence and conspicuous lack of expression among these infants (Schaffer, 1958; Schaffer & Callender, 1959). Virtually every study of hospitalized infants and children over 7 months old has noted excessive upset and other similar symptoms such as anger, acute anxiety, and protest (Douglas, 1975; Ferguson, 1979; Illingworth & Holt, 1955; Jessner et al., 1952; Mrazek, 1984; Pearson, 1941; Robertson & Robertson, 1971; Schaffer, 1958; Schaffer & Callender, 1959; Vaughan, 1957).

Some hospitalized children respond to the experience with dulled affect rather than extremes of affect. Hollenback et al. (1980), who undertook a prospective study of four hospitalized cancer patients ages 1.5 to 4 years, observed that a long period of isolation in a germ-free Laminar Air Flow Room resulted in a decided lack of affect in their facial expressions. The researchers noted, however, that isolation did not produce a blunted affect immediately, but rather over a period of weeks. The phenomenon of nonaffect-imbued facial expression is particularly significant in light of studies of face-to-face interaction between infant and caregiver that suggest that the infant expands his or her emotional repertoire through exchanges with the caregiver. Face-to-face studies indicate that affective facial expression serves as an indicator or barometer of the success of the attachment relationship being formed between caregiver and child. Lack of facial expression may then signal a withdrawal, disruption, or severance of this crucial bond.

Other research indicates that dulled affect appears as early as 3 weeks of age among hospitalized infants. Schaffer (1958) labeled the phenomenon "global syndrome" and identified it in infants less than 7 months old. Infants characterized by global syndrome typically appear silent and expressionless while scanning the room without paying attention to any single object. Nothing in their immediate environment elicits attention; they respond similarly (i.e., globally) to everything. Schaffer described their faces as blank or bewildered and characterized the infants as inactive. Spitz and Wolf (1946) documented a similar phenomenon when they wrote of children in the second half of the first year lying on their beds with averted faces ignoring their surroundings and their caregivers. They referred to a searching expression on the infants' faces. Brown and Semple (1970) noted global gazing and freezing among children 3 to 5 years old. "Freezing," as the term has been used by infant researchers, generally refers to the phenomenon of complete immobilization, including freezing of posture, motility, and articulation (Fraiberg, 1982b), and is suggestive of a manifestation of behavioral dysregulation.

A set of related symptoms—apathy and disinterest—are frequently cited in the literature. In 1942, Bakwin remarked on the degree of listlessness and apathy in hospitalized infants. Ten years later, Robertson and Bowlby (1952) observed the same phenomenon as the second phase of a child's response to separation from parents, an experience that was intrinsic to hospitalization at that time. Apathy and listlessness have both been noted from early infancy through childhood. Reichelderfer and Rockland (1963), as well as Robertson and Robertson (1971), detected these symptoms in the middle of the second year. Ferguson (1979) noted them among the 82 children 3 to 7 years old, and Kashani et al. (1981) observed low energy and disinterest in activities among 7 to 12 year olds.

Moreover, in follow-up studies on the impact of repeated hospitalization, research has shown that these affective symptoms persist. Bowlby et al. (1956) investigated a group of children who had entered a sanatorium over an 8-year period, at various ages up to 4 years old, and had remained there for considerable lengths of time. When their behavior was monitored at follow-up—the children then ranging from 6 years and 10 months to 13 years and 7 months—a much larger proportion of the sanatorium children was found to be diffident and apathetic. They lacked concentration and often withdrew into reverie. Agle (1964) and Mattsson (1972) described inactivity as one of the three major patterns of poor adjustment among children of all ages.

Not surprisingly, these changes in affect either cause or are accompanied by social avoidance, detachment, and withdrawal. Self-imposed isolation—beyond that necessitated by treatment requirements—is common, for example, among AIDS victims (Nichols, 1985). This kind of withdrawal represents the third stage of Bowlby, Robertson, and Rosenbluth's (1952) model of children's response to separation during hospitalization. Subdued withdrawal often alternated with violent protest among infants as young as 7 months old (Prugh et al., 1953; Schaffer & Callender, 1959). Weepiness among the 6-month-olds studied by Spitz and Wolf (1946) often yielded to complete withdrawal. These infants met social approaches with responses ranging from complete disinterest to outright rejection, which manifested as violent screaming. This phenomenon surfaces with particular clarity during the preschool years (Prugh, 1983). Preschoolers hospitalized over long periods tend to demonstrate not only detachment and shallow social interactions, but outright antisocial behavior.

From a review of the literature it appears that a young child traumatized by repeated or lengthy hospitalization may develop symptoms of depression, be at risk for a major depressive disorder or present a picture similar to that of children displaying suicidal behavior. Thus, when combined with other predisposing factors—loss of a significant other through death or separation, unstable family background, and communication problems—hospitalization may place a child at risk for suicide.

Indeed, such a child may be likened to a child subjected to repeated episodes of learned helplessness, which are known to cause depressive disorders in adults. The hospitalization experience, combined with other factors indicating a nonsupportive environment at home, may suggest to the child that the world offers no opportunity for mastery or escape from the debilitating effects of repeated failure. Such a child may come to view himself or herself as the cause of his or her sickness. Suicide or attempted suicide may thus represent a feeble and desperate attempt to escape from the overwhelming sense of defeat engendered by a history of learned helplessness (Trad, 1986).

Moreover, all of the characteristics that Douglas (1975) and others have cited in adults who suffered repeated and/or prolonged hospitalization during childhood—social isolation, inability to form lasting and meaningful relationships, depression, delinquency, aggression, hypochondria, impulsiveness, and rigidity—form part of the profile of adolescent and adult suicides (Adam, 1982; Bowlby, 1973). It is crucial then to assess children for the combination of factors that may heighten the trauma of hospitalization, leading to maladaption, depression, and self-destructive personality.

To summarize, the following DSM-III symptoms for major depression and dysthymic disorders frequently appear among sick children:

Feeding disturbances
Sleep disturbances

Depressed affect

Excessive crying

Apathy

Listlessness

Lack of concentration

Psychomotor agitation or retardation

Irritability and restlessness

Social avoidance and withdrawal

Suicidal ideation

While all of these symptoms can characterize children who are not well, some symptoms, such as dulled or depressed affect and social avoidance, can assume particular prominence when an ill child also requires hospitalization. (See Tables 16 and 17.)

Table 16. Behavioral Features of Hospitalized Child Compared to DSM-III Criteria

Hospitalized Child Features	DSM-III for MAJOR DEPRESSION (1980, pp. 213-14)	DSM-III for DYSTHYMIC DISORDER (1980, pp. 222-23)
Dysphoric mood (2,3,4,5,6,7,8,9,10,11)	Dysphoric mood	Dysphoric mood
Sleep disturbances (1,2,5,6,7,10,11,12)	Sleep disturbances	Sleep disturbances
Eating disturbances (1,2,5,6,7,10,11,12)	Eating disturbances	Eating disturbances
Psychomotor agitation/ retardation (1,3,4,5,6,7,8,9,10,11)	Psychomotor agitation/ retardation	Psychomotor agitation/ retardation
Loss of interest/pleasure (5,6,8,9,10)	Loss of interest/pleasure	Loss of interest/pleasure
Less compliant/difficult (1,2,4,6,7,8)		Irritable/excessive anger
Avoidant (5,9,11)		Social withdrawal
Aggression (2,3,4,5,6,7,9,12)		
Anxiety/fear (2,3,4,5,7,9,10,12)		

1. Douglas (1975)
2. Ferguson (1979)
3. Illingworth & Holt (1955)
4. Jessner et al. (1952)
5. Kashani et al. (1981)
6. Mrazek (1984)
7. Prugh et al. (1953)
8. Reichelderfer & Rockland (1963)
9. Robertson & Robertson (1971)
10. Schaffer & Callender (1959)
11. Spitz (1945)
12. Vaughan (1957)

Table 17. **Summary of Findings**

Study	Number	Age Range	Duration	Methods	Time Frame	DSM-III Symptoms	Other Symptoms
Pearson (1941)	11	2-10 years	Hospital and follow-up	Case studies	chronology not determined	Sleep disturbances	Amnesia, repression Anger, towering rage Compulsive behavior Continued masturbation Enuresis Fear of abandonment Feeling of inadequacy Psychic shock Acute anxiety, hysteria
Spitz (1945)	164*a*	0-1 year	Long-term	Tests, Filming	greater than 2 weeks	Depression "hospitalism" Disturbed cyclical changes Psychomotor retardation	Susceptibility to illness Avoidance Developmental retardation Abnormal reactions to strangers/strange objects Separation anxiety
Jessner et al. (1952)	143	2-14 years	Hospital and 3-4 years after	Interview/observation and after	greater than 2 weeks	Depression Demanding/irritable Eating disturbances Sleep disturbances Hypoactivity/restlessness Masochism/suicidal	Regression Speech/voice disturbances Abnormal anxieties and fears Threatening/aggressive Introjection/identity loss Separation anxiety
Prugh et al. (1953)	100*b*	2-12 years	4 months and after	Interview and observations	greater than 2 weeks	Depressed, withdrawn Eating disturbances Sleep disturbances Hypoactivity/restlessness	Acute fear and panic states Threatening/aggressive Abandoment, helplessness Ego regression Separation anxiety
Illingworth & Holt (1955)	181	1-14 years*c*	Up to 2 weeks	Observations	approximately 2 weeks	Irritable/negativistic Depressed, withdrawn Eating disturbances Persistent sadness	Bewildered/helpless Crying & protest Toilet disturbances Threatening/aggressive
Vaughan (1957)	40	2.3-9.9 years	Hospital and after	Observations and controls	approximately 2 weeks	Irritability/helplessness Eating disturbances Sleep disturbances Anxiety/restlessness	Easily upset Overly compliant Crying & protest Threatening/aggre
Schaffer (1958) and Schaffer & Callender (1959)	76	3-51 weeks	Hospital and after	Observations Developmental tests	approximately 2 weeks	*Global syndrome* Eating disturbances Sleep disturbances *Overdependent syndrome* Eating disturbances Sleep disturbances Restlessness/hyperactivity Subdued withdrawal	*Global Syndrome* Preoccupation w/environs Vomiting *Overdepended syndrome* Excessive crying & protest Toilet disturbances Autoeroticism Negativism Separation anxiety

279

Table 17. (Continued)

Study	Number	Age Range	Duration	Methods	Time Frame	DSM-III Symptoms	Other Symptoms
Reichelderfer & Rockland (1963)	1	18 months	greater than 2 months	Clinical observations	greater than 2 weeks	Anaclitic depression Eating disturbances Restlessness/hyperactivity Apathetic/unresponsive Subdued withdrawal	
Robertson & Robertson (1971)	13d	17 months	27 days and after	Observations Film	approximately 2 weeks	Chronic crying/despair Eating disturbances Apathy/disinterest Restlessness Withdrawn/quiet	Anger/aggression Autoeroticism Avoidance Fear of strangers
Douglas (1975)	958	0-5 years and after	26 years and after	Data collection and analysis	Long-term	Irritable/difficult Eating disturbances Sleep disturbances Restless/maladaptive	Crying protest to parent Toilet disturbances Speech disturbances Less confident in parents
Ferguson (1979)	82	3-7 years	Variable	Interview Film Controls	approximately 2 weeks	Depression Eating disturbances Sleep disturbances Apathy/withdrawal Lethargy	Aggression to authority Separation anxiety Anxiety: self-reported, behavioral, and physiological
Kashani et al. (1981)	7100	7-12 years	7 months	DSM-III BID Clinical observations	approximately 2 weeks	Dysphoric mood Eating disturbances Sleep disturbances Hypoactivity Distinterest in activities Low energy Self-reproach/guilt Cognitive disturbances Death/suicidal ideation	Somatic complaints Enuresis School refusal Separation anxiety Diminished socialization Aggressive behavior
Mrazek (1984)	55e	3-6 years	Short-term	Questionnaire Video	approximately 2 weeks	Depressed mood Sleep disturbances Unresponsive/withdrawn Low rhythmicity & intensity	Regression Negativity Noncompliant/opposing Fear/anxiety "Slow to warm up"

a 130 in two institutions; 34 controls in homes.
b 50 experimental; 50 control; 200 initial sample.
c 66% were 1-6 years.
d symptoms describe the one control subject placed in an institution for 9 days.
e 33 severe asthmatics and 22 controls.

Learned Helplessness Among Sick and Hospitalized Infants and Children

The depressive symptomatology in sick children described in the previous section corresponds more or less directly with symptoms identified in DSM-III. However, the set of symptoms described in DSM-III hardly exhausts the list compiled in the last 40 years of research on childhood illness and hospitalization. In particular, DSM-III underplays a collection of symptoms loosely associated with learned helplessness depression, a debilitating form of depression in adults. The reformulated learned helplessness theory proposes that specific affective, as well as cognitive, deficits place an individual at risk for depression. The cognitive deficits have two main components: (1) an expectation of response-outcome independence in which a belief in uncontrollability in one situation generalizes to other situations, and (2) a specific explanatory style in which bad events are attributed to internal, global, and stable causes (Abramson, Seligman, & Teasdale, 1978; Peterson & Seligman, 1984).

Several components of infants' cognitive and emotional structures generally insulate them from developing this cognitive structure that may predispose an older child to learned helplessness depression. For example, infants' ability to experience contingencies at an early stage of development (Fagen & Ohr, 1985), bolstered by illusions of control, cushion them against acquiring a feeling of helplessness in the face of aversive stimuli. Moreover, lack of a stable self-concept before approximately age 2 and attribution of failures to external rather than internal sources impede the development of full-fledged self-esteem deficits which often accompany functional learned helplessness.

Sickness and hospitalization threaten these protective mechanisms. A feeling of loss of control can be engendered both by the debilitating nature of illness and by the need to surrender one's care to parents and medical professionals. Diseases as unpredictable in their course and as grim in their prognosis as AIDS (Oleske, Minnefor, Cooper, Thomas, et al., 1983), may make the child especially prone to feelings of lost control. Limitations imposed by hospitalization can further challenge young children's illusions of control, causing them to experience control as exterior to themselves.

A clinical case of learned helplessness also incorporates a self-esteem deficit, which, it has been argued, cannot emerge until a child has acquired self-definition and attributional style capacities. Children typically do not develop a stable self-concept until the end of their second year. Even then, evidence has shown, they often blame their failures on exterior causes, typically displaying illusions of control. Sickness and hospitalization, particularly during the immediate pre-Oedipal period, can invert this attributional style and cause children to ascribe their condition to themselves. As Anna Freud (1952) observed, children often cannot distinguish between pain caused by illness and pain caused by treatment. On a more conceptual level, this might be interpreted to mean that pain and treatment blur a child's perceptions of causality—impairing his or her ability to differentiate correctly between external and internal causes. The potential for finding internal rather than external explanations for pain can be further exacerbated by the tendency of children in certain age groups to view illness and/or hospitalization as punishment for their real or imagined misdeeds. This heightened risk for self-esteem deficits is the product of a number of developmental factors, including unconscious beliefs and cognitive immaturity.

The following section will explore the manifestions of these companion phenomena—the loss of internal control and the attribution of sickness to oneself—and review the evidence demonstrating how sickness and hospitalization corrode the psychological structures that ordinarily shield infants and children from learned helplessness. As will be discussed, sickness and hospitalization can elicit a progressive pattern of symptoms betraying an infant's surrender to noncontingency and loss of control. Once this surrender has occurred—possibly as early as the third month—sickness or hospitalization can predispose an infant to learned helplessness depression.

Loss of Control Issues.   As its name implies, learned helplessness is an acquired deficit. The cognitive components interacting to produce such a depression evolve over time. Although a sick or hospitalized child reaches the peak of vulnerablity to such a depression during the pre-Oedipal period, patterns of response from early infancy can condition the child to abandon internal resources for overcoming stress. Indeed many researchers have observed that sickness and hospitalization tend to diminish infants' and children's perceptions of control over themselves and their environment.

The impact of illness and hospitalization can take several routes. Potentially one of the most damaging that has been observed is through physiological impairments that illness or hospitalization can exert on a child's cognitive abilities. Such deficits, occasioned by illness or hospitalization, may predispose infants and children to depression by disabling the processing capabilities that would ordinarily enable signalling and interpretive response to caregivers—thereby interfering with the creation of attachments through which infants begin to build a cause-effect relationship with their environment (Greenspan & Porges, 1984). According to this theory, the impact of illness or hospitalization on cognitive functioning can create a depressive predisposition as early as the third month. Bowlby (1980) offers a similar interpretation of the indirect effect of hospitalization-induced cognitive and affective deficits—and their derivative, the impaired infant-caregiver attachment—on the development of depression. Such impairments, he posits, may cause a child to experience losses later in life that are essentially reenactments of earlier failures in attachment formation.

Several studies have, in fact, detected cognitive deficits among hospital-ized infants and children. Telzrow et al. (1980) detected that full-term jaundiced infants undergoing phototherapy respond differently to visual social stimuli than do nonjaundiced infants. Although their findings are difficult to interpret, given the absense of normal visual, verbal, taste, and tactile experiences during this time, it is notable that the greatest differences occurred during periods of separation from the mother. Als (1981) found premature infants, who spend a longer time in the hospital than do full-term infants, significantly less responsive to social stimulation and generally less attentive. Prugh (1983) also noted that children who have undergone hospital isolation lose at least some, although not necessarily all, sensory capacity.

Illness or hospitalization need not actually cause a cognitive impair-ment—leading to subsequent deficits in developmental tasks—to foster a belief in response-outcome independence. This outcome may occur largely as a result of the child's perceived inability to control the course of his or her illness, particularly a chronic illness. The need to submit passively to painful treatment procedures, as well as to the possibility of separation from parents coupled with the restrictions imposed by hospitalization, may further induce this surrendering outlook in a child.

Regardless of the mechanisms that give rise to loss of control, however, sick and hospitalized children do tend to exhibit a variety of readily observable behaviors betraying their seeming relinquishment of mastery. It has been common to suggest that loss of control does not assume its full potency until the preschool years at the earliest. Before that time the reactions of children are thought to relate primarily to separation from parents—a function of hospitalization rather than of sickness (Jessner et al., 1952; Lambert, 1984). This argument fails to differentiate adequately between the unique aspects of each experience and to recognize that for the very young, with newly established attachments to parents and familiar home environments, separation from parents may represent one form of loss of control. Thus, while the outward manifestations of loss of control undoubtedly change over time, the subjective experience is available even to infants.

Much of the symptomatology described for sick children substantiates this claim. Regression to previous developmental stages has been noted among sick children of all ages (Langford, 1961). Ribble (1944) termed this phenomenon "regressive quiescence." Although the majority of the 143 hospitalized children studied by Jessner et al. (1952) were older than 5, two of those who were less than 3 years old displayed regressive signs. A 23-month-old boy displayed decreased bowel and bladder control in the hospital and a 30-month-old boy clutched a diaper constantly and engaged in head banging. Older children also regressed, with incidences of incontinence. Some children who had relinquished the bottle suddenly demanded it (Prugh et al., 1953). Mrazek (1984) also found hospitalized asthmatics between 3 and 6 resorted to immature and regressive behavior and, in some cases, regressive behavior persisted for several weeks after release from the hospital.

The phenomenon of regression commented on so frequently by independent researchers may have two possible explanations. First, the child may be attempting to resurrect earlier experiences during which feelings of security and mastery over the environment were present. In this sense, regression during the hospitalization experience may be viewed as a form of defending against feelings of uncontrollability. In addition, regressive behavior may indicate an effort to reexperience an earlier stage in order for the child to discern a method of extricating himself from the unpleasant hospitalization experience. Thus, regression here symbolizes an effort to search previous experience for a strategy of escape and mastery.

Overdependence, another precursor of learned helplessness, is also noted frequently in the literature. Schaffer (1958) describes such overdependent behavior as excessive crying when left alone by the mother, clinging, and wishing to be nursed continually. In contrast to regressive behavior, however, overdependence does not appear immediately but rather, requires the antecedent formation of a stable attachment to a caregiver. Since this does not occur until at least the sixth month, a clear reaction of over-dependence does not emerge until that time.

The literature supports this view. Schaffer (1958) traces overdependence to the seventh month, noting that it develops rapidly and reaches its full intensity almost immediately. When it emerges it can assume a variety of forms such as separation anxiety after the ninth month (Ferguson, 1979; Jessner et al., 1952; Kashani et al., 1981; Prugh et al., 1953; Spitz, 1945), fear of abandonment (Pearson, 1941), diminished confidence in parents (Douglas, 1975), overt helplessness characterized by chronic depression and detachment, shallow social relationships, and limited capacities for learning (Illingworth & Holt, 1955; Prugh et al., 1953). In Jessner et al. (1952), for example, children of all ages undergoing tonsillectomy and adenoidectomy experienced the separation of hospitalization as abandonment and exhibited a great need for their parents' protection. Overdependent and demanding behavior, particularly among young children, but also in latency-aged children, can persist for several months after physical symptoms subside (Prugh et al., 1953).

By school age, many children can verbalize this sense of loss of control. School-aged children may react most strongly to the prospect of diminished ability to compete actively, while 7- and 8-year-old boys reveal obsessive fears about damage to some part of the body (Kenny, 1975). This sense that control is slipping away emerges with particular potency in response to specific medical and surgical procedures, rather than to sickness or hospitalization per se. As Jessner et al. (1952) have shown, fear of surgery and anesthesia replace fear of the hospital as children grow older. In their study, fear of the hospital was highest in the patients under 5 years of age, but decreased dramatically by the time the children had reached 13 years old. Over three quarters of those under 5 years feared the hospital, while only 10 percent of those aged 10 to 13 expressed such fears. Older children tended to fear those experiences, such as anesthesia and surgery, that posed the greatest threats to self control. Lambert's (1984) survey of preoperative fears among children aged 10 to 12 revealed that this group feared loss of control during anesthesia. Not surprisingly, many older ill children overcompensate for their feelings of helplessness by becoming overly independent rather than overly dependent. Brown and Semple (1970) noted, for example, that chronic illness may encourage displays of bravado and risk taking.

Holmes' (1976) depiction of a 5-year-old girl's behavior after spinal surgery illustrates the significance of threats to bodily integrity and mastery during the preschool years. A young girl, Sally, was especially concerned with her mobility, seeking to walk soon after her surgery. For example, she refused to let her mother support her when she was lifted from bed to take her first postoperative walk. Holmes interpreted Sally's controlling behavior surrounding urination (e.g., insistence on immediate attention when she had to urinate) as compensation for a helpless feeling created by dysuria.

Unconscious as well as conscious fears contribute to young children's sense that they are losing control over themselves. Fears of mutilation and castration, which figure so prominently during the preOedipal period, find an avenue into consciousness when children anticipate many medical and surgical procedures (A. Freud, 1952). Although children less than 2 years old may succeed in incorporating amputation into their bodily image (Earle, 1979), and therefore not equate lost limbs with lost control, preschoolers and adolescents may experience this kind of radical surgery quite differently. During these periods, concern with bodily integrity is elevated, generating fears of disfigurement and mutilation. This phenomenon has been noted particularly among 4- to 6-year-old boys (Kenny, 1975). Jessner et al. (1952) observed that children 3 to 5 years old associate operations with multilation, disfigurement, and castration. Prugh et al. (1953) noted that boys, in particular, between the ages of 4 and 6, created more vivid fantasies of helplessness and imminent attack than other groups. These childhood and adolescent fantasies are revealed most potently among children and adolescents confronting the very real experience of mutilation as a result of amputation. In reviewing the literature on the psychological effects of mutilating surgery, Earle noted that the experience of limb loss in early adolescence often provokes grief over the loss of a complete self-image. However, Earle also observed what she characterizes as remarkable resiliency in adolescent amputees. She speculates that the bodily changes accompanying adolescence may actually facilitate integration of lost limbs into a new bodily image. Such changes may help blunt the effect of such surgery on an adolescent's sense of control.

Young children possess remarkable defensive mechanisms, commonly grouped under the rubric of "illusions of control" (Langer, 1975). That is, among young children, the tendency is to entertain illusions, sometimes fantastic in proportion, concerning their abilities to control and manipulate events. The findings in the Earle study (1979) suggest that even adolescents, in whom the defense of illusive control has receded and been replaced by more realistic cognitive conceptions of cause and effect, may resurrect these defenses when confronted with overwhelming loss. In this sense, the illusory control mustered by adolescent amputees may serve as a crucial factor in the healing process, facilitating the ability to cope with a virtually uncontrollable situation.

That illness or hospitalization should influence a child's locus of control beliefs is not surprising. However, dispositional factors or early coping successes can help preserve a strong sense of internal control. These factors, rather than the experiences of either sickness or hospitalization, may predict behavioral outcome. Children with a strong sense of internal control—a characteristic lacking among the learned helpless—present a different picture from those lacking such control. Among these children (mean age, 10 years), Gochman found an inverse relationship between potential health behavior and perceptions of vulnerability. Evidence from Lamontagne's (1984) study of 51 children (ages 8 to 12) hospitalized for minor elective surgery provides additional support for this hypothesis. In this study, children with a strong sense of internal control as measured on the Nowicki-Strickland Locus of Control Scales (1973) adopted a more active coping style than children with a weaker sense of internal control. (The Nowicki-Strickland Locus of Control scale for children involves a paper and pencil measure consisting of 40 yes/no questions. The items describe reinforcement situations across interpersonal and motivational areas such as achievement and dependency and indicate the degree of internal orientation [Lamontagne, 1984]). Notably, none of the children had been acutely ill prior to surgery. This study may suggest that some preexisting locus-of-control beliefs influenced certain children's coping more than the actual surgical event. Although these studies attest to the strong relationship between locus-of-control beliefs and adaptation to illness or hospitalization, they do not explain how these seemingly resilient children develop a sufficiently strong sense of internal control to withstand the threat presented by illness and hospitalization.

The Impact of Illness and Hospitalization on Explanatory Style. Learned helplessness depression develops not merely when an individual experiences events as independent of his or her influence, but also when bad events are perceived as being caused by factors that are internal to the individual, global in setting, and stable across time (Peterson & Seligman, 1984). This total cognitive component, variously referred to as the individual's "attributional" or "explanatory style," is an integral part of the learned helplessness theory of depression. While each of the dimensions of explanatory style need not be present for learned helplessness to develop, their presence or absence will shape the symptoms, the pervasiveness, and the chronicity of the depressive outcome. According to Peterson and Seligman, the internal-external attribution will predict the presence or absence of self-esteem deficits. The tendency to make global rather than specific attributions will predict the pervasiveness or generalizability of helplessness from one situation to another. Stable causal beliefs affect chronicity.

Children who are sick and/or undergo hospitalization often develop an explanatory style closely resembling the one described in the learned helplessness model. The dimension of a child's explanatory style that has received most comment in the literature is internality-externality. However, some limited evidence also suggests that the ill child's explanatory style matches the learned helplessness model on the globality dimension as well. Unfortunately, researchers have not yet investigated the third dimension—the stability of causal explanations—of the depressive explanatory style in terms of ill and/or hospitalized children. Therefore, this section will discuss only internality and specificity.

When reviewing the evidence with respect to illness and hospitalization, it is critical to keep in mind that explanatory style is not a static quality, but rather is developmentally determined. Moreover, developmental factors may influence each of the three dimensions of explanatory style differently. For example, a certain style on the internal/external dimension may be typical for one developmental period and not typical for another. Risk for depression is a function of the overall balance on the three dimensions taken collectively.

INTERNAL CONTROL ISSUES AND EXPLANATIONS FOR ILLNESS AND HOSPITALIZA-TION. Children's tendency to blame themselves for their illness is well documented, and even children whose attachment and self-object development have been uneventful may be prone to this type of self-attribution in the face of serious sickness (Beverly, 1936; Blom, 1958; Brodie, 1974; Forsyth, 1934; Langford, 1948; Schecter, 1961; Vanderveer, 1949). Such an explanatory style may have its roots in many facets of the child's development. For example, unconscious fantasies often cause young children to interpret sickness and hospitalization as confirmation of the punishment they expect for their Oedipal fantasies (A. Freud, 1953). Cognitive factors may further reinforce these tendencies. Piaget's (1952) model of cognitive development suggests that infants' and children's cognitive capacities may impinge on their ability to understand illness in a way that will shield them from depression. A child in the sensorimotor stage, who cannot distinguish between the self and the outside world, will view himself or herself as the author of all events, including illness (Jordan & O'Grady, 1982). Even when the child has advanced to the preoperational phase, he or she thinks concretely and in terms of adherence to, or violation of, specific rules. He or she cannot ascribe illness to rational exterior causes, but rather concretizes it by attributing the disease to his or her own violation of specific rules (Mattsson, 1972). At both stages, therefore, infants and children assume blame, rather than attribute it elsewhere. In so doing, they begin to erode the foundation of their recently consolidated self-concept.

This distorted causal attribution has been noted at many different periods throughout childhood. Children as old as 10 may view their illness, and even death, as deserved punishment (Mattsson, 1972; Orbach & Glaubman, 1978). Until this age, children may also confuse illness and injury with recent family problems, expressing the view that they deserved their illness because they were bad. Langford (1961) even links this perception explicitly with depression, noting that depression in a child is often the result of self-blame and an acceptance of punishment that he or she believes is deserved or inevitable (Langford, 1961).

In a study comparing attitudes about health in chronically ill and healthy children between the third and fifth grades, Brodie (1974) clearly illustrated this common distortion. While chronically ill children articulated a view of illness as punishment, healthy children rejected this explanation. Moreover, healthy children expected that their parents would be especially kind, rather than punitive or abandoning, if they were sick. Simeonson et al. (1979) offers additional empirical proof of this developmental progression with respect to illness causality. When these researchers tested hospitalized children 5 to 9 years old to evaluate their understanding of illness causality, they found that none of the 5-year-olds and only a small percentage of the other age groups had developed abstract reasoning that would enable them to attribute illness to rational, external causes rather than to themselves.

Children's fantasies about death reveal this attributional attitude in its most extreme form. Since children do not acquire a normative concept of death (i.e., universality, nonfunctionality, and irreversiblity) until at least age 5 and perhaps later, they defend against it by indulging in fantasies and overly concrete thinking (Ackerly, 1967; Alexander & Alderstein, 1958; Koocher, 1973, 1981). Thus they may borrow the very real experience of punishment for this purpose.

Attributing illness to one's real or imagined misdeeds, as young children frequently do, is clearly a function of age and cognitive development, as a study by Eiser, Patterson, and Tripp (1984) demonstrated. The research team compared diabetic children and a control group with a mean age of 12 years to determine whether the groups differed in their knowledge of the causes of illness. The investigators found no significant difference between the two groups, suggesting that the internal attributional style seen in younger children may diminish with growing ability to comprehend illness rationally.

GLOBALITY OF EXPLANATIONS FOR ILLNESS AND HOSPITALIZATION.   While most research on these children has focused on symptoms that might fit into the internality–externality dimension, some limited evidence suggests that the explanatory style of these children also matches the learned helplessness model on the globality dimension. According to the model, those who attribute negative outcomes to global factors are more likely to have a helpless reaction in new situations—regardless of whether the new situation is similar or dissimilar to the situation that induced helplessness. By contrast, those with a specific causal attribution will only show such deficits in situations similar to the original (Alloy et al., 1984). A global style, therefore, might predict a more generalized depressive outcome resulting from the experience of sickness or hospitalization.

Although evidence is still fragmentary and indirect, Burstein and Meichenbaum's (1979) study of children's defensiveness and anxiety levels prior to surgery, and their distress seven months subsequent to surgery, provides some important insight. Their subjects were 20 children with an average age of 7.1 years hospitalized for minor surgery. Subjects reporting the least stress after surgery tended to view the threats arising from hospitalization as discrete threats. In contrast, the less adaptive group perceived the threats as more vague and undifferentiated. In learned helplessness terms, this response may be characterized as a global attributional style that permits the inference of a more generalized risk for depression.

Summary

Symptoms reminiscent of learned helplessness depression appear even in young infants suffering from chronic illness. Chronically ill infants and children show many signs suggesting that they experience loss of control over their environment. This is reflected in regression, common at all ages, and overdependence, which emerges only after the seventh month. Full symptomatology of learned helplessness depression generally does not emerge until after the second year. Children face the highest risk for such depression between the ages of 3 and 5, when unconscious fantasies reinforced by limited cognitive capacity for understanding illness during this period make them apt to assume responsibility for their illness, rather than to attribute blame to exterior factors. These forces can promote a self-esteem deficit that is integral to learned helplessness depression.

RISK FACTORS IN ILLNESS

Although much of the research on child hospitalization and depression points to risk factors associated with the hospitalization experience, a substantial part of a child's response inheres in the experience of sickness itself. Many aspects of sickness in a global sense evoke depressive responses from infants and children. The prospects for developing psychiatric symptomatology appear to vary directly with the severity of the condition (Mrazek, 1986). Specific illnesses and the treatments they require—whether or not such treatments also entail hospitalization—also elicit specific responses that ultimately shape a child's ability to adapt to his or her condition. Diseases such as AIDS, which raise the fear of contagion, can encourage ostracism, reinforcing the sick individual's common tendency toward self-isolation and further increasing the prospects of a depressive reaction to illness (Cassens, 1985; Dilley, Ochtill, Perl, & Volberding, 1985; Nichols, 1986; Polan, Hellerstein, & Amchin, 1985). Although the Center for Disease Control has not documented the spread of pediatric AIDS horizontally within a child's household or classroom, the possibility that AIDS can be transmitted through shared food, toys, and secretions has caused the CDC to recommend that preschool AIDS victims be removed from these settings (Church, Allen, & Stiehm, 1986). Thus, sickness in the absence of hospitalizaton can deteriorate a child's defenses against depression and may even spark the onset of a depressive episode.

Illness increases risk for depression in both direct and indirect ways—through its effects on control and self-esteem as well as through its effect on cognition, temperament, attachment, and object–selfrepresentation. Although Werner and Smith (1979) argue that a child's temperament influences his or her life more than his or her medical condition, a large body of research suggests that medical condition actually shapes temperament. Rothbart and Derryberry (1981, 1982) concern themselves with the infant's self-regulatory abilities. They consider affect to be one of the contributors to self-regulation. Since illness is commonly accompanied by negative affect, the ill child is at risk for dysregulation in two ways. First, the somatic response systems which underlie self-regulation are compromised by the disease. Second, the child is unable to regulate the source of sadness (the disease) and this failure may trigger dysregulation. Research often describes sick children as having impaired adaptability (e.g., irritability), negative quality of mood (e.g., subdued), and/or impaired motor activity (e.g., restlessness, listlessness). Any of these temperamental reactions or developmental deficits resulting from illness can strain, if not disrupt, important attachments early in life. Since temperamental traits play a vital role in the subsequent development of attachment behavior and, in turn, in self-representation, which ultimately regulates affective responses, illness itself can be said to constitute a risk factor for depression and depressive-like phenomena.

Minde et al.'s (1980,1983) research on the effects of illness on parent–infant interaction offers some important insight into the mechanism by which the parent's reaction to an infant's illness can create the preconditions for learned helplessness depression. Minde et al. (1983) found that mothers of sick infants showed consistently lower levels of interaction, often for a long time after hospital discharge, than mothers of well babies. The researchers suggest two explanations for this phenomenon. Serious illness may so overwhelm the parents that they respond with emotional withdrawal. Alternatively, with preterm infants, extremely sensitive parents may fear overwhelming the behavioral capabilities of their preterm infant, who cannot tolerate the level of stimulation tolerated by fullterm babies. In either case, the result for the infant is heightened exposure to noncontingency between their actions and those of their caregivers. Notably, by using a time-lag procedure to assess the directionality of influence, the researchers found that the infant assumes the primary signalling role through decreased motor activity and that the mother takes an essentially reactive role. In Minde et al.'s terms, the infant steers the course in the interaction at this stage. Thus, by impairing an infant's signalling ability, illness poses the risk of triggering both parental withdrawal and resultant infant exposure to noncontingency. In the context of learned helplessness, this situation heightens the risk for depression.

Minde, Marton, Manning, and Hines' (1980) assessment of interactional style rather than level further confirms the relationship of illness to the possibility for development of contingency expectations in infants. When the researchers tabulated different types of social and gross motor behaviors on the part of infants and mothers, they found that mothers of infants with severe and long-lasting complications exhibited less contingent behavior— face-to-face looking and direct vocalization—than mothers of infants with short illnesses. In other words, mothers whose face-to-face interactions with their infants were less conducive to establishing rhythmicity and synchrony tended to have infants who experienced more complicated convalescent periods. Together with the findings of an earlier study (Minde et al., 1980) showing that early interaction levels predict later interaction levels, Minde et al.'s (1980) research suggests that early interactional failure can establish a persistent pattern of noncontingency that may contribute to a depressive outcome. Significantly, patterns of noncontingency may serve as a prelude or contributing factor to the development of learned helplessness depression.

These findings have been disputed by Parmelee et al. (1983). While these researchers acknowledge the importance of the mother–infant interaction in arresting possible development of behavioral difficulties arising from early illness, their research contradicts Minde et al.'s (1980) conclusion that illness diminishes the level and style of dyadic interaction. When Parmelee et al. compared 35 normal full-term infants to 35 preterm infants they, like Minde et al., found some deficits in the preterm infants. In contrast to Minde et al., however, Parmelee argues that the infant's deficiencies as a social partner actually intensified rather than attenuated the mother's interaction with the infant. This compensatory behavior may serve to promote rather than hinder contingency expectations on the part of the infant and thus actually reduce the risk for depression.

Whether or not the risk for depression is increased through the effects of illness on attachment, the attributes of the illness can have a direct impact on the child's sense of control. A number of examples are described in the literature. Illness that either temporarily or permanently impairs bodily function or severely disfigures the body can cause a child to experience loss of control, a precursor of learned helplessness. When illness interrupts the exercise of newly acquired skills, it can have a particulary devastating impact on young children, who often feel shame and even extreme humiliation when forced to depend on others in areas where they have already gained self-sufficiency (Emde et al., 1981). Illnesses that create toilet disturbances, impose mobility restrictions, or interfere with communication all challenge a child's growing sense of competence and control. Mattsson (1972) notes that prolonged or sudden mobility restraints can cause withdrawal into apathy and depression, particularly if the child lacks the verbal ability needed to express his or her feelings about the illness.

Different diseases elicit different symptomatic variations on this theme of lost control. Children with convulsive disorders may fear loss of con-sciousness or uncontrollable behavior during a seizure. Purcell et al. (1969), and Purcell and Weiss (1970) found that children with serious respiratory diseases, such as asthma, commonly fear suffocation and drowning or dying while asleep. McCollum and Gibson (1970) found similar reactions in children with cystic fibrosis. Often this loss of bodily control culminates in dysphoria, which is common among burn victims, the preponderance of whom are children under 5 years old (Stoddard & O'Connell, 1983).

Children's perceptions of internal control reveal the inverse relationship that exists between such control and adaptive health behavior. Gochman (1971) showed that among school-age children (mean age, 10.3 years), for whom health is a salient issue, those children with high levels of internal control accompanying awareness of adaptive health behavior will experi-ence lower levels of vulnerability. Sick children, whose sense of control has at least temporarily eluded them, will thus accord a more influential role to random events than to their own exertions and efforts. In short, illness obscures cause–effect thinking on which children build a contingent relationship with their environment. Although this relationship has not been studied among younger children, it may be reasonably expected that illusions of control, which have not yet receded, would promote similar ideas.

Surgery dictated by specific illnesses challenges a child's self-control more rigorously than virtually any other phenomenon of disease or hospitalization. As such, it must be regarded as a major risk factor for childhood depression. Its intrinsically invasive nature, combined with the specter of lost limbs and disfigurement, often violates a child's sense of bodily integrity, which can be particularly detrimental between the ages of 3 and 5 when castration anxiety permeates the child's unconscious thoughts (Kenny, 1975). Prugh (1983) takes a minority position when he contends that children do not react differently to surgery than to other medical or hospital procedures. Levy (1945), who studied the impact of surgery by reviewing the case records of 124 children of all ages who had had an operation, also seems to implicate other factors—such as separation from mother and from a familiar environment—above surgery per se. However, these findings may reflect the fact that half of his sample had undergone surgery prior to age 3. As Jessner et al. (1952) showed, fear of surgery increases in magnitude, while fear of the hospital diminishes, as the child grows older. Jessner et al. (1952) note that a depressive reaction to surgery can linger for as long as 10 days after an operation. Other observers have commented on the psychological risks of operating on young children, including the activation of such childhood fears as abandonment, mutilation, and death (Deutsch, 1942; A. Freud, 1953; Jessner et al., 1952; Pearson, 1941).

Surgery's inevitable companion, anesthesia, generates the same fears of loss of control. Along with surgery, fears of being "put to sleep" must therefore represent a potential risk for depression. Unfortunately, little systematic research has examined the specific reactions of children to the loss of consciousness that accompanies anesthesia.

The greatest threat of all in the context of learned helplessness depression arises from children's contemplation of death—a contemplation that magnifies the developing child's sentiments about illness. In the course of early healthy development, children focus virtually all of their efforts on attaining mastery over their bodies and their environments. The prospect of death inverts this process. As Schowalter (1970) wrote: "Instead of mastery, there is failure. Instead of growth, there is wasting. Instead of joy, there is grief" (p. 51). In effect, the prospect of death wrests from children whatever vestiges of control they may have retained through their illness.

Death represents loss of control in different ways depending on a child's developmental status. Since children under 3 years old do not have a realistic concept of death, they equate it with separation (Hug-Hellmuth, 1965; Lourie, 1966; Nagy, 1948; Schowalter, 1970). Death comes to signify the ultimate abandonment—and hence the ultimate early failure—dreaded by children of all ages. As children's ideas about death develop with age, they can succumb to other potentially depressive interpretations of death. The child's primitive representational abilities may create a risk of interpreting the death as unduly relating to himself or as punishment for his actions.

Also, the stress caused by the death of a close relative can, itself, throw the child's self-representational abilities into disarray. Similarly, a preceding depression or depressive-like phenomena puts the child at risk for misinterpretation of death issues. The cognitive deficits accompanying depression make it harder to clarify the boundaries between fantasies and realistic conceptions of death. The perception of death as retribution can persist long after the Oedipal period, perhaps as late as 10 years old, breeding guilt that can translate into passivity, withdrawal, and depression. Children who do not project guilt onto parents or medical personnel, but rather conceive of themselves as deserving the ultimate abandonment and pain symbolized by death, are primed for depression.

In sum, the degree to which any aspect of childhood illness exposes a child to risk for depression is a function of the nature of the illness and the time of onset. A review of the literature supports the view that sickness creates risk for depression through its impact on temperament and attachment, as well as through its impact on a child's sense of control over his or her environment. Most evidence suggests that sickness presents the greatest psychological peril before the age of 5 years. During this time, children have the fewest resources for controlling their environment and thus, the most tentative sense of physical and psychological competence. Moreover, illness evokes conscious and unconscious fears about the newly established self.

RISK FACTORS IN HOSPITALIZATION

Spence (1947) has noted that the first children's hospital was founded in London in 1851 by Charles West as a refuge for slum children. A century later, the model he used, that of an adult hospital, still characterized most facilities for children's care. In the past 40 years, researchers have studied this model exhaustively and it has been subject to repeated attack. As early as the 1940s, a number of researchers began investigating the impact of hospitalization on the psychological as well as the physical health of children, even questioning such hallowed practices as isolation (Bakwin, 1942). The publication of Spitz and Wolf's (1946) classic paper, in which they described several cases of what were termed "anaclitic depression" among infants less than 1 year old, further dramatized the potentially harmful consequences of childhood hospitalization. By the 1960s, pediatricians, cognizant of the previous two decades of research, began to inquire about integrating treatment of emotional reactions with treatment of children's physical ailments.

From the last four decades of research on child hospitalization one fact has emerged quite clearly: The experience of hospitalization, superimposed on the experience of illness, increases the probability that a latent depressive predisposition will evolve as a function of the sickness into a clinical case of depression.

All sick children, irrespective of their illness, their relationship to their parents, the quality of the hospital care, or their preparation for hospitalization, react at least minimally to hospitalization (Prugh et al., 1953). Despite the growing awareness of the adverse effects of hospitalization, Prugh (1983), who has studied the emotional impact of hospitalization for over 30 years, charges that hospitals still adhere to many of the same "adultmorphic" practices and policies thought to pose the most serious risks to children. Although the extreme form of hospitalism as it was described by Spitz (1945) is no doubt rare, the risks of childhood hospitalization cannot be minimized. Prugh's work and the work of other researchers, suggest that several variables factor into the probability that childhood illness and hospitalization will have a depressive outcome.

Frequency of hospitalization and length of stay represent two significant factors in determining the likelihood of depressive outcomes from hospitalization. Most research suggests that a single, isolated stay in the hospital rarely leads to long-term damage, even if the emotional distress is acute and persists after discharge from the hospital (Douglas, 1975; Quinton & Rutter, 1976; Rutter, 1979). In contrast, evidence indicates long-term, significant effects on the child who has been hospitalized repeatedly at an early age (Bowlby, 1969; Douglas, 1975; Quinton & Rutter, 1976).

In a recent review of children's and parents' reactions to hospitalization, Prugh (1983) cited a variety of restrictive practices that can be loosely called "forced immobilization": confinement in cribs, restraint for specific medical procedures such as intravenous infusions, and excessive use of sedatives. Some of these factors, however, are a function as much of illness as of hospitalization per se. One phenomenon, however, is unique to hospitalization: separation from parents. Indeed, many of the earliest studies on infant and childhood depression—whether or not in the context of hospitalization —point to prolonged separation from the mother as the driving force in the development of infant and childhood depression. During the period when Spitz (1945) and Spence (1947) conducted their studies, long-stay hospitals lacked adequate facilities for providing the relationship and companionship of personal attachment. This led many early researchers to conclude that separation, more than any other aspect of hospitalization, constituted the preeminent risk factor for infant and childhood depression (Bowlby, Robertson, & Rosenbluth, 1952; Spitz, 1945; Spitz & Wolf, 1946). More recent observers have upheld the view that early separation through hospitalization may cause childhood depression (Beck et al., 1963; Blumberg, 1977; Langford, 1961; Pilowsky et al., 1982; Prugh, 1983). Prugh (1983) even concluded that separation from the mother may, in some cases, be more significant than the medical and surgical procedures undergone by the child.

Previously, hospitals justified limiting visitation as an attempt to reduce the high incidence of infant mortality, and mortality of hospital patients in general (Klaus & Kennel, 1976). This concern was so significant that during the 1940s, parents' visiting hours in major children's hospitals were commonly limited to 30 to 60 minutes per week.

Even today, hospitals separate parents and children in many ways. They often impose restrictive visting hours despite open ward settings. Closed wards, which severely limit children's interaction with the outside world, also hinder the establishment or perpetuation of intimate and secure parent-child relationships. Other practices such as isolation and reverse isolation, indicated in the most extreme cases, inhibit essential parent-child physical contact.

Separation, and the lack of stimulation that ensues, exert a ripple effect on young children, first influencing their ability to send and receive stimulation (Als, 1981), then their affect (Lowrey, 1940), and ultimately their attachment (Klaus & Kennell, 1970; Leifer, Leiderman, Barnett, & Williams, 1972). Lowrey described the impact as "affect deprivation" and Bakwin (1949) called it emotional deprivation. Others, such as Provence and Ritvo (1961), posit a more direct relationship to depression, arguing that the deprivation of human contact prevents normal integration of a child's ego and therefore jeopardizes its capacity to adapt to the environment. We might expect—although the phenomenon is so new that there is not yet data to support this assertion—that infants born with AIDS will face a particularly great risk, given the general phobia about AIDS that appears to be spreading throughout many communities and the fear of infection that exists even among health-care professionals (Polan, Hellerstein & Amchin, 1985).

Bowlby (1958, 1960) delineates three stages of reaction to separation in young children: protest, despair, and detachment. These reactions parallel the experience of mourning for adults, and as such, there appears to be widespread agreement that separation can lead to depression among hospitalized infants and children. Illingworth and Holt (1955) isolated parental visits as the single most important factor in preventing depression and other disturbances.

Further evidence of the strong link between early hospitalization and the development of depression has been supplied by a study of adult psychiatric patients and patients referred to chronic pain and rheumatology clinics. In this retrospective study, Pilowsky et al. (1982) found that diagnosed adult depressives recalled early hospitalization far more frequently than did the rheumatology control group. While the study used an adult sample, it suggests that the separation which may have subsequently manifested in a form of adult depression, had its antecedents—whether causal or merely predispositional—in childhood hospitalization.

While these studies draw a direct link between separation and depression, most research has approached this issue in an indirect and somewhat fragmented way, by focusing on isolated mechanisms or correlates of infant and childhood depression. Research posits a two-step sequence in the development of this pathological outcome. First, separation reduces mutual parent–child stimulation, thereby diminishing the quality of attachment. Second, interactional failures in the form of precarious attachments can undermine an infant's sense of competence, threaten development of self-concept, and set a pattern for social isolation and, hence, depression. Much of the empirical research to date has focused on one or the other of these steps, examining either the relationship between separation and attachment formation or the relationship between attachment and depression. Tracing the impact of separation on depression, therefore, requires a large quantum of inference from the existing literature. Fortunately, each step in the sequence of events potentially leading to childhood depression has been studied extensively, and researchers have reached a general consensus on the two questions central to any discussion of separation and depression among hospitalized infants and children: (1) how does separation at different stages of development affect attachment? and (2) how does attachment affect depression?

Addressing the first question, Rutter's (1979) review of the literature on maternal deprivation, although not limited to deprivation necessitated by hospitalization, confirms the role of physical contact in attachment. He concluded that intimate and open mother–infant relationships depend on early physical contact and that lack of such contact presents a serious risk to early attachment. Hospital policies that limit such contact are invidious to attachment. Klaus and Kennel (1970) believe that there is a critical period during the first hours of the infant's life when the mother must nurture the child herself in order to establish a subsequent attachment. These researchers claim that the bonds of affection between mother and infant are extremely fragile during the first days of an infant's life and that interference with them can be catastrophic. Similarly, Clancy and McBride (1975) observe that early initiation of the bonding process is necessary for normal development and that meddling with this process by separating mother and infant may result in a pattern of behavior that reduces the mother–infant interaction and diminishes the relationship. Lozoff et al. (1977) echo this view in a review of the literature on the mother–newborn relationship. They warn that hospital procedures that interfere with early maternal involvement with a child may strain human adaptability.

Preterm infants exemplify best the impact of early separation and attachment formation. Researchers interested in the impact of early separation have, in fact, studied such infants extensively. Since they experience lack of physical contact with their parents while isolated in a nursery, preterm infants often appear significantly less responsive to social stimulation (Als, 1981) and often do not form attachments as easily as do normal infants (Klaus & Kennell, 1970 ; Leifer et al., 1972). Separation as a result of preterm birth not only removes the infant from the mother and deprives it of essential physical stimulation, but also taxes the mother's ability to attach to the infant. Thus, such separation has a compound, negative effect on the formation of a successful mother-infant attachment.

These arguments notwithstanding, some evidence challenges the critical nature of physical contact—impeded by early separation of infants suffering perinatal complications—during the so-called sensitive period. Rode, Chang, Fisch, & Sroufe (1981), for example, contend that the cumulative pattern of infant-caregiver interaction during the first year, rather than the initial contact, determines security of attachment and, hence, adaptations that depend on it. While admitting that data from a prospective study on bond formation and neglect are tentative because of imprecise measures for bonding failure, Egeland and Vaughn (1981) also question whether separation immediately following birth undermines mother-infant bond formation, causing what they call disorders of mothering, from which the infant can suffer many outcomes including abuse, neglect, and depression. Rejecting the notion of a sensitive period advanced by Klaus and Kennel (1970), they also view the development of attachment as an evolutionary process occurring over the entire first year of the child's life. According to this line of reasoning, long-term illness that affects the interaction throughout the first year would pose a greater risk for depression than a brief period of hospitalization. Further investigation of the relationship between early separation and bonding will, as Egeland and Vaughn urge, require more objective definitions of bonding and bonding failure.

Even if an early period of hospitalization in the first year does not irreparably damage attachment, both sides of the sensitive period controversy concur that hospitalization resulting in prolonged interference with parent-child interaction will threaten attachment. The next question is how such attachment disruption may result in depression. The literature provides rather conclusive findings on the relationship between attachment and depression among hospitalized infants and children. Research has tended to focus on whether secure attachments lead to adaptive behavior in response to hospitalization, rather than on whether insecurely attached children become depressed. Bakwin (1949) has observed that children adapted most successfully to hospitalization when they enjoyed secure relationships with their parents. Similarly, Mason (1965) found that children traumatized by separation anxiety from one episode of hospitalization can overcome their fear if hospitals take corrective measures, such as jointly hospitalizing a healthy parent with the sick child. Unfortunately, a dearth of well-designed studies on the impact of joint hospitalization prevents us from drawing firm conclusions on the reactions of hospitalized children when they are not, in fact, separated from their parents (Rau & Kaye, 1977).

The risks of separation are far from limited to preterm infants, as Hollenbeck et al. (1980) have shown. These researchers carried out a prospective study of the effects of isolation on four children, ages 1.5 to 4 years, who were undergoing chemotherapy in a germ-free, protected environment provided by a Laminar Air Flow Room. Hospital staff and family maintained sterile procedures including the wearing of rubber gloves. Behavioral assessments, covering role, behavior, communication, and affect, were made four times each week. Although the children remained physically and vocally active during the initial few weeks of the isolation, by the later weeks they displayed a lack of affect in facial expressions and a depressed demeanor. The researchers concluded that this reverse isolation fostered changes in affect ultimately leading to depression.

Some research suggests that separation does not even achieve its full impact until after the child is at 6 least months old and has established an attachment with his or her mother. Schaffer and Emerson (1964), Bowlby (1969), and Ainsworth (1967) all describe the period up to 6 to 7 months as one of undifferentiated attachment behavior, when the infant will demonstrate attachment behavior toward any adult. Schaffer (1958) and Schaffer and Callender (1959) contend that the seventh month marks the point when infants show the most pronounced effects of maternal deprivation. Institutionalized infants over the age of 7 months studied by Schaffer and Callender displayed the impact of separation with a variety of symptoms, including clinging to the mother after returning home from the hospital, excessive crying when left alone, a wish to be nursed by the mother, and fear of strangers. Infants younger than 7 months showed none of these symptoms.

Enforced separations during the developmental period, when the young child is in the process of establishing his or her physical and psychological autonomy from the mother, may pose a particularly significant risk for the development of depressive symptomatology. According to Mahler's (1972, 1975) chronology of object relations, young children between the ages of 15 and 24 months experience a natural depressive reaction to the recognition of their own separateness from their mother. This reaction, part of the rapprochement subphase of separation–individuation, can take the form of helplessness, dependence, and loneliness resulting from the toddler's realization that his actions can no longer invoke an instant response from the mother. Not surprisingly, these shifts in self-object relations create ambivalence and conflict in the young child's feelings about the primary libidinal object—generally the mother. With maternal empathy and acceptance, the naturally occurring depressive reaction ebbs. However, if the child is deprived of the opportunity for contact and identification with a loving parent, these feelings may intensify into acute helplessness, moodiness, and aggression against the self (Anthony, 1983).

Disruptions in object relations, necessitated by hospitalization, may ultimately impair the definition of the self. Insofar as the self is initially defined in relation to a primary caregiver (Ainsworth, 1967, 1973),

interferences, such as those occasioned by hospitalization, in the development of this relationship, may present a risk to the process of self-matura-
tion. The ability to represent the self mentally—a capacity that is vulnerable
in the face of extremes of emotion (Greenspan, 1981)—may regress or fail to
develop if the strangeness of the hospital environment and the intermittent
disappearances of the caregiver cause a child to panic. (Pain and fear of
different medical procedures, which are more a function of the experience
of illness than of hospitalization, may have similar consequences for the
development of the representational capacities that underly self-definition.)
Greenspan (1981) has identified the period between 30 and 48 months as the
period of greatest vulnerability to such failure, but stress even later in
childhood may bring about regressions in representational ability.

Although the weight of opinion clearly ties maternal separation to
depression among hospitalized infants and children, some theorists have
questioned whether the two are intrinsically linked. Howells (1955, 1956,
1963) argues that the quality of the care received, rather than the separation
itself, dictates the impact of hospitalization on a child's mental health.
Separation, according to the researcher, does not necessarily equal
deprivation. Furthmore, Howells claims that separation for the child
deprived of proper parenting may actually serve a prophylactic role. In
those instances, when the child's home environment has created a
preexisting depression or depressive predisposition (e.g. when there is a
depressed or abusing parent in the home), the separation occasioned by
hospitalization may not represent a totally negative factor. Access to care by
competent medical personnel may more than compensate for the separation
from parents, especially when the interchange between parent and child
confers a vulnerabiity to the development of depression.

Even children from healthy home environments often display remarkable
resilience, provided adequate measures are taken to blunt the effect of the
separation. Substitute mothering, even in an alien environment such as a
hospital, can apparently cushion the depressive impact of maternal
separation. In an experiment to evaluate the impact of providing adequate
substitute mothering for hospitalized children, Robertson and Robertson
(1972), whose theories have long emphasized the role of maternal
deprivation in the etiology of childhood depression, found that such
surrogates could prevent children separated from their mothers for 10 to 27
days from responding with distress and despair. The Robertsons studied 14
children, ranging in age from 17 to 29 months, whose mothers were going to
the hospital to have a second baby. They took four of the children into their
own home; nine others were cared for in their respective homes by a familiar
relative, and one control, a boy of 17 months, was kept temporarily in an
institution. All of the subjects were only children and lived with both parents.
None had previously been separated from his or her mother, except for
intervals of a few hours when he or she was attended by a familiar person.

All four of the children residing in the Robertsons' home transferred cathexis to their substitute mother and continued to function and relate well in varying degrees that reflected their different levels of object constancy and ego maturity. Similar responses were observed in the nine other children fostered in their own homes by familiar relatives. By contrast, the 17-month-old control, who was observed simultaneously in an institutional setting for 9 days, where he was without continuity of mothering, suffered during the experience and deteriorated in all areas. While at the institution, apathy, withdrawal, eating disturbances, and chronic crying marked the boy's behavior. At reunion with his mother, he rejected her by struggling and crying desparately. The Robertsons (1972) concluded that this behavior related directly to inadequate substitute mothering in a strange environment. Although this study dealt with healthy rather than sick children, and did not examine the potential for adequate substitute mothering specifically in a hospitalized setting, it nonetheless offers valuable insight into the possibilities for surrogate mothering in strange environments. Prugh et al. (1953), however, noted that when the hospitalized children they studied began to establish parent–surrogate relationships, pregenital, primitive gratifications often diminished and ceased to interfere with the children's adjustment.

Children's resilience with attentive hospitalization is highlighted most dramatically by the case of the young child who lived from birth in reverse isolation. Researchers who followed this child's progress during the first 52 months of his life concluded that reverse isolation need not thwart affective development despite the fact that the child had been deprived of many experiences thought to be essential for normal development, including smelling and touching of another's body, ventral clinging to the mother, consistency in caregiving, and quality of mothering (Freedman et al., 1976; Williamson et al., 1977). They found that reverse isolation had not impeded the processes of internalization, the establishment of object representation, or the structuring and regulation of drive manifestations. Researchers studying the impact of reverse isolation on a set of young German twins did, however, find significant intellectual impairment. They attributed these deficits to the circumscribed existence that limited the development of ego autonomy, imitation, and self-directed activity. It is possible, however, that differences in the parent's socioeconomic, educational, and psychiatric backgrounds accounted for some of the deficits detected in the German children (Simons et al., 1973). Observers of both the German twins and the American child concede that the full effects of early reverse isolation may not manifest themselves until later in the children's lives.

In sum, several aspects of hospitalization—beyond the experience of illness—expose a child to greater risk of depression. These aspects include separation from parents, isolation, and lack of stimulation. Such factors can promote depressive outcomes by dulling both a child's and mother's

Table 18.   Hospitalization Population Compared with Three Risk Populations

Abuse/Neglect	Maternal Depression	Handicapped
Maltreated children have more illnesses, especially in the first six months. (1)	Hospitalized child is at greater risk with an emotionally disturbed parent. (2)	Handicapped child tends to be more chronically hospitalized. (3)
Birth complications are associated with increased risk for maltreatment. (4)	Depressed mothers have better chance of recovery if not separated from infants (5)	
	Depressed hospitalized children had high incidence of loss and parental depression. (6)	

1. Sherrod et al. (1984)
2. Mason (1965)
3. Barbero (1984)
4. Elmer & Gregg (1967); Hunter et al. (1978); Klein & Stern (1971)
5. Douglas (1956)
6. Kashani, Barbero & Bolander (1981b)

responsiveness in the dyad and creating insecurity in the attachment. Although some evidence suggests that maternal deprivation as a result of hospitalization can damage attachment and thereby predispose a child to depression from the earliest days of life, other evidence traces such interactional failures only to the seventh month. Some research suggests that parent surrogates and other techniques such as joint hospitalization, can prevent hospitalization from leading ineluctably to depression. (See Table 18.)

PARENTAL REACTIONS TO THE ILLNESS AND HOSPITALIZATION OF THEIR CHILDREN

Clearly, perceptions of illness figure significantly into the depression equation. By at least age 10, children have progressed sufficiently to have realistic perceptions of illness and, by extension, realistic perceptions of their vulnerability to it (Natapoff, 1978). Distortions in perception of illness, therefore, alter their sense of control and weaken their defenses against depression. Such distortions can arise in many ways. Failure on the part of medical professionals to convey to children a clear picture of their condition or of the difficult and painful treatment procedures they may undergo leaves children confused and anxious.

Parents, however, share responsibility with medical professionals. In fact, parents generally have the greatest impact on their children's perceptions of their own vulnerability. Adaptive coping attitudes on the parents' part thus underlie successful treatment of the child (Mattson, 1972). Illness and hospitalization evoke parents' ego strength and nurturance in devising an appropriate reaction to their child's condition. Often, however, these systems fail a parent whose child is either ill or hospitalized. Such experiences, as well as the surrender of certain responsibilities to medical professionals, may seem to parents usurpations of their caregiving role at a time when their child needs them most. Parents may thus react with feelings of helplessness, which they can easily transmit to the child.

Some parents react with oversolicitous, controlling, or fearful behavior that can impart to the child an enhanced sense of vulnerability (Green & Solnit, 1964). Overprotectiveness is common among parents of children who are ill, yet it deprives children of the opportunity to participate actively in the management of their own health. The ability of parents to master their initial fear and guilt, arising from feelings that they may have been in some way responsible for the child's illness, is critical for avoiding overprotection and the transmission of maladaptive coping attitudes to children (Solnit, 1960).

Constructive parental involvement can be difficult to obtain under the best of circumstances. When parents themselves suffer from guilt about their child's conditions, as may occur with pediatric AIDS, or when they suffer from depression or other pathology, the hospitalized child faces an even greater risk of developing depressive symptoms. Research has documented a comparatively higher incidence of depression among the parents of hospitalized children suffering from depression. Of those children who met both the BID (Bellevue Index of Depression) and DSM-III criteria for depression in Kashani et al.'s (1981) study of depression among hospitalized, school-age children, well over half had parents with a positive history of depression. The BID includes 10 major categories of psychopathology (Petti, 1978). The first two categories—dysphoric mood and self-deprecatory ideation—are prerequisites for inclusion in the diagnostic category of depression. The process whereby parental depression relates to children's hospitalization and to their own depression is no doubt complex. Whether parental depression, rather than hospitalization, actually causes the depression seen among hospitalized infants and children, is still unclear. What is clear, however, is that through healthy relationships with their parents, infants and children find the security and sense of control to forestall the possible onset of depression. Parental psychopathology can rob them of this protection.

INTERVENTION STRATEGIES

Given the wealth of evidence on the harmful effects of early hospitalization, it is apparent that unnecessary hospitalization presents a high risk for the development of infant and childhood depression. It should, therefore, be avoided. The medical community has subscribed to this admonishment in theory, but the reality leaves room for improvement. Various studies indicate that as many as one third of child hospitalizations before the age of 5 could have been avoided (Haggerty, 1968; Prugh, 1983). Field and Miller (1969) charge that an estimated 36 percent of hospitalized preschool children could safely be treated at home. Stocking et al. (1975) called for greater pediatric day hospitals to treat such children. Although tonsillectomy and adenoidectomy are recognized as potentially traumatic to young patients, they are still performed too often, according to Prugh (1983). Haggerty (1968) concluded that of the 30 to 40 percent of Rochester children who underwent tonsillectomy in 1968, the operation was medically necessary for less than 5 percent. Moreover, the proportion of children undergoing "long and repeated" hospitalization has not declined. This finding led Douglas (1975) to conclude that despite the overwhelming consensus on the potentially serious impact of hospitalization on children, it is still not being discouraged.

The manner in which children's medical and psychological treatment, whether in a hospital or at home, is managed will clearly influence the psychological impact of the illness and/or hospitalization on them. Appropriate intervention requires early identification of risk for depression. However, the clinical signs of depression or self-blame in an infant or child are frequently easy to overlook because the depressed child rarely causes trouble or protests treatment, particularly since unconscious fantasies may lead to acceptance of treatment as punishment for bad thoughts or bad deeds. Ironically, at the moment when a child seems most compliant, he or she may actually be masking depression. Moreover, in the early stages of certain diseases, such as AIDS, it may be difficult to distinguish certain psychological symptoms, such as psychomotor retardation, from physical symptoms related to central nervous system dysfunction (Holland & Tross, 1985).

Emde et al. (1981) described such a diagnostic failure in the case of a 3-year-old boy who had been accidentally burned over the lower extremities, and was referred for psychiatric evaluation because of increased withdrawal. The child psychiatrist immediately noted that the boy was severely depressed. He had fallen prey to a vicious cycle: after separation from his parents for treatment, he seemed irritable unless left alone. This was the depressed child's way of engaging his environment, the only way his depression permitted. Unfortunately, the hospital staff misconstrued this irritability and left him alone for long periods of time. Such misinterpretations of irritability among depressed children and infants are all too common, according to the researchers.

Unfortunately, in contrast to the child described by Emde et al., many sick infants and children never get the benefit of psychiatric consultation. When presented with a concrete and treatable physical ailment, physicians often fail to suspect or detect psychopathology, especially in infants. Stocking, Rothney, Grosser, and Goodwin's (1970) study of 80 children, ages 0 to 16 years, confirmed the magnitude of these oversights on the part of pediatricians. During a 10-month period, two child psychiatrists evaluated each of these children on admission to a pediatric hospital. Their objective was to determine whether psychiatric consultation might enhance the child's overall medical treatment. In almost two thirds of the cases, they determined that psychiatric consultation was indicated because of significant psychopathology or difficulties in emotional adaptation. They did not share these recommendations with the pediatric staff which, by contrast, sought psychiatric consultation in only about one quarter of the cases identified by the interviewing psychiatrists. Notably, the psychiatrists found that all 12 infants under 2 years old—the group at highest risk for depression—demonstrated overt difficulty adapting to their mothers. As this study suggests, reducing the risk for depression will clearly require better screening to identify high-risk children—those with chronic and debilitating conditions and those with little family support structure to buttress them against defeatism.

The medical community must be persuaded to improve techniques for identifying high-risk infants and children earlier. It will also have to refine methods of managing both parents' and children's reactions to illness and hospitalization. When treating sick children, the medical community typically permits them little reaction to their illness or to the procedures they are undergoing. Sick children are too infrequently given the opportunity to vent their anger. Lacking such an outlet, they often submit passively, turning their anger on themselves in anxiety, guilt, masochism, or depression. Encouraging children to express such feelings while maintaining self-control enables them to dissipate self-destructive guilt and to turn their energies toward convalescence.

A large body of literature has pointed to the importance of preparing families for difficult medical procedures and for hospitalization. Researchers and clinicians emphasized home preparation, honesty, and decreased waiting time prior to a procedure or hospitalization. Others focus more exclusively on the value of preparation. Pearson (1941) and Langford (1961) argued that preparation is a major factor in preventing emotional problems stemming from hospitalization and surgery. In the classic film, "A Two Year Old Goes to the Hospital," Robertson (1970) also called for greater preparation to cushion the blow of hospitalization. Kenny (1975) noted that lack of preparation can lead to a negative reaction by both parent and child. With proper preparation, Jensen (1955) contends that hospitalization can even foster maturity and development in some children. In short, most researchers agree that preparation must direct itself both to the child and to the parent.

Empirical evidence seems to confirm these observations concerning preparation. Vaughan (1957) compared the inward and postdischarge behavior of 20 children (mean age, 5.9 years) who had been prepared for surgery using a simple schematic explanation, and 20 children who received no preparation. Although the prepared children showed slightly more disturbed behavior during hospitalization, Vaughan (1957) found that preparation led to reduced disturbances one week after discharge. Use of simple preparation is critical, the researcher noted.

A number of techniques have shown particular promise. Modeling films, describing a prospective operation, appear to work effectively with preschoolers, according to a study performed by Ferguson (1979). This investigation measured children's fear and adjustment while in the hospital, as well as their behavior after discharge—both in relation to the type of preparation they received. In assessing the children after discharge, Ferguson used the Post-Hospital Behavior Inventory devised by Vernon, Schulman, and Foley (1966), which considers a number of behavioral indices of significance to depression, including general anxiety and regression, separation anxiety, anxiety about sleep, eating disturbances, aggression toward authority, apathy, and withdrawal. According to the study, older children appear to respond equally well to modeling films and home visits in which a nurse visits the child to explain upcoming medical procedures and answer the child's questions. Ferguson hypothesizes that the increased verbal abilities of the older children allowed them to assimilate information provided in the home visit better than the younger children.

Children also require consultation and clarification about death. In the absence of such consultation, competition between normative thinking about death on the one hand and contradictory fantasies and immature beliefs on the other can increase children's anxiety and predisposition to interpret illness and death as punishment. Although children do not reach a full comprehension of death until they reach about 12 years old (Speece & Brent, 1984), they can assimilate and take advantage of straightforward information even at an early age (Furman, 1964).

Hospitals face perhaps the biggest challenge of all in devising strategies for reducing the potentially depressive impact of early hospitalization. Accommodating the special needs of infants and children may require hospitals to revise some of their most time-honored practices. Control over the patient—whether through visting policies, isolation, or any of the many other restraints imposed on patients and their families—is rooted deeply in the hospital mentality. Lozoff et al. (1977) made a provocative recommendation that any aspect of peripartum care not based on verified scientific evidence should be left to parental choice. While their comments referred explicitly to the neonatal period, their conclusions apply throughout childhood. They support abolition of all hospital routines that separate mothers and infants, calling for early and extended contact for the dyad.

To minimize the potentially depressive risks to children, hospitals should exercise far greater discrimination before deciding to place a child in isolation or reverse isolation. Although hospitals have employed isolation to reduce the spread of infection and ultimately reduce infant mortality, Lozoff et al. (1977) suggest that these practices may immutably alter the mother-infant relationship and precipitate potentially devastating consequences. Bakwin (1949) noted that the benefit of freer cuddling of hositalized infants far outweighs the liability of infection due to such interaction.

Hospitals are merely tools, as Spence (1947) correctly observed. Their structure and their operating policies have attempted to express state-of-the-art knowledge of physical disease. Pediatric hospital management has not, however, kept pace with growing understanding of hospitalization and children. The alarming incidence of infant and childhood depression within this hospitalized population testifies to this fact. Reducing the risk to children must start with a reevaluation of hospital routine in light of these realizations.

Despite the potential for undermining a child's sense of control, illness and hospitalization need not lead inexorably to helplessness. A number of investigators have found that children can grow to adulthood without helpless dependence—and that they can even convert a potentially regressive experience into one of growth—if they are taught to deal realistically with the limitations imposed by their illness and are given the opportunity to assume some responsibility for the medical management of their disease (Langford, 1961; Mattsson, 1972; Prugh et al., 1953).

Parmelee (1986), who has extensively studied children with illnesses, even makes a convincing argument for the beneficial impact of illness on children's behavioral development. Although his argument is based on clinical impressions of the reactions of children with comparatively brief and moderate illnesses, such as respiratory infections and gastrointestinal upsets, it may have broader applicability than is currently recognized. He suggests that these recurring illnesses actually promote development of the self by expanding children's awareness of changes in their physical and psychological selves. Moreover, increasing awareness of the unique character of certain recurring illness may improve children's ability to identify the source of discomfort correctly, potentially alleviating the self-recriminations that often result from the novel experience of illness. Children who can understand the emotional and physical causes of distress and changes in internal states—of themselves and others—may also be better equipped to engage in the kind of prosocial behavior that helps fortify social relationships and relieve the guilt arising from empathic distress that they may suffer (Trad, 1986).

CONCLUSION

Sickness and hospitalization serve as twin examples of noncontingency: An infant or child previously accustomed to receiving nurturance from the caregiver is suddenly removed from a familiar milieu and placed in a strange environment without his or her parents. Disease itself exacerbates the sense of noncontingency, representing an uncontrollable force in the child's life. These dual phenomena, of hospitalization and illness, contribute to the feelings of helplessness often experienced by infants and children who are ill and/or hospitalized. Literature on the debilitating effect of "hospitalism" has been reviewed, from Spitz' classic work to present studies, and recommendations for ameliorating the debilitating effects of these conditions have been proposed.

CHAPTER NINE

Handicapping Conditions as a Risk Factor for Infant and Childhood Depression

Not too long ago, the words "handicap," "impairment," and "disability" were absent from everyday conversation and indeed, such labels were not a part of familiar vocabulary. Individuals with handicaps were generally relegated to institutions or were kept close to home, their conditions sequestered in secrecy. But the liberating spirit of the past few decades, coupled with dramatic advances in medical technology, have enabled those with physical handicaps and deformities to emerge into the world of mainstream America.

With this new integration of the handicapped population, however, has come an acute awareness of the types of problems—particularly emotional problems—experienced by individuals with impairments. Moreover, it has become increasingly apparent that much of the psychopathology encountered among handicapped adults can be traced back to the experiences of childhood and perhaps even infancy.

This chapter contends that a handicapping condition can present a unique risk for the development of subsequent depression and depressive-like phenomena, particularly when the condition affects an infant or young child. Such an "imperfect" infant or child may have difficulty, due to an organic defect, in manifesting the temperamental repertoire of a normal infant. Moreover, caregivers may experience unique frustrations in interacting with such infants and may graft their own feelings of disappointment, inadequacy, guilt, or anger onto the attachment behaviors they display toward their infant. Thus, by the advent of a full-fledged sense of self, such an infant may already perceive of himself or herself as a stigmatized individual. This stigma, in turn, can become part of his or her internal perception or self-image and can set the stage for depressive symptomatology.

Nonetheless, this unfortunate scenario is far from inevitable. As this chapter will discuss, early attunement to the needs of these infants and children can avert the experience of noncontingency, distorted attachment behaviors, and overexposure to stress. Ultimately, this chapter suggests that the handicapped population is one in which the challenge of circumventing the downward path leading to depression and depressive-like phenomena can be addressed.

Investigations into physical disorders of any kind have typically served as a vehicle for gaining insight into the normal course of development and normal behaviors. Not surprisingly, therefore, studies of handicapped populations have proven to be a popular topic of research. These studies have generated a wealth of data on critical developmental tasks such as the dynamics of attachment formation (Blacher, 1984a; Cicchetti & Serafica, 1981; Stahlecker & Cohen, 1985; Thompson & Cicchetti, 1985) and the evolution of representational thought (Fetters, 1981; Mans, Cicchetti, & Sroufe, 1978) among impaired populations.

Moreover, research into development among handicapped populations has yielded greater understanding of the sequence and chronology of many developmental processes and is appealing as a basis for theoretical modeling. The tendency to study handicapped populations as a means of understanding nonhandicapped populations has, however, often obscured the importance of treating the developmental processes of the handicapped as worthy of investigation in their own right. Nowhere has this been more apparent than in the literature on the handicapped as a population at risk for depression.

Various avenues of research during the past two decades have hinted at the importance of studying psychopathology in general, and depression in particular, among the handicapped. One of the initial studies to highlight the comparatively high prevalence of psychopathology among the handicapped was the Isle of Wight study (Rutter et al., 1970b), which found far greater rates of psychiatric impairment among the mentally handicapped than among the nonhandicapped. Similarly, the handicapped number significantly among some of the well recognized risk populations for childhood depression. The high incidence of abuse observed by Elmer and Gregg (1967) among premature infants suggests that some of the handicapped—those born prematurely—may be at risk for depression through abuse or neglect. Other handicapped groups have been implicitly included among risk populations by virtue of their frequent need for hospitalization.

Thus, while there is no scarcity of data on many of the important underlying developmental processes related to depression, or on handicapped populations, most research has evaded direct discussion of the topic of depression among handicapped children. Although the last decade of research on the handicapped has supplied detailed accounts of mother-infant interaction comparable to those that have helped researchers trace the etiology of depression in normal infants and children, these valuable studies have been largely overlooked as a source of understanding of depression. Research has dealt in depth with the difficulties in face-to-face interactions between handicapped children and their caregivers, but has for the most part stopped short of discussing such interaction in the context of noncontingency—the experience of which often lies at the root of depression. Similarly underutilized have been studies of temperament among handicapped populations.

In the past, researchers have displayed a tendency to view a handicapping condition as a rigidly determining factor in such developmental phenomena as attachment formation and temperament expression. This has been true despite the prevalent view that physiological and environmental factors interact to determine infant psychology. To a large extent we have, perhaps unwittingly, accepted rigid characterizations of different types of handicapped children and, as a result, are implicitly expected to treat as "given" certain aspects of handicapped children's affects and behaviors—for example, the lack of sparkle in the social encounters of Down's Syndrome infants (Emde et al., 1978) and their higher threshold for arousal (Cicchetti & Serafica, 1981; Sorce & Emde, 1982), the lack of differentiation in the responses of severely handicapped children (Blacher, 1984a), and the impulsivity, hyperactivity, rigidity, and suspiciousness of the deaf child. There is a tacit assumption that these characteristics, which are typically seen as the initial impediment in building effective mother-child interaction, are a function almost exclusively of the handicapping condition. Consequently, researchers have adopted a quiescent attitude in speculating about alternative meanings for the behaviors they have carefully documented.

This chapter will question whether, in fact, such behaviors can be legitimately viewed as "given" by the handicapped condition or whether they also express other aspects of a handicapped child's early development. It will be asserted that the various depictions of early emotional development in many handicapped children must also be viewed, as they would be for nonhandicapped children—as derivative of the early infant-caregiver interaction, not of the handicapping condition per se. Thus, for example, the muted quality of a Down's infant's social smile may also serve as an important index of the infant's affective state, perhaps a product of the infant-caregiver interaction, rather than as a totally predetermined expression of organic disorder. Considered in this light, many of the studies of attachment behavior must be reanalyzed for what they indicate about the prevalence of depressive symptomatology in the early lives of many handicapped children. When the various depictions of handicapped children are reinterpreted from this vantage point, the affective expressions and behavioral characteristics of many handicapped children reveal as much about the physical expressions of organic disorder as about a strong depressive symptomatology often resulting from handicapping conditions.

While it would be naive to contend that none of the characteristics just noted reflect actual biological impairments, the tendency to resort to such rigid characterizations has long disguised other potential interpretations of these phenomena. Viewing these characteristics as manifestations of underlying depression is one such interpretation. This chapter generalizes from the advice of Chess and Fernandez (1980), who, in their study of deaf children, urged abandonment of the notion of the typical personality of such children. It will question existing research to demonstrate that when the handicapped child is no longer conceived of as an organically fixed and invariable participant in early development, but rather as a dynamically determined affective being, data from studies of attachment, temperament, and self-representation among handicapped populations provide compelling evidence of a population whose risk for depression has long gone underrecognized (Trad, 1986).

Several recent investigations have sought to clarify the relationship between depression and symptomatology heretofore viewed as intrinsic to handicapping conditions. Colbert, Newman, Ney, and Young (1982) have argued that many purported learning disabilities are actually manifestations of an underlying depression that depletes a child's energy and attention, leading to poorer school performance. They contend that adults often prefer to conceive of poor performance as a learning disability rather than as depression, since the former does not appear to imply neglect. In their study, over half of the child population (under the age of 15) admitted to a family unit of a Canadian hospital—almost two-thirds of whom were above average in intelligence but underachieving—were diagnosed as depressed. Ironically, as the investigators noted, underachievement often leads to segregation in special classes, which may worsen a depressed child's self-image and further increase depression.

While other researchers do not go as far as Colbert et al. (1982) in claiming that symptoms of depression are often mistaken for symptoms of handicapping conditions, they do document a great deal of depressive symptomatology among the handicapped. A review of the last six decades of case literature led Sovner and Hurley (1983) to reject the theory that the mentally retarded lack the psychological capacity to experience affective disorders. Of course, retrospective case reviews may be subject to serious methodological questions. Incomplete data often prevent the reviewer(s) from making reliable diagnoses, particularly by DSM-III standards. This problem is confounded in the cases reviewed by Sovner and Hurley, since the relationship they were examining—that between affective disorders and mental retardation—requires diagnoses of both disorders. These obstacles notwithstanding, the researchers argued that a sufficient number of clearcut cases exist to justify the conclusion that the mentally retarded cannot be considered invulnerable to affective disorders. The authors suggest, however, that the presence of mental retardation may distinguish the expression of affective disorders. For example, hallucinations may be more common in both mania and depression.

Whether the mentally handicapped are more or less vulnerable than populations with normal intelligence could not be determined from their review. Inpatient studies evaluated by Sovner and Hurley (1983) yielded widely varying estimates of the prevalence of affective disorder among the mentally retarded. According to the authors, however, the methodological problems no doubt responsible for these differences probably have caused them to underestimate, rather than overestimate the incidence of affective disorder among the mentally retarded. Such problems included failure of some studies to identify psychotropic drugs (which may obscure affective symptomatology) in use by the populations they studied, the focus on institutionalized mentally retarded individuals and the implicit omission of those who may be symptomatic but may not require hospitalization, and the reliance of these studies on case material compiled by clinical staffs inadequately trained to recognize possibly masked affective symptomatology.

Silver (1984) studied severely emotionally handicapped children between the ages of 8 and 14—the large majority of whom had some biological defect—and found that almost a quarter of them were depressed. Dosen (1984) found 16 percent of 194 mentally handicapped children studied were depressed. The portrait of the depressed child presented by Dosen does not bear some of the characteristics, most notably dysphoric mood, typically prominent in depression. This atypical expression of depression may help explain why depression, while possibly prevalent, has remained perplexing to diagnose in handicapped children. Difficulty in diagnosing depression was also raised by Breslau (1985)—whose research demonstrated more than twice the level of severe psychopathology among the handicapped than among controls—as a possible explanation for the failure of her study to prove that handicapping conditions confer risk specifically for depression. She notes that symptoms of depression may not be obvious to parents, who may misconstrue these manifestations as indications of excessive anger or irritability.

DEFINITION OF THE HANDICAPPED POPULATION

Despite an abundance of research data on the handicapped, scant effort has been devoted to specifically delimiting the population. Diagnoses for some of the largest handicapped populations—the learning disabled and the developmentally delayed—are still difficult to obtain, and criteria for assessment are often imprecise. The research has reflected this imprecision. Investigations that have recognized a possible risk for psychopathology when brain damage comprises part of the handicap have differentiated between handicapped populations with mental impairment and those without (Breslau, 1985). This distinction, however, is one of the few that has been acknowledged. In many cases, handicapping conditions have been viewed on a continuum with conditions that are thought to cause less extreme disturbances in a child's overall development. Some research, for example, includes the chronically ill (Barbero, 1984; Steinhausen, 1981). Children with undiagnosed developmental delays or learning disabilities have also been included in the handicapped population (Brooks-Gunn & Lewis, 1984; Greenberg & Field, 1982; Van Tassel, 1984). Some investigations have included the severely emotionally handicapped, since a large portion of such children also have some biological defect.

THE SCOPE OF THE HANDICAPPED POPULATION

The breadth and diversity of the handicapped child population has made it difficult to obtain comprehensive estimates on the overall size of the population and of the different subgroups within it. Fortunately, enactment of the Education of the Handicapped Act in 1975 has encouraged the collection of reliable statistics to help identify the many handicapped children who, since the passage of this legislation, have been assured access to public education. Public school enrollment figures may fail to include some handicapped children, such as those in institutions and those educated in private schools. However, since most handicapped children are now cared for in homes rather than in institutions, these figures may provide a reasonable low-end estimate of the handicapped population as a risk group for depression.

The most recent figures released by the U.S. Department of Education (DOE) reveal that in 1983–1984, over 4 million handicapped children received services through the Education of the Handicapped Act. Learning disabled children represented the largest category, consisting of over 1.8 million children. Speech-impaired children accounted for slightly more than 1 million handicapped children, and three quarters of 1 million handicapped children were classified as mentally retarded. None of the other subgroups of handicapped children—the hearing-impaired and deaf, the orthopedically impaired, the visually handicapped, the deaf-blind, or the multihandicapped—consisted of more than 75,000 children.

Overall trends, rather than absolute figures, may signal important developments in this risk population. According to DOE statistics, the number of mentally handicapped children, who represent a significant portion of the handicapped child population, has appeared to decline since 1976–1977. However, it is possible that many children formerly called mentally retarded are now described as learning disabled in an attempt to reduce the pejorative connotations and potential for bias in the label "retarded." This phenomenon may, in fact, be reflected in the doubling of the number of learning disabled that occurred during this time. Moreover, this doubling is particularly significant in light of one recent suggestion (Colbert et al., 1982) that parents and clinical professionals may mistake depression for learning disabilities.

Al was born with multiple anatomical handicaps, including a cleft lip and palate, hypospadias, and a patent ductus arteriosus. He was placed under special observation at the hospital and discharged two days after his mother. Despite his physical problems, Al was an affectionate infant with large eyes and an active disposition.

Following his birth, his parents—particularly his mother—displayed obvious hurt and disappointment when gazing at their disfigured son. Mrs. A, an overweight woman who looked exhausted after the birth of the infant, had hoped for a little girl. Initially, Mrs. A did not want to see her son. She began crying after she was told of his deformities, saying that she felt ashamed of herself for having produced such a baby. In contrast to Mrs. A, Mr. A expressed immediate concern for his son. He coaxed his wife into holding Al, trying to convince her that he was a cuddly infant.

During the first 2 months of Al's life, Mrs. A manifested a marked ambivalence to her son. The attachment behaviors she exhibited toward him in face-to-face interaction reflected her feelings of negativity and her not well-concealed belief that Al was a burden. She looked tired and disheveled at her weekly visits to the clinic with her son, asserting that she was angry at the situation and felt overwhelmed at times by guilt, helplessness, and depression. When she took Al out into the street, she would cover his face with a blanket claiming that she was trying to protect him and also noting sheepishly that she was embarrassed by his appearance.

Mrs. A's ambivalence toward Al was especially reflected in her attitude toward her son at night. She insisted on sleeping in his room, and would pick him up at the slightest sound. She also commented that when she bathed him, she was afraid of drowning him. Nevertheless, despite these outward displays of apparent concern, Mrs. A also referred to Al by disparaging nicknames, like "The Monster" and "The Rat." She reported feeling sorry for Al, but often was observed acting aggressively and intrusively during interaction.

With time and therapy, however, Mrs. A's behavior toward her son began to modify. Most notably, by the end of the third month, she referred to the child as "Little Pumpkin." She began to relinquish her feelings of injured self-esteem, noting that she was beginning to give up the vision of the "perfect" child she had expected.

Beginning at approximately 4 months, surgical repair designed to fix Al's lip was initiated. Both parents visited their son frequently at the hospital, although Mrs. A occasionally expressed such emotions as confusion, anger, avoidance, and self-blame. The hospital staff was supportive and ultimately both parents experienced great pleasure at the outcome of the operation, which improved the infant's physical appearance and for the first time, enabled Mrs. A to feed her infant in a more traditional manner.

Over the next few months, Mrs. A's ambivalence toward her son continued to recede. She began taking pride in her appearance and when she returned from a weekend of visiting relatives, she was delighted to discover that her son had "missed her." Al faced a further series of operations in the upcoming months, and this time both parents displayed concern and support for their son, rather than focusing on their own emotions.

At Al's 9-month check-up, Mrs. A was able to speak maturely about her feelings for Al and her sense of anger at having a handicapped child. She seemed more attuned to Al's needs, and she and her husband had slowly begun to reconstruct their social life.

By the 20-month evaluation, most traces of Mrs. A's self-pitying attitude were gone, although she still looked tired and expressed the often frustrating feelings that can be associated with nurturing a handicapped child. Al too, had progressed well, but he walked and ran with severe awkwardness and his social development lagged behind other children of his age. He appeared happy and playful. However, he evinced some degree of shyness and reticence at playing with new toys and meeting strangers. Both parents implied that they were aware of Al's developmental lags, noting that they intended to have him fully evaluated in the near future. They appeared able to accept the fact that Al might be mentally disabled as well, but preferred to allow themselves to "wait and get accustomed to the idea."

The transitions in attitude experienced by Al's parents reflect a familiar pattern of parental ambivalence often encountered with handicapped children. Al's mother was able to overcome this ambivalence primarily because of a supportive therapeutic team that consistently allowed her to ventilate her anger, fear, resentment, and anxiety (Mintzer, Als, Tronic, & Brazelton, 1984).

DEPRESSIVE SYMPTOMATOLOGY AMONG HANDICAPPED CHILDREN

Before addressing the issue of how depression manifests itself in handicapped infants and children, it is important to accept the proposition that even those with severe handicaps are developmentally capable both of participating in the experiences that can produce depression and of experiencing depression per se. The portrait that emerges varies with the specific type as well as the severity of the handicapping condition. Chess and Fernandez (1980), for example, found that behavioral profiles of children whose sole handicap was deafness differed dramatically from children with multiple handicaps. However, research to date indicates quite conclusively that handicapped *infants* are equipped for social interactions at a very early age and that they can provide caregivers with rather unambiguous signs of their needs. Despite severe mental and visual handicaps, many such infants can engage in the face-to-face interaction that is critical for building a mutually satisfying relationship with a caregiver.

For example, all of the infants studied by Stahlecker and Cohen (1985) had neurological impairment, but were nonetheless able to demonstrate clear attachment behavior. This finding suggests that even conditions that may inhibit signal processing do not necessarily impede effective infant-caregiver interaction and the attainment of developmental hallmarks dependent on such interaction. Furthermore, the latter study demonstrated that for those handicapped infants who were classifiable, severity of the handicap did not discriminate in terms of the quality of attachment. Blacher and Meyers' (1983) review of the attachment literature noted that severely impaired children such as those with Down's syndrome can maintain eye contact, appear to remember attachment figures, and can respond selectively—all critical skills for developing attachments through the third stage of attachment delineated by Ainsworth (1973). An infant who has reached this stage has progressed substantially toward object constancy. Such an infant knows that the mother exists, though she may be absent, and can recognize many of the mother's features, such as her voice and face, at a distance. According to Ainsworth's conceptualization, at the fourth and final stage, a child, generally 4- to 5-years-old, has established a fully trusting and reciprocal relationship with his or her mother. Separation distress no longer exists and the child has some ability to take the mother's perspective. Even blind children, who lack visual capacity, a characteristic generally deemed critical for sociability, display attachment behavior comparable to nonhandicapped children (Blacher & Meyers, 1983).

Strong support for the apparent readiness or preparedness of handicapped infants to engage in social interaction is furnished by two studies that Sorce and Emde (1982) performed to determine whether mothers recognize the affective expressions of their 3- to 4-month-old infants and how their degree of recognition influences caregiving behaviors. The researchers studied four categories of emotion—enjoyment, interest, drowsiness, and distress—and explored how these emotions stimulated such behaviors as play, soothing, physical caregiving, and attentiveness. Photographs of the infants' expressions were taken in a naturalistic setting and the biological mothers were asked to identify what the children were feeling in each photo. Although the mothers' descriptions revealed significant differences in the absolute arousal level of normal and Down's Syndrome children, the same patterns of response between categories of emotions and caregiving behaviors prevailed. When these same photos were shown to other mothers of similarly aged normal infants, these nonbiological mothers achieved comparable success in identifying expressions of both the normal and Down's syndrome infants, and the expressions elicited similar responses. The second part of the study adds compelling evidence of the ability of even severely handicapped infants to participate in contingent relationships with caregivers. Sorce and Emde interpreted the results of these studies as evidence of what they called a "natural language" for caregiving.

To the extent that children are capable of such development as indicated by existing research, they may also be capable of experiencing deviations from this developmental course. The same data documenting readiness for reciprocal interaction can be used to illustrate behavioral deviation—most significantly, depression. If such children are equipped to communicate their needs to caregivers, they are also equipped to experience the effects of failure at such interaction. Indeed, although there are pronounced individual differences in the affects of many handicapped infants and children, some of the descriptions of these children closely resemble those of children exposed to persistent experiences of noncontingency. The dulled affects and higher threshold for arousal described by researchers such as Thompson and Cicchetti (1985) recall the descriptions of the muted and undifferentiated facial expressions noted by researchers such as Field (1984a) among the offspring of depressed parents and those described by Spitz (1945) among hospitalized children. Dulled affects may thus reflect less of an intrinsic genetic quality than a learned-helpless response to asynchronous infant–caregiver interaction. Researchers who interpret the muted responses of Down's syndrome children to alternating sequences of stressful and nonstressful events as evidence of delayed attachment development (Serafica & Cicchetti, 1976) may be overlooking important evidence of affective dysregulation—and potentially depression—arising from a reciprocally determined noncontingent situation.

Methodological obstacles have made it difficult to relinquish many of the traditional theories about the affective expressions of handicapped children. As noted elsewhere, researchers interested in infant and childhood depression have, for at least the last decade, found themselves in the midst of unabated controversy about how best to detect depressive symptomatology in the earliest stages of life. The difficulties encountered in diagnosing depression at a very young age are further compounded by the presence of handicapping conditions. Greenberg and Field (1982) question the applicability of several dimensions of the Infant Temperament Questionnaire for studying mood and responsiveness of handicapped infants and children. Other standard measurement devices, such as the Ainsworth Strange Situation, that have proven reliable for evaluating attachment patterns of the very young rely to a certain extent on behaviors that some handicapped children may be physically unable to display. For example, searching and reaching are behaviors used to measure attachment, but these manifestations may be outside the repertoire of infants with certain handicaps.

There remains a great deal of controversy about whether such well-accepted barometers of affective development as the Strange Situation can be used reliably among handicapped infants. Blacher (1984a), for example, used a variation of this paradigm to evaluate the attachment behaviors of 50 severely to profoundly retarded children, and concluded that the lack of discrete and differentiated behaviors made it impossible to classify these children in the standard categories. Furthermore, Blacher concluded that there was no evidence to demonstrate attachment beyond the second stage described by Ainsworth. (By the time an infant has reached this stage, he or she has learned to differentiate the mother or another caregiver from others and directs attention selectively to that person. During this stage, absence of the attachment figure evokes anxiety and distress.)

These findings would appear to confirm conclusions from Blacher and Meyers' (1983) earlier review of the literature that the demonstrated validity of the Strange Situation for handicapped populations still remains limited. However, tests of the Strange Situation on handicapped infants within the recommended age range do provide some positive results about its ability to tap critical development information about handicapped children. Stahlecker and Cohen (1985), for example, found that while a small percentage of handicapped infants—perhaps those whose handicaps were of a degree comparable to those infants studied by Blacher (1984a)—cannot be described in conventional terms because of their inability to orient, reach, cling, and follow, 80 percent were fully classifiable using the procedure. Based on the results of this study, then, it appears that even when studying severely handicapped infants and children, one can rely on many of the observations of studies undertaken with standard measurement devices. Whether or not current instrumentation can fully measure early emotional development among handicapped children—that is, whether researchers can designate such children as securely or insecurely attached—these and other studies provide valuable raw data from which we can determine the general course of development of such children and infer signs of depressive symptomatology.

Throughout the last decade, research has documented that the most notable characteristics of several categories of handicapped children relate to their interactional difficulties (Blacher & Meyers, 1983; Chess, 1978; Cicchetti & Serafica, 1981; Emde & Brown, 1978; Emde, Katz, & Thorpe, 1978; Mordock, 1979; Thompson & Cicchetti, 1985). Since their facial expressions, which are considered critical for effective face-to-face interactions, have typically been viewed as part of their natural endowment for social engagement, a popular view has emerged that handicapping conditions result in homogeneous and inalterable infant facial expressions and arousability. Empirical support for this thesis would appear to require demonstration of a greater degree of response homogeneity within and across handicapped groups described in the literature. Although some research has compared attachment behaviors and temperaments of handicapped and nonhandicapped children, there has been minimal large-scale controlled research to test this hypothesis with subgroups of handicapped children. The little research that does exist, whether exclusively on depression among the handicapped or on their affective development in general, suggests that their emotional expressions are probably as varied as those of nonhandicapped infants and children. Depression itself, where it has been identified among handicapped children, presents a heterogeneous picture comparable to that found among nonhandicapped infants and children. Common depressive symptoms such as dysphoric mood may or may not be evident (Dosen, 1984). Poor school performance (which is included in some criteria, but not DSM-III, for childhood depression) may appear in some cases but not in others (Colbert et al., 1982). Finally, the nature of the handicapping condition—whether it is acquired or congenital—may determine whether self-concept is altered.

Particular types of depressive symptomatology thought to be common, if not intrinsic, to certain handicapped populations are by no means uniformly

infant's ongoing experience. The fact that Bridges and Cicchetti (1982) could find little stability in their temperamental measures provides some limited support for the plasticity of these behaviors.

Temperament studies are also useful for identifying the clusters of traits that may coalesce to exacerbate parent–child interactional difficulties, ultimately producing a degree of noncontingency that results in depression in the infant or child. Describing an infant's or child's temperament as "easy" or "difficult" says little about the origins of that classification. As Crittenden (1985a) demonstrated among abused children, temperament is responsive to environmental changes. However, an understanding of the various influences on parent-child interaction can help determine whether strains in this interaction, rather than other forces, are shaping the child's affective state. From the temperament literature, it is clear that temperamental difficulty, whatever its origins, may contribute far more than previously recognized to the interactional failures underlying early learned helplessness depression.

The Bridges and Cicchetti (1982) study, for example, showed a relatively equal distribution of infants among the several categories of "easy" and "difficult" temperaments. These findings tend to refute the stereotype of the Down's syndrome baby as a placid and easy infant (Gunn, Berry, & Andrews, 1983). Van Tassel's (1984) study of temperament among mildly developmentally delayed infants (ages 3 to 16 months) confirms this picture. Mothers who completed the Revised Parent Perception of Baby Temperament questionnaire (Pedersen, Zaslow, Cain, Anderson, & Thomas, 1979) indicated that they perceived their infants as less positive in mood—a dimension that embraces happiness, irritability/fussiness, self-comforting, and response latency to soothing. (See Table 19.)

Attachment

Some of the attachment literature suggests that there is no "biologically" fixed affective profile of handicapped children and that signs of blunted affect should not be accepted in an unqualified manner. Rather, they should be examined for what they indicate about the infant's or child's affective states. Chess's (1978) comparison of parent–infant interaction between deaf children with deaf parents and deaf children with hearing parents offers a particularly good illustration of the plasticity of development in an interactional framework. The observation that deaf offspring of deaf parents adapted better than deaf children of hearing parents (Meadow, Greenberg, & Erting, 1983) suggests that most handicaps are not necessarily deterministic and that characteristics of caregivers are important variables in influencing a child's developmental outcome. Meadow et al. studied the attachment behavior of 17 profoundly deaf preschoolers who were exposed to a 30-minute separation–reunion sequence. Only one child less than

Table 19. Temperament Studies of Handicapped Risk Population

All Handicapped

Found Deaf and Blind and cerebral palsied children were rated (ITQ) the most difficult compared to normals, Down's Syndrome, and retarded.

Negative emotions, mood swings, absence of smiling, and temperamental difficulty were correlated with degree of mental and physical handicaps.

Suggested the ITQ, designed for use with normal children, needed to be broadened for use with handicapped.

In temperament rating of difficulty, mothers rated their handicapped offspring easiest, observers next easiest, teachers most difficult.
(1)

Developmentally Delayed

Using ITQ, found at 3 to 16 months less positive mood and approach, more withdrawing.
(2)

Down's Syndrome

Using ITQ, found at 6, 9, and 12 months less smiling and laughter, more duration of orienting, fear, and startle.
(3)

Using ITQ, found less stability of temperamental dimensions (except for rhythmicity and mood), which suggested a heterogony in the developmental profiles of Down's Syndrome profiles.
Also, these infants tended to move from difficult to easy classification (which might reflect a decrease in maternal anxiety).
(4)

Using ITQ, found at 6 months, only slight insignificant differences from normal temperamental profiles; slightly less persistent and approaching, and lower threshold for stimulation.
Also, less stability of temperamental dimensions, tendency to move from difficult to easy classification.
(5)

Using ITQ, found greater measures for distractibility and less persistence.
(6)

1. Greenberg & Field (1982)	4. Gunn, Berry, & Andrews (1983)
2. Van Tassell (1984)	5. Bridges & Cicchetti (1982)
3. Rothbart & Hanson (1983)	6. Greenberg & Field (1982)

Table 19. Temperamental Studies of Handicapped Risk Population (Continued)

Attachment Studies of Handicapped Risk Population

Confirmed the usefulness and acuity of the Strange Situation paradigm for use with even severely handicapped children.
(7)

Study of attachment in 50 severely handicapped children (3 to 8 years) showed attachment bond always present although more muted and less complex, provocative, and differentiated than in normals.
(8)

Deaf

Attachment study with deaf clearly showed attachment behaviors at 24 months.
(9)

Social responsiveness and communication competence determined level of attachment in deaf.
(10)

Down's Syndrome

More attachment studies of Down's Syndrome (DS).
Review suggests that Down's Syndrome children experience the same stages of attachment but at delayed sequence and often diminished intensity, for example, less separation anxiety.
(11)

In DS infants found a lag in attachment behaviors with delays in affective and cognitive growth, but normal sequence, and quantitative differences only in response to strangers and novel stimulation.
(12), (13)

In DS infants found diminished eye contact, smiling, and overall social responsiveness.
(14)

7. Stahlecker & Cohen (1985); Blacher & Meyers (1983)
8. Blacher (1984a); Stone & Chesney (1978)
9. Meadow et al. (1983)
10. Stahlecker & Cohen (1985); Greenberg & Marvin (1979)
11. Blacher & Meyers (1983)
12. Berry, Gunn, & Andrews (1980); Cicchetti & Serifica (1981); Thompson et al. (1985)
13. Serafica & Cicchetti (1976); Cicchetti & Sroufe (1976, 1978); Emde, Katz, & Thorpe (1978)
14. Emde & Brown (1978)

3 years old agreed to a brief separation for which the mother had prepared the child, and half of the children under 3 experienced distress upon separation. The majority were sociable upon reunion, with only 20 percent exhibiting resistant/avoidant behaviors. These behaviors are remarkably similar to those found in nonhandicapped children.

Emde and Brown (1978) found similar results in the attachment behavior of families with Down's syndrome infants. In the cases they studied, for example, they found that certain characteristics of the parents' adaptation to the birth of a handicapped child differentiated among the attachment behaviors of the infants studied. A young blind infant observed through the first 1.25 years by Als, Tronick, and Brazelton (1980) further testifies to the competence of infants in developing the behaviors which, despite the limitations of their handicap, bind them in mutually gratifying, reciprocal relationships with their parents. By 3.5 months of age, the infant they studied could control her level of arousal and was demonstrably available for interaction. Severely handicapped children studied by Blacher (1984a) demonstrated a progressive decline in neutral responses during successive episodes of the Ainsworth and Wittig (1969) paradigm administered in their homes. Children in this study were severely to profoundly retarded and the majority had additional handicaps such as cerebral palsy, seizure disorders, visual impairments, and neurological impairments. This study suggests that varying stimuli can elicit differentiated responses from even the most severely handicapped and that neutral affect may be a selectively employed response to emotional confusion or dysregulation.

Multidimensional scaling used by Emde et al. (1978) in one of the earliest attempts to compare the emotional expressions of Down's syndrome infants to normal infants revealed a variety of individual differences in the interactional styles of the infants. Sorce and Emde's (1982) studies on expressiveness among Down's syndrome infants demonstrate a range of readily discernable expressions at the disposal of the infant.

Within this variety of attachment behavior, however, there is still a frequently noted quality of affect reminiscent of depressive-like response in handicapped infants and children. Emde et al. (1978) observed the lack of sparkle, lack of eye contact, general lack of facial participation in smiles, and an overall dampening of affect in Dawn, the young Down's syndrome infant they studied. They described a feeling of disappointment at not experiencing what they hoped (and expected most parents would hope) would be a "sun-filled" social encounter with the infant. Muted early crying and less intense and engaging social smiles than might be expected were also noted. While the researchers accept these phenomenon as intrinsic to the development of the Down's syndrome infant, the evidence presented on the heterogeneity of affective expressions even within a Down's syndrome population casts doubt on whether these behaviors can be accepted as developmentally expected. (See Table 20.)

Table 20. Behavioral Profile of Handicapped

Phys. Handicapped	Developmental delays in language, social skills, and affective regulation at 24 months (1)
	Developmental delays in language, hyperkinesis, and conduct disorders (2)
	Delay in separation-individuation (3)
	Psychopathology, especially with brain-involved lesions (4)
	In girls, increased levels of guilt and anxiety (5)
	Depression, withdrawal, and lower self-image (6)
	Nonorganic feeding problems from birth (7)
	Abuse/neglect (8)
Blind	Hostility, passive aggression, compulsive solitary play (9)
Deaf	Impaired communication competence (10)
Mentally Retarded	Blunted/atypical positive affective responses (11)
	Avoidance, withdrawal, more crying (12)
	More disturbing cry (13)
	Psychopathology (14)

1. Wasserman, Allen, & Solomon (1985)
2. Reid (1980)
3. Mordock (1979)
4. Rutter (1970a,b); Seidel et al. (1975); Breslau (1985)
5. Shindi (1983)
6. Glaser et al. (1964)[a]; Lawler, Nakielny, & Wright (1966)[b]; Schecter (1961)[c]
7. Weir (1979)
8. Friedrich & Boriskin (1976); Frodi (1981)
9. McGuire & Meyers (1971)
10. Wedell-Monnig & Lumley (1980); Greenberg (1980)
11. Emde & Brown (1978)
12. Greenberg (1970)
13. Otswald & Peltzman (1974)
14. Reid (1980)

[a] congenital cardiac defects
[b] cystic fibrosis
[c] physically handicapped

Self-Concept

The literature on self-concept presents an equally varied, but nonetheless distressing picture of the handicapped child. Negative self-concept need not always accompany a handicapping condition, as the research of Molla (1981) has shown. In a comparison of self-concepts among physically handicapped and nonhandicapped latency-age children, Molla found no significant differences in their self-concepts. Whether this is attributable to a small sample size, or to distortions arising from the self-report instrument used (the Piers–Harris Self-Concept Scale, 1969) or from the children's denial, is unclear. Nevertheless, the absence of a negative self-concept when it might intuitively be expected should alert investigators to its potential significance if such negativity subsequently surfaces. When considered along with other symptoms, such as the dampened affect frequently noted among the handicapped, a negative self-concept may signal depression.

It has been suggested that among certain populations, such as the mentally handicapped, self-esteem deficits may not be developmentally possible. Dosen (1984), whose description of depression among a mentally handicapped population resembles the "masked depression" thesis of Cytryn and McKnew (1974), questions whether this population has a sufficiently defined identity for self-esteem deficits accompanying depression to be a meaningful concept.

That self-concept is a meaningful concept to discuss even among the cognitively impaired has been demonstrated by Mans et al. (1978) in a study of Down's syndrome infants and children. These researchers selected 55 Down's syndrome infants and children between the ages of 15 and 48 months to determine what impact their cognitive deficit might have on abilities to demonstrate self-recognition in the standard mirror and rouge paradigm. Their results indicate that although comparable numbers of handicapped and nonhandicapped children could demonstrate such recognition by the end of the second year, self-recognition among most Down's syndrome infants lagged behind nonhandicapped populations by 6 months to a year. Nevertheless, the Down's syndrome children all recognized themselves during the third year, and thus must be considered as capable of possessing an integrated self-concept and hence susceptible to self-esteem deficits.

Many studies have demonstrated differences in self-esteem between normal and handicapped populations and among different subgroups of the handicapped. Harvey and Greenway (1984) observed that latency-age children with congenital physical handicaps had lower self-esteem than nonhandicapped controls. Those in special schools fared somewhat more favorably than those who attended normal schools and encountered constant comparisons with nonhandicapped children. This observation was made several years earlier by Van Putte (1979). Low self-esteem may figure prominently in some of the social passivity described earlier (Wasserman & Allen, 1985). The vulnerability of self-esteem to social pressures again attests to the malleability of handicapped children's affective states and the need to probe behind seemingly predetermined expressions.

Important differences also exist in the self-concepts of children with different handicapping conditions. Visibility of the handicap to others is particularly important. When Steinhausen (1981) compared self-esteem among groups of physically handicapped, chronically ill but not visibly handicapped, and nonhandicapped teenagers, he found the most significant differences between the physically handicapped and other groups. The physically handicapped had less ego strength than the other groups, as measured on a modified version of the Junior Eysenck Personality Inventory (Eysenck & Eysenck, 1969). Handicapped teenagers studied by Shindi (1983) showed differences in self-esteem that appeared related to the age of onset of the handicap. Those with acquired handicaps measured higher on self-esteem than those with congenital conditions. Such findings may appear counter-intuitive given that those with acquired handicaps are forced to confront emotions such as shame and loss, which may result from an alteration in self-concept. However, Shindi suggests with some plausibility that those with acquired handicaps can view themselves as victims of cirmcumstances, such as a car accident, whereas those with congenital conditions often inherit their parents' guilt and self-blame. This hypothesis may represent another way of saying that those with congenital handicaps can find external attributions for their condition whereas those with acquired handicaps ascribe them to internal causes. Such an explanatory style is consistent with certain dimensions of the learned helpless attributional style, which results in feelings of impotence in the face of uncontrollable forces. (See Table 21.)

RISK FACTORS FOR DEPRESSION AMONG THE HANDICAPPED

Research that accepts the theory that certain characteristics of handicapped populations are relatively "fixed" has tended to treat the child as a constant variable and to view the family environment as a function of the child. But when the child is viewed in a more fully interactional framework, it becomes clear that risk factors for depression inhere both in the child—his or her neuroendocrine, cognitive, and affective make-up—and in the family setting. Clearly, there is a dynamic interaction between the two types of factors, but for simplicity, this section will devise an arbitrary division between risk factors inherent in the child and those that are part of the environment. The caveat remains, however, that no single source of risk can be considered in isolation from the others.

Table 21. Developmental Trends in Handicapped Children Compared to Normal Children

Object Permanence	Normally person permanence develops at 12 months; and object permanence at 24 months; determining later cognitive gains and capacities for representation. (1)	Sensorimotor handicapped children were NOT delayed in object permanence as measured by VISUAL (non-traditional) means. (2)
Self-Recognition	Normally self-recognition is achieved at 15-22 months and is critical to: fixed categories of self-representation (e.g. gender); empathy & the emergence of complex emotional expression, language, complex means-ends, symbolic representation. (3)	In handicapped DS children pattern of self-recognition was normal but delayed: 23-24 months. (4)
Self-Concept	Normally self-concept is generally established by about 24 months, and is critical to subsequent development. (5)	Both physically handicapped and premature infants tend to be delayed in self-concept after 24 months. At 24 months they tend to show more distractibility, social passivity, depression, and less positive affect. (6)
Object Constancy	Normally the stages of Object Constancy and separation-individuation are variable but generally occur between 5-36 months and reveal appropriate levels of separation anxiety and self-image. (7)	Suggested that handicapped children are delayed in their separation-individuation process due to psychomotor and sensory impairments. (8)

1. Bell (1970); Simoneau & Decarie (1979)
2. Fetters (1981)
3. Lewis & Brooks-Gunn (1979)
4. Mans, Cicchetti, & Sroufe (1978)
5. Kagan (1981); Piaget & Inhelder (1969)
6. Wasserman, Allen, & Solomon (1985)
7. Mahler (1958); Mahler et al. (1975)
8. Mordock (1979)

Characteristics of the Handicap

We have argued that a handicap is not deterministic, but it need not follow that a handicap is insignificant. Many characteristics of a child's handicap will, indeed, influence whether or not a depressive outcome will ensue and how that outcome will be expressed. Perhaps one of the most significant factors to be considered is the developmental period of the child when the handicap is diagnosed. Receiving a diagnosis of impairment may set in motion a chain of reactions which will almost inevitably expose a child to the depressive symptomatology experienced by his or her parents. Handicaps, such as Down's syndrome, which are generally diagnosed immediately, would thus present the greatest risk to the child since the parental reaction would coincide with a critical bonding process thought by some investigators (Klaus & Kennel, 1976) to occur in the period immediately following birth.

According to this theory, infants with acquired handicaps and handicaps such as developmental delays that are not typically detected until later in the first year may face reduced risk, since they can benefit from early attachment behaviors. Even those who do not concur with Klaus and Kennel (1976) as to the importance of postnatal bonding, accept the idea that the child's first attachment is formed during the first year of life. Thus, the quality of attachment may be affected by any change in parental attitudes during that time. There have been no empirical studies as yet investigating how the timing of diagnosis affects early attachment.

The timing of the handicap, whether at birth or later, may also affect the child's ultimate sense of self-esteem. There is still dispute about whether one type of handicap, either congenital or acquired, can be more damaging to self-esteem than another, and therefore presents greater risk for depression. While the sense of loss associated with the alteration in bodily image occurring with an acquired handicap may produce a depressive reaction, Shindi (1983) contends that the fortuitous events that often cause such handicaps actually may help children to accept such impairments. According to Shindi, preadolescents and adolescents can view themselves as victims of circumstances, whereas those with congenital handicaps have no acceptable causal explanation for their condition.

The degree of impairment, in addition to the timing, will clearly affect the infant or child's development in many respects. At the most basic level, the handicap will influence the decision about how best to care for the infant—at home or in an institution. Even if a handicapped child is not institutionalized, he or she may face recurrent hospitalization. The need for hospitalization may disrupt attachment formation if it occurs early in a child's life. Many of the more common diagnoses of congenital handicaps are made only after repeated evaluative hospitalizations during the first year of life, which is a critical period for attachment formation.

Even acquired handicaps, such as those that result from accidents, often necessitate long periods of acute care followed by prolonged rehabilitation. Hospitalization experiences can rapidly obliterate progress in many facets of development—physical, emotional, and intellectual—and can potentially damage self-esteem (Trout, 1983).

Since the majority of handicapped children will be cared for in the home, it is imperative to examine how specific characteristics of the child's handicap may interfere with certain routine activities and possibly contribute to depression in the child. Severity of a handicap, in particular, may have a significant impact on the development and evolution of attachment relationships, which provide infants with their first opportunity to experience a sense of competence, the lack of which may underlie depression. The degree of handicap may, to some extent, limit a child's ability to communicate his or her needs to a caregiver, or to interpret the caregiver's responses. Impairments in an infant's ability to read a parent's facial expressions may deprive the infant of valuable confirmation of the effectiveness of interaction (Trad, 1986).

Severe handicaps may also interfere with attachment by creating a more difficult temperament (Bridges & Cicchetti, 1982) that may thwart caregiver initiatives. Handicaps may intensify an infant's or child's frustration to limitations and make it difficult to adapt to changes in the environment. Chess and Fernandez (1980), for example, have observed that although children whose sole handicap was deafness did not fit the classic portrait of a deaf child—rigid, impulsive, hyperactive, and suspicious—the large majority of those with multiple handicaps did display those characteristics. Of the five groups of infants studied by Greenberg and Field (1982)—developmentally delayed, Down's syndrome, cerebral palsied, audiovisually impaired, and normal—those with the least severe handicaps received the least difficult temperament ratings by teachers. Even among the mildly handicapped, significant differences from nonhandicapped infants may occur in the dimension of approach, a temperament trait reflecting response to new people and new objects (Van Tassel, 1984). Although Rothbart and Hanson (1983) did not detect differences between Down's syndrome and normal infants in their distress to limits, it is possible that infants who repeatedly experience frustration adopt a resigned, helpless style that the investigators interpreted as lack of frustration. Despite the evidence of the relationship between severity of a handicap and difficult temperament, no studies have taken this finding a step further to determine how severity affects attachment. Most studies, unfortunately, either focus on infants or children with a single type of handicap, or their samples are too heterogenous to measure the impact of severity on parent–child interaction in a controlled way.

Research on the impact of handicapping conditions has focused largely on limitations in attachment formation. Mordock (1979) turned his attention to the impact of the handicap on the separation/individuation process, during which a young child's early self-concept is formed. He hypothesized that limits in ambulation and vision may interfere with early exploration, as the child may not feel secure in his or her ability to venture far from a caregiver while still retaining supportive contact. Failure to attain this developmental hallmark may not only damage a young child's self-esteem, but may also create continued demands of parents expecting greater independence of their child, amplifying their disappointment in their child's failure to meet their expectations, and possibly communicating this sense of inadequacy to their child.

Finally, the extent of a child's handicap may also dictate certain practical decisions, such as educational choices, that may have profound consequences for the child's self-concept. Paradoxically, with respect to educational setting, those with more severe handicaps may be somewhat more protected against challenges to their self-esteem. Since these children are generally segregated into special classes, they do not face constant comparisons with nonhandicapped children. Mainstreamed latency-age children have, with some consistency, shown lower self-concepts than children segregated in special educational settings (Harvey & Greenway, 1984; Van Putte, 1979). (See Table 22.)

Parents' Reactions to Handicapped Children

The adjustment of parents to a child's handicap has been described repeatedly in the literature (Blacher, 1984b; Emde & Brown, 1978; Murphy, 1982; Trout, 1983). Because, as we have seen, certain aspects of the child's emotional development are often treated as invariant, the literature has dwelled on the impact of the child on the family, and has often stopped short of examining the impact of parental adjustment on the child's affective development. As noted in the chapter on the impact of parental depression, infants and children readily perceive and even absorb their parents' affective states. Thus, the ability of parents to adjust to the birth of a handicapped child or to accept an acquired handicap may represent a critical source of risk for a depressive outcome in the child.

Investigations on how infants' and children's affects may reflect an internalization of their parents' reactions to their handicaps are extremely limited and impressionistic. These studies tend to focus on the impact of the parent on the child's self-esteem rather than on attachment or temperament. Parents' low expectations of their handicapped infants' performance, and their awareness of their child's failure to attain normal developmental hallmarks (Smith et al., 1985), may translate into low expectations and a sense of inefficacy in the infant.

Parental shame may compromise an older child's self-image. Lussier (1980) described the case of a 12-year-old boy, Peter, who had a severe congenital defect. Lussier concluded that the child's emotional insecurity

Table 22. *Handicapped Population Compared with Three Risk Populations*

Abuse/Neglect	Maternal Depression	Hospitalization
Handicapped children are more likely to be maltreated. (1)	Hospitalized child is at greater risk with an emotionally disturbed parent. (2)	Handicapped child tends to be more chronically hospitalized. (3)
Birth complications are associated with increased risk for maltreatment. (4)	Parents of handicapped children are more likely to be depressed. (5)	
Parents of handicapped children experience heightened stress. (6)	Parents of handicapped children experience heightened stress. (7)	
Handicapped child is more likely to be "difficult," which may lead to maltreatment. (8)	Parents of handicapped children show more depressive symptoms, but not more MDD. (9)	
Handicapped child is more likely to have a more disturbing cry. (10)	Depressed, hospitalized children had high incidence of loss and parental depression. (11)	
Handicapped child is more likely to suffer from poor dyadic relationship and experience less positive attachment behaviors. (12)		

1. Blacher & Meyers (1983); Freidrich & Boriskin (1976); Jaudes & Diamond (1985); Lynch & Roberts (1977); Meyers, Zetlin, & Blacher-Dixon (1981)
2. Mason (1965)
3. Barbero (1984)
4. Elmer & Gregg (1967); Hunter et al. (1978); Klein & Stern (1971)
5. Burden (1980); Cummings (1976); Cummings, Bayley, & Rie (1966)
6. Bernheimer, Young, & Winton (1983)
7. Bernheimer, Young, & Winton (1983)
8. Frodi (1981); Steinhausen (1981); Shindi (1983)
9. Breslau & Davis (1986)
10. Otswald & Peltzman (1974)
11. Kashani, Barbero, & Bolanger (1981)
12. Blacher (1984); Emde & Brown (1978); Helfer (1975); Stone & Chesney (1978)

334

stemmed not from a sense of his own limits but from the shame and discouragement of his mother. As Lussier noted, Peter related to his body in the same way that his mother did. Although an infant would be unable to experience parental shame, he or she might experience a parent's ambivalence. The parent-child interaction thus fails to help the infant learn to represent itself in an unambiguous way.

A more systematic demonstration of the relationship between parents' affective states and their handicapped child's self-concept is provided in a study by Harvey and Greenway (1982). When they measured parents of latency-age handicapped children on six Primary Mood Factors (on edge-uneasy-tense; discouraged-guilty-unhappy; angry-annoyed-furious; lively-energetic-cheerful; worn out-fatigued-weary; and confused-bewildered-uncertain), they found that ambivalence in the parents correlated with a lowered self-concept in the child.

While the limited literature relating parental adjustment to depressive symptomatology in handicapped children focuses on the child's self-concept, parents' reactions may create risk for depression in a handicapped child long before a sense of self has emerged. This is particularly true of parental responses to the birth of a child with a handicap. As noted previously, establishment of mutually adaptive, synchronous interactions between the parent and infant gives the young infant his or her first opportunity to control the environment and those in it. How, exactly, the conditions for synchrony are established are not yet known (Izard & Buechler, 1982). When synchrony fails, however, the infant can experience a state of noncontingency, which can degenerate into a form of learned helplessness, manifestation of which is evident in the emotionally dysregulated behaviors and affects seen in attachment studies reviewed in the early part of this chapter. Throughout other clinical chapters of this book, numerous instances of interference with this delicate system have been described.

From the parent's perspective, a child's handicap may introduce unique obstacles to the development of synchronous interactions. A child's physical or mental handicap can reduce the repertoire of behaviors at his or her disposal for communicating internal states to the caregiver, augmenting the stress of what is already a challenge for the parent—understanding the internal states of an infant unable to communicate verbally. The inability of a child, because of physical limitations, to produce an expected response to a parent's caregiving initiative can cause parental confusion and frustration which may, in turn, breed a sense of ineffectiveness and futility. Indeed, a number of researchers have confirmed the sensitivity of maternal responsivity to both a child's level of functioning and his or her responsivity. Brooks-Gunn and Lewis (1984), for example, found that maternal responsivity varied with the child's handicapping condition and mental age. They compared the responsivity of mothers of infants (3 to 36 months) in three groups: Down's syndrome, cerebral palsy, and developmental delays. Mothers of infants with developmental delays were found to be the most responsive, presumably because their children had the highest mental age and the largest behavioral repertoire. On the other hand, in Wasserman and Allen's (1985) longitudinal study of maternal withdrawal from handicapped toddlers, they attributed the mothers' reactions neither to low mental age nor to a decline in mental age, but rather, to the cosmetic nature of the handicap. They studied mother-child interactions in three groups of toddlers, one group with facial or orthopedic deformaties, one group of premature toddlers, and a group of controls. At 24 months, significantly more of the mothers of handicapped children showed signs of ignoring their children in a free-play observation. Moreover, all of the ignored children had facial deformities and over half of those with facial deformities were ignored.

The results of Sorce and Emde's (1982) research, however, are more consistent with those of Brooks-Gunn and Lewis (1984) in assigning a more prominent role to unimpaired perceptual capacities. Their study of emotional expressiveness and its consequences for caregiving also indicated that mothers would stimulate their infants more in response to higher-intensity signals. A lower sense of parental efficacy, combined with lower expectations of the child, may create a self-fulfilling prophecy by which the infants and children perform below their ability (Smith et al., 1985). Infants may experience this cycle of expectations as noncontingency in a parent-child interaction. Later in childhood, it may be reflected in the child's damaged self-esteem (Trad, 1986).

Parents' perceptions of certain aspects of a child's temperament may further diminish their sense that caregiving efforts have been effective. For example, Van Tassel's (1984) depiction of developmentally delayed infants may stress the parent-infant interaction. The irritability and fussiness these children can display, combined with their long latency of response to soothing, may increase an infant's dependence on a caregiver without necessarily satisfying the needs of the caregiver. Withdrawal from arousing stimuli, a characteristic that is captured in the temperamental measurement of approach, may limit the types of interactions a caregiver can have with such an infant. The seemingly strained interactions often observed may reflect the parent's perception of the overall ease or difficulty of his or her infant's temperament.

While the notion of certain handicapped children as temperamentally easy has been advanced frequently in the literature (Greenberg & Field, 1982; Gunn et al., 1983), there is also some evidence that handicapped infants and children may have more difficult temperaments than popularly believed (Beckman, 1983; Bridges & Cicchetti, 1982). Even Greenberg and Field's (1982) study, which found that mothers of various groups of handicapped infants rated them as less difficult than did teachers or observers, noted that certain severely handicapped infants were extremely difficult as measured by their scores on the ITQ. (A score summarizing nine dimensions of temperament—activity, rhythmicity, adaptability, approach, threshold of response, intensity, mood, distractibility, and persistence—was used to determine temperamental difficultness. Ratings ranged from 1, which signified an easy temperament, to 4, which signified a difficult temperament.)

These frustrations may limit the gratification a parent derives from interactions with his or her handicapped infant, and in combination with other factors, produce depression or depressive symptomatology in the parent. Such reactions are well documented—more by clinical observation than empirical study (Blacher, 1984b)—and should be seen as presenting a significant risk for depression or depressive-like phenomena in the child. For example, nearly half of the mothers of severely handicapped children between the ages of 1.5 and 3 years were considered depressed in a study done by Burden (1980). It is not yet clear exactly how this parental depression is communicated to the handicapped child, except when it is accompanied by behaviors such as abuse and neglect. However, as noted in Chapter Six on the offspring of depressed parents, the capacity for empathy may serve as a conduit through which infants and children come to share the distress of their depressed parent(s).

Theories of empathic development have not been tested with handicapped populations to determine whether the sequence and chronology of growth is similar to that of nonhandicapped populations. It seems more probable that empathy plays a role in the early stages of development, when the handicapped infant has yet to differentiate physically and psychologically from his or her mother and might, according to Hoffman's (1977) model of empathic development, experience the depression of others as if it were his or her own. Since certain types of handicapped infants (e.g., those with Down's syndrome) may take longer than nonhandicapped infants to achieve self-recognition (Mans et al., 1978) and to differentiate themselves from their mothers, the developmental period during which they are at risk for experiencing undifferentiated, empathic distress may be extended in relation to nonhandicapped children. On the other hand, handicapped children with severe cognitive deficits may never attain the highest levels of empathic development, which ordinarily make a child vulnerable to a multiplicity of new and more subtle distress cues (Hoffman, 1977, 1982b). When, for example, a normal child reaches the final stage of empathic development described by Hoffman (1977, 1982b), his or her capacity for empathic distress can reach beyond the immediate situation and can be triggered by an ability to understand the complexities of another's general life situation. Handicaps that compromise a child's ability to fathom another's mental state may thus provide some insulation from the variety of additional distress cues to which he or she may be subject.

Despite what might be conceived as a possible arrest in empathic development, such children still remain capable of empathic distress, albeit in a more limited and undifferentiated way. These children may still experience their parents' distress, but they may lack the usual outlet, prosocial behavior, for such distress. The expression of their depression may thus assume an atypical character more akin to conduct disorders than to depression. Indeed, the emotional lability of the handicapped children studied by Greenberg and Field (1982) is reminiscent of the dysregulated emotions and behavior of the children of bipolar parents studied by Zahn-Waxler et al. (1984a). The latter, at risk for depression, showed the combination of a high level of empathic distress and antisocial rather than prosocial behavior.

The way that a parent's depression evolves—in conjunction with how a child's own development enables the child to experience his or her parent's psychological states—will clearly influence how the child experiences the depression. Debate continues about how parental depression unfolds in response to the birth of a handicapped child—whether parents proceed through sequential stages culminating in acceptance, or whether they experience chronic sorrow. Many descriptions, however, emphasize depression at the outset. Although the depression may not reach the syndrome level, parents of handicapped children may experience significantly more depressive symptoms than parents of nonhandicapped children, according to Breslau and Davis (1986), whose study measured major depression by administering the Diagnostic Interview Schedule to parents in their homes. Their investigation tapped the level of depressive symptomatology through a depressive symptom scale, developed by the Center for Epidemiological Studies, that incorporates 20 questions selected from the most widely used depression scales including the Beck Depression Inventory (Beck & Beck, 1972), the Minnesota Multiphasic Personality Inventory, and the Zung Depression Scale (Zung, 1965). Nearly one third of the parents of handicapped children reported depressive symptoms, a level twice as high as that reported by the parents of nonhandicapped children.

Stage models, which have gained a broad—although not necessarily empirically demonstrated—base of support, suggest that parents' reactions may unfold over time. A parent's initial response to his or her child's diagnosis may include a range of emotions such as grief, detachment, and bereavement (Blacher, 1984b). Blacher's review of the literature on parental adjustment rarely detected a positive parental reaction on learning of a child's handicap. Grieving for the lost "ideal" child narcissistically invested during pregnancy may make overwhelming adaptive demands of the parents and deprive them of energy for attachment (Emde & Brown, 1978). Since many types of handicaps are not likely to be diagnosed until well into the first year, the first stages of grieving may not interfere with initial bonding and subsequent attachment formation. However, some of the more frequently occurring handicaps, such as Down's syndrome, are generally diagnosed within several days of birth, and for such infants, parental grieving is likely to hamper early attachment. Emde and Brown (1978) have underscored the importance of completing the grieving process before parents can free their energy for attachment. Although parents may ultimately succeed in completing the grieving process, the time required may account for some of the delays observed in measuring attachment behaviors in infants such as those with Down's syndrome.

Parental reactions even after the initial crisis has passed may continue to expose children directly to depression associated feelings such as guilt, disappointment, and anger (Blacher, 1984b). Other commonly expressed parental reactions, such as feelings of defectiveness, may undermine parental self-esteem, diminish their pride as caretakers (Blacher, 1984b; Trout, 1983), and ultimately detract from their parenting. When these affects prevent parents from responding consistently and predictably to their infant's needs, the infant may, in turn, develop a sense of futility and helplessness that renders him or her vulnerable to depression. In extreme cases, a parent's sense of futility in caring for a handicapped child may find an outlet in abuse and neglect. Murphy's (1982) review of the literature notes that child malteatment is more common among premature and sick children—many of whom are likely to be handicapped.

The degree to which many of these parental reactions abate and parents ultimately accept their child's handicap will clearly affect the depressive risk to the child. Blacher (1984b) writes of a period of reorientation and reconstruction in which parents adjust to their handicapped child. The timing of this acceptance is obviously critical, especially to self-esteem, since children appear to experience an age-related response to disability. Ryan (1981) has observed that children are particularly rejecting of disability during the periods of early childhood. Physical attractiveness forms a major part of a child's perception of other people at this developmental stage, and children during this period may construe negative traits as indicative of a bad person. Because young children cannot understand the subjective perspective of others, they may confuse their own reactions to others with others' reactions to them—thereby developing an aversive reaction to themselves.

Increasingly, investigators have commented that some parents may never reach a stage of acceptance. Rather than experiencing time-bound grief, they may feel chronic sorrow as they are continually reminded of the differences between their expectations of their child and the reality they confront (Blacher, 1984b; Murphy, 1982). (See Table 23.)

In one of the first studies to use direct observation in order to subject the underlying hypotheses of stage models to empirical proof, Wasserman and Allen (1985) have shown that interactions between mothers and their handicapped children grow progressively worse, not better, over time.

Table 23.   Handicapped and Risk for Depression

Developmental delays in language, social skills, and affective regulation at 24 months.
(1)
Depression, withdrawal, and lower self-image
(2)
Hostility, passive aggression, compulsive solitary play
(3)
Blunted/atypical positive affective responses
(4)
Avoidance, withdrawal, more crying
(5)
More disturbing cry
(6)

1. Wasserman, Allen, & Solomon (1985b)[a]
2. Glaser et al. (1964)[b]; Kolin et al. (1971)[c]; Lawler et al. (1966)[d]; Schecter (1961)[e]
3. McGuire & Meyers (1971)[f]
4. Emde & Brown (1978)[g]
5. Greenberg (1971)[g]
6. Ostwald & Peltzman (1974)[g]

[a] physically handicapped
[b] congenital cardiac defects
[c] spina bifida
[d] cystic fibrosis
[e] physically handicapped
[f] blind
[g] mentally retarded

Rather than adapt to the birth of a handicapped children, many mothers may "burn out" with the continuing stress of caring for such a child. When the interactive behavior of mothers of handicapped toddlers (24-months old) was compared at four different times (9, 12, 18, and 24 months) to that of mothers of premature and control children, Wasserman and Allen found that although maternal ignoring was rare before 18 months, by 2 years of age, the mothers of handicapped children ignored their children significantly more than did the other mothers.

Wikler et al. (1981) have proposed that there are 10 critical periods in the life of a handicapped child that may reevoke feelings of grief and disappointment. Several of the periods are associated with general developmental hallmarks such as walking, talking, starting school, advent of puberty, and reaching the age of 21. Others relate to experiences confronted by families with handicapped children—the initial diagnosis of a handicap, comparisons to siblings of the same mental age, discussions of the child's placement, periods of behavioral disturbances, and discussions of care and guardianship. Bernheimer et al. (1983) outline similar episodes.

The potential for chronic parental depression, arising from the attempt to cope with important decisions in their handicapped child's life and the emotions that such decisions evoke, may continually jeopardize children's ability to engage parents in reciprocal interactions and use those interactions to form a positive representation of themselves. Since mental representations of the self in relation to others are functions of the earliest patterns of interaction (Main et al., 1985), through which a child forms a model constructed from a history of the parent's responses to its actions, parental depression—by attenuating responsiveness—must be regarded as a major risk factor for depression among handicapped children whose parents are depressed.

Surmounting some of the obstacles to communication with a handicapped child may prove difficult for many parents, and asynchrony may be the inevitable result. But special intervention can help circumvent the limitations posed by the child's handicap, forestall parental depression and perhaps reduce depressive risk to the child. Burden (1980), who sought to determine whether the birth of a handicapped child would lead ineluctably to parental depression, found that regular, weekly home visits to the mothers of severely handicapped infants reduced maternal depression by nearly two thirds. In contrast, depression among mothers who received no home visitation declined by only one third during the course of the study.

Child-directed interventions have also yielded promising results. Als et al. (1980) achieved success helping the parents of a young blind infant provide their baby with special tactile and auditory stimulation that promoted healthy and satisfying interaction. The comparatively greater success with which deaf parents, as opposed to hearing parents, interact with their deaf children also highlights the importance of competence in communication in general rather than in any specific form of communication (Chess, 1978; Chess & Fernandez, 1980; Meadow et al., 1983).

CONCLUSION

This chapter has explored the premise that handicapping conditions in infancy and childhood serve as a risk factor enhancing susceptiblity to depression and depressive-like phenomena. As the statistics revealed, handicapping conditions—running the gamut from visual impairment to mental retardation to orthopedic infirmities—are widespread among the childhood population. These conditions often interact synergistically with such developmental hallmarks as temperament, attachment, and self-concept, placing the child at a heightened risk for depression. Overall, the two most pertinent factors to consider when dealing with this population are the characteristics of the handicap and parental response to the infant's or child's disabling condition. Careful analysis of these variables, along with parental education, can avert or ameliorate instances of noncontingency experienced by the handicapped child, thus bolstering his or her defenses against the onset of depression. In short, the handicapped infant and child needs more than ordinary attention to prevent his or her handicap from becoming a factor contributing to dysregulation and lack of synchrony with the environment.

CHAPTER 10

Therapeutic Approaches for Affective Disorder in Infants and Children

THE AIMS OF INTERVENTION

The therapist dealing with an infant-caregiver dyad strives to achieve an interaction personified by harmonious and synchronous exchange, from which the infant can eventually extrapolate skills of mastery and competence necessary for the formulation of high self-esteem. When the therapist is confronted with an older child whose behavioral manifestations already belie a damaged sense of self, efforts may be geared toward repairing the negative parent-child interaction, and toward instituting more optimal communication. Regardless of the specific treatment situation that the therapist encounters, however, he or she is cautioned against applying theoretical models too rigidly to practical application. Whatever the treatment model, the therapist must take into consideration the developmental level of the infant's or child's affective and cognitive abilities.

Minde and Minde (1981) comment that the overall goal of therapy remains the enhancement of the infant's or child's attachment relationship with the caregiver, coupled with the optimal development of object relationships. These researchers note that recent observational investigations of infants have dramatically increased understanding of the complex contribution the caregiver makes to the infant's development. Despite this new data, however, researchers have only begun to clarify the most efficacious strategies for communicating this information to parents.

In keeping with the dictates of a developmental perspective, the Group for the Advancement of Psychiatry (1982) has noted that since affective disorders occur in the context of specific phases of development, the therapist must be aware that such disorders may present differently in conjunction with different developmental phases. This awareness has implications for both diagnosis and treatment. Developmental variables include biological maturation, mental changes, and the ever-widening social sphere of the child. One of the therapist's initial tasks is to assess each of these variables in terms of the developmental status of the patient.

Developmental analysis has been stressed by numerous researchers as a key for evaluating any infant or child case. Glenn et al. (1978) have argued, for instance, that the child's development will inevitably affect his or her relationship with parents, and thus the familial interaction represents, in a sense, one artifact of the developmental process. Glenn (1978) has also observed that parents must be capable of tolerating a child's developmental advances if optimal results are to be achieved. Finally, Anthony and Benedek (1975) have noted that the clinical depression encountered in adolescents often tends to evolve from the developmental phases of childhood, rather than from adolescent experience itself—although the latter may well add inflections to the disturbance. Thus these researchers concur that in order to achieve optimal results from interventive strategies, patient evaluation must begin by comprehension and assessment of developmental status.

DEVELOPMENTAL APPROACH TO THERAPEUTIC INTERVENTION

Introduction

The developmental perspective, as observed in previous chapters, offers the therapist a highly flexible instrument for discerning abnormalities, deviations, and irregularities in infant and childhood maturation. Developmentalists advocate no single, uniform approach to the treatment of disorder or incipient disorder. Rather, developmental psychopathology strives to tailor a therapeutic program to each infant's or child's specific psychopathology, in the context of his or her overall phase of development.

Developmentalism works as a therapeutic approach in cases of overt psychopathology and incipient manifestations of disorder; additionally, recent efforts have been devoted toward guidance at a stage when bona fide aberrations have not yet surfaced. Thus, developmental psychopathology may be conceived of as a useful tool of interventive strategy designed for prevention of subseqent disorder. According to Bond (1982), preventive tactics are designed, first, to enhance the coping skills of both children and caregivers and, second, to alter or eliminate stressful environmental agents. Belsky (1985) has articulated these goals more specifically by noting that therapeutic strategies should activate parental awareness of newborn competencies. This heightened awareness, according to the researcher, will result in more sensitive caregiving with the fostering of concomitant positive affect toward the infant. In this manner, the quality and range of infant–caregiver interaction will be improved. This form of intervention provides caregivers with a new perspective or, as Belsky phrases it, with "windows" through which to view their infants' behavior, as well as with "handles" or specific phenomena to focus on during the interaction.

For Bond (1982), the value of these guides to infant behavior is that they give parents insight into the motivations inherent in their infants' adaptive interactions with the environment. Preventive strategies can also ward off feelings of interactional failure, which can contaminate behaviors between caregiver and infant by generalizing to infuse the entire relationship, as Donovan and Leavitt (1985) have emphasized. Preventive strategies, of course, do not imply abandonment of concern for infant and child populations who are at increased risk for psychopathology. Instead, as several researchers have argued, early intervention can benefit ostensibly normal infant–caregiver dyads as well as dyads known to be at high risk (Bond, 1982; Donovan & Leavitt, 1985).

Regulation is the ability to coordinate adaptive responses. The therapist should be alert to the infant's or child's capacity to regulate his or her affective responses, and the therapist must be aware of his or her own role in facilitating the patient's regulation. For instance, Glenn (1978) reports that very young children disclose their sense of physical sensation and bodily image to the therapist in a variety of ways, including through direct statements, play behavior, and drawings. By "listening" for these insights from the child, the therapist can help the child organize and exert more restraint over affective manifestations. In addition, the therapist can guide the child to an understanding of buried conflicts and can coach a mutual regulation of affect. Affect regulation must be achieved in the domain of the therapeutic session, but it is also essential that parents be alerted to instances of improper affect control in their children and be tutored in methods of ameliorating maladaptive response to the environment. Glenn, Sabot, and Bernstein (1978) note that the parent-child interaction is not simply one in which adults influence the child, provoking pathology. Nor, as Anna Freud (1971) has written, should the parents be considered "innocent" bystanders to the child's seemingly spontaneous psychopathology. Instead, the relationship between parents and child is one of mutuality, with both members of the dyad viewed as active forces in shaping the outcome of its fate—whether normal or pathological (Glenn, Sabot, & Bernstein, 1978).

To facilitate and reinforce the notion of an interactive dyadic relationship, Glenn et al. (1978) urge that caregiver and infant or child be observed together by the therapist. The ability of the mother to empathize with and understand the child will be enhanced when she sees him or her acting out conflicts and when the therapist's responses are observed as a paradigm of nurturing behavior. Bond (1982) is even more insistent on maternal presence and involvement during intervention, because she views the efficacy of the dyadic partnership as the chief goal of therapy. Bond suggests that caregivers must feel an ongoing responsibility for their infants and a sense of complete involvement in the nurturing process. Parents must come to view themselves as virtual "curriculum designers" (p. 29) for their infants, whose curriculum will be subject to constant revision as new skills are acquired. This view of the dyadic exchange, instituted during the first months of life, will foster the eventual development of the infant's "self" as a competent problem solver, geared toward mastery of the environment.

Discussion

As we are concerned here with using the developmental model for therapeutic purposes, it is appropriate to reiterate the ultimate goals that may be achieved through therapy. Within the context of the infant-caregiver system, the final goal remains the enhancement of feelings of efficacy. Such feelings both grow out of and foster adaptive behaviors in the infant-caregiver dyad. Thus the goal of therapy may also be described as the emergence of an effective dyad with capacities to adapt to the changes of development (Trad, 1986).

The model of intervention proposed here is, however, significantly different from other prescriptions for the infant's development in both subtle and complicated ways. Since the main goal of intervention is an effective dyad, the means to achieve this end will be through the establishment of a continual, mutual regulatory system within the dyad. Bond (1982) has observed that harmonious interaction of this type is possible only when both infant and caregiver simultaneously recognize each other's uniqueness. She has added that a dyad that is efficacious or "competent" is likely to sustain itself. Competence additionally includes the caregiver's comprehension that he or she exerts an overwhelming impact on the infant's development of self-concept and attitude toward the world.

Chess and Hassibi (1978) have emphasized that psychiatric intervention, through initial consultative and/or subsequent periodic therapy, is particularly well suited to examining any maladaptive patterns of behavior and to confronting, clarifying, interpreting, and deciphering such patterns. By suggesting alternative strategies of interaction, the child psychiatrist can ameliorate dysfunctional interpersonal exchange and provide more mutually fulfilling modes of interaction. Other researchers have also pinpointed the dyadic relationship and have suggested that by increasing caregiver awareness and attunement skills, infant development can be shaped and molded. Bond (1982) indicated that if the child psychiatrist hones parental skills, parents in turn will develop the confidence and skill necessary to become "curriculum designers" for their infants. Beyond observing the caregiver-infant interaction, the therapist can focus on the child's play activities to glean information about the quality of the infant and child's incipient sense of self. Klein (1932) was the first to argue that play activities, because they are free from the censorships of reality, may be valuable tools for the psychotherapist. The nurturance of a competent, directed caregiver helps the infant to evolve a sense of competence and mastery that will culminate in a positive self-image and high sense of self-esteem.

It should be noted that the developmental model permits intervention not only in cases of overt maladaptive dyadic exchange, but also in cases of "normal" or merely problematic interaction. Indeed, strategies may be suggested for almost any caregiver-infant pair to enhance what may be an adequate mode of communication and to elevate this relationship to its optimal level. Thus pediatricians, teachers, and others who deal with infant-caregiver dyads outside the context of overt psychopathology should be attuned to potential dysharmonious interactions and should be tutored in methods of effective intervention.

Preventive Intervention Strategies

In a study designed to assess the effects of early intervention in the dyadic relationship on subsequent development, Morris (1973) isolated a group of children from poor socioeconomic backgrounds. Since children from these backgrounds have been shown to display lags in development in the areas of reading and related cognitive skills, the researcher attempted to determine whether direct and early intervention within this group could result in averting such lags. The study focused on honing maternal interactive skills, particularly in the realms of language, perceptual development, and problem solving. The researcher found developmental improvement in cognitive abilities, as well as the related finding that once mothers witnessed improved performance in their children, a positive change in their attitude was detected.

Such studies affirm the contention that early intervention strategies can exert a marked impact on infant and child development, and may circumvent the process leading to subsequent behavioral disorders. Hourcade and Parette (1986) reported similar positive outcomes as a result of intervening in cases of developmentally disabled (handicapped) infants. The researchers found that intervention did in fact result in developmental gains in both mental and physical skills; significantly, interventions among the youngest children achieved the greatest gains on both the Bayley Mental Development Index and the Bayley Psychomotor Index, both of which measure a child's cognitive and psychomotor development.

Sander (1983), reporting on a 25-year longitudinal research project, noted that evaluation of data of such extensive duration has provided some clues to the types of intervention strategies that can be utilized by developmentalists. Sander found that significant variables have predictive value for individual behavior patterns. These variables include such factors as sources of ego strength within the family structure, family organization, and the particular characteristics of one or more parents or grandparents with respect to values or idealizing perspectives of culture and family tradition. Sander concludes that these variables that affect behavior contain both genetic and environmental factors, both of which the developmental framework must define and separate. Sander's review also suggests that early intervention strategies may eventually be devised, geared to norms articulated from developmental studies.

One recent study involving early intervention was conducted by David (1983). Drawing on an "at-risk" population of parents and infants who participated in a Day Home Care Unit, the researcher noted that parents involved in the study, the majority of whom were diagnosed as emotionally disturbed or psychotic, exposed their infants to three sorts of dangers. First, such parents could be fostering early pathology in their infants that might not manifest itself overtly until the infant had reached a more mature developmental stage. This pathology the researcher labeled as "silent pathology." Second, the prevalence of somatic illnesses during the first months of life in their infants led to repeated hospitalization, which in and of itself placed the infant at risk for experiencing disruptive discontinuity. Finally, marital difficulties among the parents placed these children at risk for abuse and neglect. These factors combined to create a portrait of potential early emotional deprivation that might coalesce in depression. Given the extreme risk of these infants, the researcher opted for systematized early intervention. The approach involved the entire family, but the therapeutic team focused energy on the infant. Interactions between infants and their families were observed and evaluated, and the infants were given a supportive emotional milieu in which they could establish meaningful contact with the therapists, while still maintaining continuity with parental figures. The problem behavior that the infant acted out within the context of the therapeutic relationship was viewed as part of transference phenomena. In addition, parents also received individual and group treatment. David reported that while continuation of treatment is difficult in this type of situation, it is nevertheless essential in order to sever the cycle of repetitious, compulsive disruption that the parents impose on these children. Current evaluation of the children in this study reveals that they remain in a vulnerable emotional state, but because of early intervention techniques they are functioning at the norm for their developmental age.

Fineman and Boris (1983) conducted a follow-up study of infants who had received early intervention techniques during infancy in order to assess the effectiveness of this sort of strategy. Two to three years after cessation of a relationship with the intervention therapist, the research team assessed the developmental level of this group of children. Ten out of eleven of the children assessed were not below their age-expectable level in the areas of development, object relationships, ego functioning, and instinctual expression of modification. This finding contrasts favorably with studies of at-risk children of insecure or anxious mothers who have not received intervention. Second, the researchers noted that the efficacy of infant intervention can be reliably measured by a relatively uncomplicated play assessment.

Ramey and Gowen (1984) conducted a longitudinal study involving a group of families whose infants were in a high-risk category (i.e., low socioeconomic status) for developing mild mental retardation. Isolating a group of children from low socioeconomic backgrounds, the researchers devised a series of intervention strategies that included attendance at a day-care program, improved pediatric care, and family social work services available on request. Throughout the study, a control group of children from similar, low socioeconomic backgrounds was compared with the experimental group. It was found that infants who did not participate in the intervention displayed normal intellectual functioning during the first year of life, as measured by the Mental Development Index (MDI) Bayley Scales of Infant Development (Bayley, 1969). However, during the second year of life, the intellectual performance of these infants precipitously declined. Ramey and Gowen note that it is at this developmental threshold when symbolic function, language skills, and other complex cognitive capacities begin to emerge. In contrast to the control group, infants subjected to intervention strategies performed within the normal range on intelligence tests. These data suggest that the effect of early environmental deprivation, which either causes or exacerbates cognitive deficits, may not be revealed until a later phase of chronological development.

Belsky and Benn (1982) suggest that strategies of intervention can coincide with various "sensitive periods" in the life of the infant. These researchers note that certain life events, such as onset of parenthood itself or the child's entry into school, are examples of periods when the caregiver-infant dyad comes to the attention of external support professionals, such as pediatricians and teachers. These sensitive periods offer the occasion for evaluation and, if dysharmonious interaction is encountered in the dyad, possible intervention. Professionals should be alert to factors including impoverishment of stimulation, inability of the infant to sift out distinctive features from irrelevant stimulation, selective attention, and perceptual motivation skills of the infant (Gibson, 1969).

Broussard (1976) has given enhanced credibility to the notion that observation and analysis of early dyadic interaction—particularly early maternal initiating behavior—is vital for determining patterns of optimal development, as well as for predicting dyads that may be at risk for subsequent emergence of emotional disorders. Using the Neonatal Perception Inventories (NPI), which measure maternal perception of her neonate as contrasted with maternal perception of the average infant, Broussard longitudinally charted developmental progress in a group of children from infancy through 10 to 11 years of age. The NPI involved six behavioral items on which mothers were asked to comment with regard to their infants, as distinguished from average infants. These behaviors included crying, spitting, feeding, eliminating, sleeping, and predictability. Mothers were scored on both the first or second postpartum day and when their infants were 1 month of age. As a result of these scorings, two groups were identified. The high-risk group included mothers who did not perceive their infants as being better than average, while the low-risk group consisted of dyadic pairs in which mothers rated their infant as being higher than average.

Following long-term assessment of the groups after 10 and 11 years, it was found that the initial characterization of the dyad into either a high- or low-risk group had high predictive validity for determining subsequent emotional development. In fact, only 7.7 percent of infants who were perceived negatively by their mothers at 1 month of age were found to have no mental disorder at age 10 or 11. Thus, as Broussard stresses, a dyad that receives a high-risk classification on the NPI warrants "top priority" attention for early preventive intervention.

In a more recent study, Broussard and Cornes (1981) used data from NPI studies of mother-infant dyads to derive an early intervention model. During the study, high-risk dyads were observed in a group setting, and this group milieu was maintained for 2.5 years. The group setting provided a means whereby mothers provided each other with a supportive network enabling them to become more attuned to their own perceptions. The therapeutic team provided additional support for the mother. For example, mothers with depression or low self-esteem were encouraged to ventilate frustrations and to find support within the group setting. Therapists also provided an empathic cushion for the mothers' struggles and a system of praise for maternal successes. Most significantly, therapy was designed to assist the mother in developing a model of optimal caring behavior that could be transposed into the dyadic interaction.

When the infants in the study were 2.5 years old they were assessed by an evaluator who did not know the group membership of the children or their NPI risk rating. It was found that adaptation of the high-risk intervention group was more optimal than the high-risk non-intervention group, and more nearly resembled adaptation in the dyadic pairs considered to be at low risk.

These researchers' work raises two points worth future investigation. First, since a caregiver's low perception of his or her infant has been correlated with impaired development, one implication is that the caregiver may be transmitting negative affective and cognitive cues to the infant that the infant integrates in some manner. If this is in fact the case, the possibility of intervening to restructure maternal perception is raised. Through such intervention, the negative feedback system between infant and caregiver may be broken and a more positive form of dyadic exchange instituted.

Secondly, the underlying premise of Broussard and Cornes's (1981) work—that the quality of the caregiving environment is related to the child's level of development—has been substantiated by numerous studies (Sigman, 1982). One research team has labeled the relationship between infant and environment (in this sense, the primary caregiver may be considered the infant's environmental universe, at least during the first few months of life) as a common reciprocal system (Brazelton, Koslowski, & Main, 1974). Other phrases used by researchers to describe this relationship are infant-caregiver "synchrony" and dyadic "dialogue" (Bond, 1982). Bond also observes that infant development is, above all, transactional in nature, with the infant and environment perpetually in a condition of mutual influence and regulation. Such regulation, certainly on the part of the infant, may be the outcome of experiences of contingent stimulation, during which the caregiver exposes the infant to cause and effect relationships that the infant is able to digest and process at his or her convenience. These information engrams can later be retrieved from memory for use in similar situations. Development of this ability implies that the caregiver is uniquely attuned to the requirements of the infant.

Insight into the dynamics of a mutual regulatory system between infant and caregiver is particularly valuable for the therapist and permits therapeutic strategies of a nonintrusive type. (Further explanation of this regulatory system is given in Chapter Four, on Regulation and the Development of the Self.) That is, if the therapist appreciates the intricacy of the mother-infant exchange and the potential for using this system to enhance a positive sense of self, he or she can create strategies for subtly altering flawed interaction.

Ultimately, the goal of the therapist must be to foster development of an infant who can emerge from the dyadic relationship of infancy and early childhood to the independence of self-regulation and optimal functioning characteristic of late childhood and adulthood. Since well-adjusted children and adults require an intact information processing system, this system must be installed during the dyadic period of infancy (Gibson, 1969). In addition to information processing, the period of infancy is crucial for the development of other psychological characteristics. Broussard (1982) identifies a sense of continuity of self, expectability of satisfactions, regularity of events, and the ability to tolerate frustrations as vital components of a sense of self that must be fostered during infancy within the matrix of the caregiver-infant exchange.

Kestenberg and Buelte (1983) emphasize that the caregiver's implicit respect for the child's abilities, conveyed through numerous responses, enhances the infant's positive self-esteem by developing his or her capacity to remember and anticipate events. The researchers also point out that when the child comprehends that his or her intentions are understood by the adult, feelings of autonomy are promoted. Moreover, these investigators stress that the child's ability to control adults with his or her intentions is a prerequisite for subsequent skills at representing self and others in an internal schema.

PREPARATION FOR TREATMENT

Effective therapy begins with evaluation. Prior to any successful treatment, precise diagnostic and prognostic evaluations of both the infant or child and the caregiver must be conducted (Anthony & Benedek, 1975). As a seminal part of the evaluation process, Kramer and Byerly (1978) advocate an initial interview with the parents to obtain the infant or child's full history. Equally as important is an assessment of the parent's psychological status.

These researchers further identify specific parental resistances that may be encountered during the interviewing process, as well as during subsequent treatment. For example, a parent's narcissism may surface in the form of resistance when the therapist is able to ameliorate the child's conflicts, thereby providing a form of relief that the parent may perceive he or she failed to provide. Or, as the child becomes increasingly more independent as an outgrowth of treatment, parents may feel threatened and respond with anxiety, depression, or anger. Parents may also respond negatively to a child's assertiveness or his or her "acting out" of analytic material in the home environment. Finally, a parent may feel "cheated" that he or she is not receiving the attention and care a therapeutic relationship provides.

Despite these resistances, to which the therapist should be keenly alert, Glenn (1978) and others have emphasized the significance of parental participation during the therapeutic process, particularly in cases involving latency-age children. Indeed, Glenn et al. (1978) note that a working alliance with parents is a prerequisite for treatment success and that parents can be especially effective allies in maintaining the therapy when crises are reached. The therapeutic alliance—forged between child and therapist and parents—will help sustain the treatment, enabling the child to weather any dysregulatory responses or inner conflicts evoked by the therapy.

Therapists also need to be sensitive to other factors that may create impediments to the forging of a dynamic alliance. Socioeconomic and cultural variables, prior experience with professionals and social agencies, family situation, and personal history and psychology of the parents are all factors that can impinge on the rapport the therapist attempts to establish with caregivers (Seligman & Pawl, 1983).

Furman (1957) has proposed yet an additional rationale for focusing on the caregiver. If caregiver and child use the same defense mechanisms, if they suffer from similar symptomatology, or if the child exhibits symptomatology the caregiver experienced during childhood (e.g., thumb-sucking, separation anxiety, or bed-wetting), caregiver capacity to help the child may be seriously impaired. Additionally, in some cases the child's disturbance may have a significant, but unconscious, meaning for the parent. Evaluation of the caregiver, therefore, becomes implicitly vital before the commencement of any treatment regime. Furman also notes that caregivers must be monitored throughout the treatment, since some caregivers, although capable of cooperating during the treatment process, cannot sustain the requisite degree of child care once therapy is interrupted or discontinued. Such caregivers may be chronically unsuited to the parenting role until their own pathology is resolved.

Caregivers may also bring nonpathologic fears and anxieties into the therapuetic relationship. Reporting on phenomena occuring in a baby clinic, Daws (1985) has written that, particularly with first-born infants, parents may harbor fears that they will be unable to care for the infant adequately or that the infant will not survive. These anxieties are allayed for many parents when they are involved in a program of bringing the infant to the clinic on a weekly basis. Such visits can offer the parent validation that he or she is providing sufficient nurturance for the infant. In cases where the mother herself did not experience a good relationship with her own mother, such weekly confirmations can provide her with the confidence that she is capable of being a good caregiver.

The mother's own psychology, then, assumes overriding significance during the entire evaluation process. Donovan and Leavitt (1985) have noted that if a mother has experienced feelings of helplessness prior to the birth of the child, such debilitated affect will likely color her perception of her infant, who may, by virtue of her own psychopathology, be characterized as a "difficult" child. These researchers conducted a study in which learned helplessness was artificially induced in a group of mothers and maternal categorizations of infants were then assessed. It was found that mothers who were pretreated with infant cries which were incapable of being controlled and mothers who received the experimental instruction indicating that the cry was attributable to a "difficult" infant, both exhibited debilitated performance when given an opportunity to stop the cry. The results of this experiment suggest that maternal perceptions of competence can alter the mode in which the mother relates to the infant and that feelings of helplessness can easily be transposed into the dyadic exchange.

Another manifestation of psychopathology to which therapists must be attuned is the fact that while depressed patients may feel very dependent on the therapist, they may not experience closeness to the therapist in the sense of an emotional rapport (West, 1975). Particularly when an infant or young child has been brought in for treatment, maternal depression may lurk in the background. The phenomenon of dependency without genuine attunement may be present in the relationship between therapist and mother.

Idealization of the therapist by a depressed mother and the inevitable sense of defeat accompanying such idealization can also create problems for the therapist in seeking to devise effective treatment strategies. Anthony and Benedek (1975) propose a strategy for short-circuiting the unproductive effects of idealization. They note that some patients establish a transference in which the therapist assumes the role of ideal parent, but shortly is transformed into the image of a rejecting, disapproving, or overly critical authority figure. To avert this process, the researchers suggest revealing the idealization to the patient early during the phase of positive transference and cautioning the patient about the disappointed feelings that may be experienced in the future. The expectations of a depressed mother should also be addressed by the therapist, according to these researchers. Through the process of idealization, for example, such mothers may overrate the people on whom they become dependent, unrealistically expecting them to give and do more than they can in the situation. Ironically, for the depressed mother, the therapist may become both a glorified ego ideal, the "perfect" parent she would like to be, and simultaneously a critical and overbearing superego whose approval is desperately sought.

For effective therapy to occur, however, these unrealistic expectations must be modified. The therapist should attempt to shift focus from himself or herself to the arena of the dyadic exchange between caregiver and infant. Thus parents—particularly depressed parents—must be tutored in feelings of responsibility and involvement in their infants' care. Ultimately, the therapist seeks to establish a mutually regulated dyad, and his or her primary assignment remains channeling all parental energies in the direction of such a relationship.

VARIABLES RELATING TO DEVELOPMENTAL PARAMETERS

The therapist's standard of optimal development for infant-caregiver interaction needs to be articulated at this point. Bond (1982) notes that the goal of development is to acquire skills necessary to behave in a manner most apt to elicit reciprocal, synchronous interaction between infant and caregiver, which ultimately will be used as a model for interactions with others. Such interactions are mutually gratifying and reinforcing, in that the sense of efficacy grows with the development of interaction. The therapist can thus evaluate infants by the degree to which exchange with the caregiver is mutually satisfying and facilitates further interaction.

Temperament

By temperament is meant the individual differences in behavioral style manifested by each infant. Temperament measures offer one means of analyzing the infant-caregiver interaction. Thomas et al. (1963) have outlined checklists that highlight nine specific dimensions of temperament of which therapists should be aware. First, *activity level* should be assessed. Activity level is the motor component of the infant's functioning. *Rhythmicity,* manifested by the regularity and predictability of functions such as hunger-feeding patterns, elimination, and sleep-awake cycles should also be evaluated. Whether the infant *approaches* or *withdraws* on presentation of new stimuli, such as a new toy, a new person, or a new food, is yet another temperamental barometer. Withdrawal, occurring coextensively with negative *mood,* another measurable dimension, may hint at a greater vulnerability for psychopathology. The speed or ease with which behavior can be modified in response to environment represents the infant's capacity for *adaptability,* yet another temperamental trait. Thomas et al. also advocate that the therapist gauge the infant's energy level of response, otherwise referred to as *intensity of reaction,* as well as the infant's *threshold of response.* High intensity, coupled with negative mood or withdrawal, presents occasions for evoking parental anxiety or hostility, and therapeutic intervention may be appropriate for these situations. *Distractability* from environmental stimuli and the converse trait, *attention span/persistence,* are further characteristics to be evaluated. Moreover, Thomas et al. emphasize that these traits should be assessed both individually and in terms of patterns or clusters of traits that combine to create temperamental profiles of "easy," "difficult," or "slow-to-warm-up" infants.

Carey (1983) has suggested three ways in which temperament data may be used by the therapist. First, a discussion of temperament between parents and therapist will help them both to gain a perspective on the infant as a unique personality with numerous individual, distinctive traits. Such a discussion can be especially helpful to parents who, although they may be aware of the individual temperamental characteristics of their infant, may also be unaccustomed to articulating these differences within the framework of personality. Caregivers will become attuned to how their own behavior can affect the infant and alert to typical infant behavior displays. Finally, a temperamental profile is useful for the therapist, who may gain insights into methods for enhancing caregiver-infant interaction. Knowing that an infant has a "difficult" temperament, for example, can suggest to the therapist the types of strategies that would be most effective for optimizing dyadic exchange. Thomas and Chess (1980) also observe that if the parent harbors any ambivalence toward his or her new caregiving role, infant behavioral style may be seized on as a factor aggravating interaction. That is, the parent's dissatisfaction with his or her own role may be displaced onto the infant, in the form of dissatisfaction with the infant's predisposition.

The significance of understanding the individual infant's temperament has been stressed repeatedly by Thomas and Chess (1980). These researchers emphasize that it is often the reactive characteristics of the child, not the attitude of the caregiver, that determines subsequent developmental course. That is, the infant's temperament may be a key initiator in shaping whether the dyadic relationship that evolves will be mutually regulating and fulfilling or mutually stifling and frustrating. The blend of infant characteristics—in a word, temperament—and general parental attitude are the main ingredients of the dyadic relationship. Thus, in cases of dyadic dysfunction that appears attributable to the infant's temperamental uniqueness, parents can often be reassured when the therapist explains that unexpected or difficult phases of the infant's development are due to temperamental manifestations, rather than to faulty parenting. Indeed, the therapist can be extremely helpful here in assuaging guilt, dissipating parental hostility, and restructuring the dyadic interaction into one in which the caregiver is attuned to the unique requirements of the infant's disposition.

Chess (1970) has delineated the risks associated with parental misperception of the infant's temperament. Indeed, Chess notes that certain temperamental patterns are more likely than others to predispose the infant to damaging interaction with his or her environment. Chess is careful to point out, however, that it is not temperament per se that causes the behavioral disorder, but rather, the "misfit" between certain temperamental traits and an environmental milieu unresponsive or unaccommodating to these traits.

Thomas et al. (1963) stress that temperament is manifested through each infant's individual pattern of reactivity. Such patterns are identifiable in early infancy and persist through later periods of life. As a consequence of temperament, according to these researchers, different infants will respond differently to the same environmental stimuli. Implicit in this realization is the notion that no single set of rules is or can be appropriate for all infants. Instead, the environment impinges on the infant in such a way that response is mediated by the particular combination of temperamental traits possessed by that infant. The therapist must first identify the infant's primary pattern of reactivity—his or her temperament—before designing an appropriate treatment plan.

Call (1974) has written extensively about the effects that temperament exerts on the character of infant interaction with the environment. Advocating a plan whereby the infant's temperamental disposition is integrated into the therapeutic scheme, he notes first that individual behavioral variability must be identified for each infant as soon as possible. Once identified, a knowledge of infant temperament can suggest specific types of stimulation that can be tailored to the individual infant's needs. Caregivers should be made aware of external signs of coping on the part of their infants, and therapists can provide blueprints of the landmarks of normal psychological development.

This researcher also stresses that from 3 to 6 months of age, infants should be presented with sufficiently varied stimulation geared to increasing eye-hand coordination and the social smile. He adds that strangers should be introduced to the infant in the context of secure relationships with a stable, but not overly possessive maternal figure. During the latter part of the first year, the infant is capable of engaging in play activity, and through such activity, patterns of activity and reactivity, manifestations of stranger-anxiety, and other behaviors become manifest. All of these responses are affected by infant temperament.

Thomas et al. (1963) have commented that although no overall rules can be devised for nurturing every child, some "optimal practices" facilitate development for the majority of infants. In infants whose patterns of reactivity are somewhat variant, however, custom tailoring of these optimal practices may be necessary. Thomas et al. stress that merely because an infant's temperament, as displayed through behavior, is unlike the average, does not mean that such an infant is pathologic. Treatment plans should, therefore, be designed to account for individual differences and to coach caregivers in the implications of these temperamental differences for infant behavior. The fact that the infant's individual patterns of reactivity will affect parental attitudes presents another reason for identifying temperamental traits as soon as is feasible.

Two temperament profiles have been identified as creating vulnerability for future maladaptation. Chess (1970) has explained the implications of infants with the "difficult" and "slow-to-warm-up" temperament clusters. Infants with difficult temperaments are characteristically irregular in their biologic responses, display negative affect when presented with new stimuli, adapt in a lagging fashion to environmental change, and exhibit a high degree of negative mood expressions and intense reactions. Sleeping and feeding schedules for such infants are "unpredictable and erratic," and caregivers are often hard pressed to accommodate to the special demands of these infants. In a different era, such infants might have been labeled "colicky."

Difficult infants have been demonstrated to be particularly prone to manifesting behavior problems. Chess (1970) observes that the reason for this is that the social demands on the infant to conform to the standards of the external world are enormous. No evidence exists suggesting that caregivers of such infants are the cause of the infant's difficult patterns of reactivity. Nevertheless, parents with difficult infants may be more stressed than caregivers of infants with more regular and predictable temperaments, and as such, maternal guilt, resentment, or feelings of impotence at handling the infant may develop.

"Slow-to-warm-up" children present a behavioral portrait characterized by a potpourri of negative, though mild, responses to new situations, coupled with gradual adaptation to repeated stimuli. The hesitation of response typical of such infants may provoke them to withdraw, which in turn activates a pattern of dysfunctional caregiver-infant interaction.

The early infant evaluation to detect infant temperament should therefore focus on the infant's degree of regularity, withdrawal response, predominance of negative mood, high or low intensity, and extreme levels of persistence or distractibility. Using the portraits of the difficult and slow-to-warm-up child as a guide, therapists can begin to develop strategies for accommodation to enhance caregiver-infant interaction.

As one example of how an infant's temperament may exert debilitating pressure on the dyadic interaction, Thomas, Chess, Birch, Hertzig, and Korn (1963) comment that it is relatively easy for a mother to interact harmoniously with a responsive, highly adaptive, rhythmic infant who displays an amiable disposition, but it is another matter when the infant exhibits hyperactivity, negative response, or arhythmia during periods of dyadic exchange. The caregiver may eventually abandon hope of interacting effectively with her child. Fortunately, recognition that the infant possesses a characteristically "difficult" or "slow-to-warm-up" temperament may be sufficient for the therapist to reeducate the caregiver in more effective strategies for coping with infants of this type. Caregivers may also be reassured by learning that such temperamental typologies are not unusual nor are they symptomatic of disorder. As a consequence, caregivers may experience a resurgence of energy in communicating with infants displaying these temperamental styles and this new found energy will inevitably find its way into an enriched dyadic interaction.

Interactional Style

Perhaps the most potent guide for framing a treatment model is the interactional style of the infant-parent dyad. At the time most dyads are seen by either a pediatrician or child psychiatrist, a distinctive mode of interaction has generally been forged by the dyadic pair. This mode of interaction, although identifiably unique to each caregiver-infant dyad, shares certain identifiable features with other caregiver-infant dyads and thus some behavioral patterns can be classified as being "typical" responses likely to be encountered at a particular developmental phase. The therapist must, therefore, be familiar with the patterns of rhythmic interaction demonstrated by dyadic pairs that have been diagnosed as clinically normal, as well as attuned to the less apparent behaviors that distinguish a particular infant–caregiver pair. Only by being acquainted with these two types of patterns can the ultimate goal of intervention—mutually satisfying and responsive interaction—be achieved.

In determining the specific patterns of interaction within any infant-caregiver dyad, it is necessary first to isolate the components of interaction. By breaking down interaction into discrete units of behavior, the therapist is able to identify behaviors which emanate from the infant, those which are primarily attributable to maternal initiation, and those which are a product of the rhythms of response between the two partners.

Focusing on the infant's capacity for interactive response, Lozoff et al. (1977) have outlined various elements of the sensory system intact among newborns. In addition, these researchers have noted that neonates utilize their sensory equipment to express preferences and aversions to specific stimuli encountered during social interaction. For example, forms of perception (e.g., "visual pursuit" or "visual alertness") have been observed in neonates. For example, a crying neonate is capable of being soothed when lifted to the caregiver's shoulder, resulting in a visual alertness which Lozoff et al. suggest is indicative of a readiness for interaction. Visual ability in general is another primary capacity neonates bring into the interactive milieu. This visual capacity reveals that neonates express distinctive fascination with face-like configurations as contrasted with other types of stimuli. Such visual capacities are crucial for the development of early interaction.

Auditory and motor capacities are further aspects of the infant's innate equipment that facilitate responsiveness to the caregiver. Moreover, Lozoff et al. (1977) observe that these faculties are organized in a manner designed to aid the development of responsiveness. As evidence of such organization, these researchers point to infant alertness and attentiveness to speech sound patterns, rather than to pure tone sounds. Indeed, infants appear to be able to distinguish the sounds of language from gibberish vocalizations during the earliest months of life.

The neonate, however, is capable of more than a simple response. Specific forms of initiating behavior, designed to provoke interaction and response, have also been observed. The ordinary manifestation of crying may, in fact, not be ordinary at all and as several researchers have noted, may represent an intricate form of signaling or communicating a wide variety of both physiological and psychological needs. Wolff (1969), for example, has identified four distinct neonate cries indicative of hunger, anger, frustration, and pain. The infant's initiating behaviors serve as a catalyst triggering a response in the maternal partner.

In summary, Lozoff et al. (1977) note that within the first week of life, the newborn infant shows preferences for the mother's smell, voice, and recognized appearance. From these capacities, two conclusions may be drawn. First, the infant is in a state of readiness or preparedness for interacting with the environment; as a corollary, neonate capacity is geared to motivate the development of a mutual system of interaction.

The findings of Brazelton et al. (1974) are in accord with those of Lozoff et al. (1977). Focusing on infants of 3 weeks of age, Brazelton and associates noted that infants display distinctively different behaviors when interacting with a human participant as opposed to an object stimulus. Moreover, through microanalysis of videotaped sessions between infants and caregivers, these researchers identified specific approach–withdrawal cycles, with separate phases of attention and turning away on the part of the infant.

Both Brazelton et al. (1974) and Lozoff et al. (1977) also stress the caregiver's role during dyadic interaction. Indeed, Lozoff et al. emphasize that the caregiver plays the pivotal or determining role during interactive sequences. These researchers emphasize that while the infant may possess capacities for response and initiation, infants are both new to the nuances of interaction and far less sophisticated than adults. As a consequence, it is the caregiver who, through modification, regulation, and pacing of his or her behavior, compensates for the initial limits of the infant's responsiveness. Caregivers must be flexible enough to engage in this form of behavioral modulation in order to refine the parameters of infant response. Through this process of modification, a synchronous rhythm develops whereby both members of the dyad mutually adapt to one another and evolve expected patterns of response.

Brazelton et al. (1974) also commented on the key role the caregiver plays in shaping infant response. During optimal face-to-face interactions between clinically healthy dyads, for example, infants displayed distinctive rhythmic circular patterns, which were in part composed of attentive phases. These attentive phases were brief periods of punctuation when the infant was observed to wait for maternal cueing. If the maternal initiation of interaction was consistent, infants cycled between attentive behaviors and interactive response in a harmonious rhythmic pattern. In contrast, when caregivers violated the expectancies of infant interaction, by behaving nonresponsively and presenting a still face, infants became visibly concerned, engaged in jerky motions, averted their gaze, and finally attempted to reinitiate interaction. This finding underscores the significance of the maternal role in shaping early interactive response.

Clarke-Stewart (1973) suggests that infant-caregiver behaviors may be viewed in terms of complex patterns or clusters. The optimal mother, for example, engages in a repertoire of behaviors designed to enhance stimulation and fulfill the infant's physiological and psychological needs. In this manner, maternal behaviors may be categorized into clusters, including behavior designed to minister to physical needs (optimal care), behavior designed to enhance infant responsiveness to stimulation (effectiveness), and behaviors geared to cuddling, intellectuality, and restrictiveness. Moreover, an additional sign of maternal efficacy during interaction is the ability of the caregiver to recognize the infant's increasing capacity for independence and with it, the concomitant requirements that the caregiver modulate physical contact and social stimulation (Trad, 1986).

Solnit and Neubauer (1986) have discussed another goal implicit within the mutual dyadic interaction. These researchers observe that through interaction with a caregiver who supplies nurturing, gratification, and stimulation, the infant eventually develops a sense of object constancy. These researchers explain that the early dyadic exchange results in object-relatedness, which is the cognitive and affective awareness of a connection of behaviors and response between caregiver and infant. Object-relatedness signifies the process whereby the infant internalizes the figure of the caregiver and develops representational schemata. These researchers also allude to the process of differentiation during which the infant initially responds to maternal cues, subsequently incorporates these cues into an internal schematic design, and finally develops a form of identifying and interacting with maternal behaviors and responses. Thus, object constancy, a key developmental parameter, emerges from the matrix of interactive behaviors forged between caregiver and infant.

The work of each of the researchers discussed in this section serves to accentuate the importance of early identification of infant behavioral manifestations, maternal initiating patterns, and capacity for modulation. Further the rhythmic or arhythmic form of mutual interaction exhibited by the dyad must be examined before determining an appropriate mode of intervention.

Attachment

Attachment refers to an affective tie between infant and caregiver and to a behavioral system, flexibly operating in terms of set goals, mediated by feeling, and in interaction with other behavioral systems. (Sroufe & Waters, 1977, p. 1185)

Fraiberg (1982a) notes that the attachment and detachment disorders of caregivers are generally mirrored by the infant. In fact, this researcher has suggested that unresolved maternal conflicts of the maternal figure impede the nurturing behavior of mothers towards their own infants. Maternal depression, for example, can be reflected in the quality of attachment that develops. Cherniss, Pawl, and Fraiberg (1980) have found that by working with the mother, a dramatic change can be initiated in the attachment behaviors exhibited during the dyadic exchange. It should be pointed out at this juncture, that there is a distinctive difference in perspective involved when discussing attachment behaviors, as opposed to infant temperament traits. Within the realm of temperament, as observed earlier, the unique endogeneous traits of the infant determine subsequent caregiver-infant interaction. While caregiver response to the infant's temperament will be significant, infant proclivities are accentuated as shaping development. In contrast, studies involving attachment behavior stress the maternal factor as the seminal determinant of adaptive outcome. The caregiver, by transmitting attitude, perception, and perhaps psychopathology, shapes infant response.

Despite this distinction, however, therapists must realize that *both* temperament and attachment may, at varying times and in varying situations, function as decisive determining factors of infant development. That is, therapeutic strategies should be based on the developmental approach, which can accommodate temperament and attachment under the rubric of interaction. With this in mind, we are able to discuss the specific intervention strategies which have been devised by focusing on attachment behaviors.

Blacher (1984a) suggests that intervention efforts should concentrate on developing maternal sensitivity to subtle infant cues. For example, mothers should be sensitized to the fact that gaze-aversion on the part of the infant may represent a form of communication indicating overstimulation.

Development of this sensitivity is particularly important in the case of a handicapped infant, who may possess limited methods of physically interacting with the caregiver.

Another technique for facilitating optimal interaction involves the targeting of parental perceptions and attitudes. The therapist may be able to change or modify parental attitudes toward the infant, fostering more realistic appraisal of infant capacities. The value of early therapeutic intervention to modify attachment behavior and its potential for shaping infant development has been borne out by recent research in pediatrics, which indicates that the first months of life are a vital period during which caregiving can exert a positive influence.

Focusing on an at-risk population of institutionalized infants, Lyth (1985) has noted that the lack of consistent, one-to-one caregiving often experienced by such infants leads to the lack of a consistent attachment for the infant. This lack sets the stage for subsequent psychopathology, which may be exhibited in depressive-like manifestations. To break this degenerative chain reaction, Lyth advocates the creation of small, intimate units, resembling the family model, within the institutional setting. Since the therapeutic goal remains the development of meaningful contact between an infant and adult, therapists must be aware of the negative implications of multiple, indiscriminate caregiving and must seek to establish models within the institutional setting that avert the impact of such sporadic caregiving.

Development of the Self and Self-Regulation

One reason why sporadic, indiscriminate caregiving may be so detrimental to infant development is that such relationships may thwart the healthy development of a sense of self. The caregiver spontaneously imparts attitudes and expectations to the infant, as well as reacting to infant cues. Within this system, a rhythm of regulation develops, whose elements include the infant's capacities to discriminate stimuli, to comprehend contingency relationships in the environment, and to harbor anticipations pertaining to future events as either controllable or uncontrollable. Development of the latter regarding lack of controllability may culminate in depression or depressive-like phenomena, and with time a self-concept characterized by incompetence, helplessness, self-blame, and guilt. It is suggested that the process of differentiation of the self creates pervasive attitudes toward the caregiver and the world in relation to the infant. The world may appear as a supportive environment with many opportunities for the exercise of one's abilities, or it may seem a hostile, basically uncontrollable environment.

To avert this downward process, Belsky and Benn (1982) recommend that the therapist work to bolster the infant–caregiver relationship within the interactive process. Thomas et al. (1963) contribute the notion that an awareness of the infant's temperament is crucial for intervening at a point when the degenerative process of a negative self-image can be avoided.

Chess and Hassibi (1978) suggest that the tools of psychotherapy can be borrowed to devise strategies of intervention geared toward enhancing a positive sense of self in the infant. For example, infant patterns of maladaptation and parental modification can be identified through confrontation, clarification, interpretation, and presentation of alternatives; these methods can all be used when treating the caregiver–infant dyad. The targets of the interventions are more realistic parental attitudes and expectations. Ultimately, it remains the psychiatrist's responsibility to discover maladaptive behavior patterns through observation of infant behavior and through uncovering parental anxieties that may be transmitted to the infant. Whether the therapist works directly with the infant or child, deals primarily with the caregiver, or treats the dyad as a unit, efforts need to be directed in every instance towards age-appropriate corrections in the development of infant self-awareness, interpersonal skill, enhanced sensitivity to the environment, and reality testing.

Bond (1982) has noted that the infant-caregiver dyad embraces a "changing pattern of mutual perceptions" (p. 11). The behaviors manifested within the dyad, therefore, may be broken down and attributed to either the infant or caregiver, but in the final analysis the therapist must recognize that each behavior actually contains a fused response incorporating elements from both members. Moreover, Sigman (1982) has pointed out that one way of viewing the dynamics of infant-caregiver exchange is to conceive of maternal response as being contingent on infant behavior and, conversely, to interpret infant behavior as the accumulated contingent reaction to maternal cues.

Focusing on the significance of the contingency of dyadic interaction, Bond (1982) has noted that early contingency experiences permit the infant to transfer feelings of competence readily from one task to another and from one behavioral setting to another. Indeed, contingency experience shapes every facet of the infant's development by enabling him to achieve a sense of competence or mastery over his or her environment.

White (1959) proposed that infants possess an intrinsic motivation system geared toward the goal of competence, which was defined as effective interaction with the environment. He dubbed this characteristic "effectance motivation." White noted that effectance motivation manifests itself through such characteristics as curiosity and exploration, giving the infant the impetus to interact with the environment. Through such interactions, the infant's capacity for competence and efficacy is continually reinforced. Lewis and Goldberg (1969) noted that caregivers play a vital role in enhancing their infant's sense of competence by responding promptly and contingently to the infant's behavioral manifestations. In this manner, the mother can instill and promote expectancies of contingency, which in turn bolster feelings of efficacy.

Gibson (1969) has pointed out that evidence of the infant's intrinsic motivation system emerges through the manifestation of exploratory forms of behavior. These behaviors include: fixation of the eyes, scanning, and head-turning, all of which are forms of selective perception.

Once again, Bond's (1982) notion of mutual perception between infant and caregiver within the dyadic scheme is crucial here to devising intervention strategies. It is not enough that the therapist attunes himself or herself to the variations of infant perception. The subtleties of infant perception must be contrasted with maternal perception to facilitate optimal interaction.

Gibson (1969) notes that perception is vital to learning and thus may be modified. Perception is defined by the researcher as the process whereby information about the external world is gleaned. Perception, according to Gibson, involves both an awareness of events—the phenomenological aspect of perception—and a discriminative response to stimuli—the responsive aspect of perception.

The term "perceptual learning," then, implies an ability to extract data from the environment selectively and to focus on particular sources of stimulation. Thus perceptual learning, as defined by Gibson, is actually a form of self-regulation, because the infant must modify input from the environment in a selective fashion. Underlying selectivity is the premise that the infant is continually seeking a goal, which may be articulated as the achievement of competency over the environment.

Much of the intrapsychic conflict revealed in the treatment of depressive disorders suggests impairment of the dynamics involved in perceptions, mental representations, and attachments to objects. By "object constancy" is generally meant the perceptual capacity to recognize, organize, and generalize visual stimuli into stable and unvarying precepts (Burgner & Edgcumbe, 1972).

Day and McKenzie (1977) note that evidence for three types of perceptual constancy are apparent during the first year of life. These include visual egocentric constancies, visual object constancies, and visual identity-existence constancies (also labeled object permanence). Egocentric constancies, according to these researchers, involve an object's position in space in relation to the observer. Object constancies refer to the constancy of object properties and traits. Identity-existence constancies focus on the constancy of an object's identity as the object's position in space or time varies. This latter form of constancy also embodies the perceived permanence of the object, even when it is absent from view. Since these various forms of constancy may be conceived of as adaptive patterns of behavior, the infant's perceptual capacities serve as a barometer of adaption at various stages of development. For example, Bornstein and Sigman

(1986) report that infants who encode visual stimuli more efficiently or who recall visual or auditory stimuli more adeptly tend to exhibit greater proficiency on traditional psychometric assessments of intelligence and language during childhood.

Once the infant perceives that certain stimuli in his or her environment have permanent properties, and once he or she has achieved the hallmark of object constancy, he or she is able to adapt and modify his or her behavior. Many developmentalists have described this outcome as being the result of infant capacity to perceive variations in size, shape, and color, and to associate temporally contiguous events. Perceptual learning is ultimately promoted and facilitated by easing the process whereby the infant can integrate a coordinated structure of stimulation. That is, infant experience of the world should be one in which stimuli can be readily discriminated and contingency relationships are sufficient in quantity and quality.

Belsky and Benn (1982) emphasize that the first months of life may be a particularly appropriate time to instill skills in the infant for optimal perceptual learning capacity. Referring to this time as an "opportunity for enhancement," these researchers stress that the therapist's efforts should be devoted, during the first months of life, to optimization, rather than remediation. Intervention during this period, moreover, should focus on treating the family as a "system" of interdependent relationships. By directing parents' attention to the myriad of skills they have at their disposal and to the capacities possessed by their infants, the therapist can facilitate an increase in "parental fascination with, sensitivity to, and involvement with their infants" (p. 297).

Returning to Gibson's (1969) theme of perceptual learning, certain therapeutic procedures have been developed for improving or optimizing perceptual learning. For instance, use of detection experiments, in which the presence or absence of stimulation is indicated by the subject, may be valuable aids. These include tests geared to assess the infant's level of visual acuity. During such tests, the therapist should be alert to the existence of certain infant thresholds. Thresholds, Gibson explains, are the upper and lower limits of sensitivity. Visual acuity tests are also useful in detecting the infant's capacity to "search" his or her environment for distinguishing features that enable him or her to discriminate among stimuli and aid the process of selectivity. Increased eye scanning is generally considered to be the external manifestation of searching behavior. Searching behavior is a particularly important sign for the therapist because it is through such displays that evidence of the capacity for exploration can be gleaned.

Discrimination experiments, which test the infant's ability to notice differences between two or more stimuli, are also useful to the therapist. If discriminatory ability is high, perceptual learning will likely be facilitated. Recognition experiments, during which a subject is shown stimuli, and later asked to recognize similar or identical stimuli, indicate the level of infant contingency awareness—another prerequisite for optimal perceptual learning.

In keeping with the theme of recognition of stimuli, Bond (1982) has reported that parents whose contingent responsiveness to their infants is enhanced by therapy are better able to "read" infant cues, and that infants who are congenitally blind and who subsequently experienced coaching in contingency awareness responded more effectively to parental stimulation.

Gibson (1969) has also suggested that curiosity and fluidity are key components for developing optimal perceptual capacities. In this vein, she notes that infant stimulation should be geared to enhancing the infant's sense of "intermodal similarity"—defined as the ability to match for equivalence—and "intermodal transfer"—described as the transmission of discriminatory capacity across tasks.

The final outcome of perceptual learning, according to Gibson (1969), is the development of the infant's autonomous self-regulation. Indeed, although early infant intervention focuses on the dyadic relationship, the therapist must continually envision the day when the infant will function independently. The child's regulation and coping capacities reflect the degree to which the earlier lessons of the dyadic exchange have been successfully integrated. Self-regulation finally means that the infant or child has learned to function without the need of special intervention or prodding by the therapist.

Self-regulation may be measured through an assessment of perceptual learning responses and is symbolized by an automatic, self-regulated, and highly functional capacity for processing information (Gibson, 1969). To gauge the degree of the infant's self-regulatory abilities, therapists should look for such characteristics as infant capacity to interact effectively with minimal external reinforcement, infant adaptive capacity, and infant speed and agility at incorporating and responding appropriately to new stimuli. The absence of such qualities suggests that the infant may be experiencing some sensory deprivation in the form of low stimulation or frustrated stimulation. Infants deprived in this way are at increased risk for developing subsequent psychopathology.

Using the deprivation model as a guide for discerning poor perceptual learning capacities in infants, Gibson (1969) has noted that a deprived environment has been correlated with specific deficits. These deficits may be exhibited through impaired maternal attention to the infant or may be displayed more blatantly through infant impairment itself. Thus, an unchanging environment can result in a lack of perceptual curiosity, stimulus hunger, timidity, and lack of responsiveness when exposed to new stimuli and an inability to filter out relevant data. Each of these deficits created by deprivation may utterly bombard the infant, stifling virtually all channels of synchronous response.

To combat the effects of deprivation, therapeutic intervention focused on monitoring the environment of the infant-caregiver dyad and restructuring the relationship is mandated, often for prolonged periods of time.

Broussard (1982) counsels that during an assessment of dyadic functioning therapists should concentrate on evaluating maternal self-regulation skills in isolation, as well as in the context of the dyadic exchange. After screening a group of high-risk infants, the researcher noted that mothers of such infants lacked confidence in themselves, had poor self-esteem scores, and seemed depressed and anxious. Moreover, such mothers often lost their infants from their perceptual field.

Lyth (1985) identifies "boundary control," a concept related to self-regulation, as a key element for optimal functioning. This researcher observes that effective control over boundaries exerts a positive effect on the development of identity, because the infant evolves a keener sense of the universe inside of himself or herself. From this internal universe, a sense of self is ultimately derived. Poor mastery of boundaries has been linked by Lyth to impaired abilities for introjecting stimuli and projecting responses, as well as to the projection of false identifications during the development of the self. Broussard (1982) echoes these findings by explaining that the caregiver, as the infant's first "mirror," can impart high self-esteem and empathy, resulting in good boundary control, or conversely, can convey negative images that the infant will similarly introject.

FORMS OF TREATMENT

Keeping in mind the paradigm of maturation provided by the developmental perspective, the therapist can employ techniques borrowed from a number of different treatment models.

Interpersonal Psychotherapy

Recently, interest has been generated in therapeutic models that are of shorter duration than more traditional modes. Among the models of relatively short-term therapy that have gained a degree of credibility in the past several years is the paradigm of interpersonal psychotherapy.

Essentially, interpersonal psychotherapy is premised on the hypothesis that depression evolves from a defect in the interpersonal relationships established by the patient. Indeed, interpersonal therapy postulates that a flaw in the first and primary interpersonal interaction—that of mother and child—represents the matrix from which depressive symtomatology arises. In general, this mode of therapy is brief, often lasting only 12 to 16 weeks, and focuses on restructuring the patient's prevailing interpersonal functioning. The therapy is flexible in that it may be applied by a variety of health care professionals, including psychiatrics, psychologists, and social workers, and may be used in conjunction with adjunctive measures such as psychopharmacologic agents.

Discussing the theoretical underpinnings of interpersonal psychotherapy, Klerman and Weissman (1982) explain that psychiatric disorders, including depression, may be viewed as manifestations of the patient's efforts to adapt to the environment. Moreover, early developmental experiences in the family milieu will determine the manner in which the patient responds to current events in his or her life. Because of this emphasis on the early developmental environment of the patient, interpersonal psychotherapy implicity relies on the attachment theory of bonding between caregiver and child to explain subsequent psychopathology in the patient's later life. Thus, it is not surprising that attachment theorists like Bowlby (1977) have advocated a form of psychotherapy similar to interpersonal psychotherapy. Bowlby (1977), for example, has observed that therapy should be designed to assist the patient in scrutinizing current interpersonal relationships in order to understand how these relationships may derive from the patient's earlier experience with attachment figures in childhood, adolescence, and adulthood.

Since the interpersonal model focuses on relationships, it is recommended first that the therapist assess the types of roles the patient plays during interaction with others. Moreover, the therapist should explore the types of perceptions and cognitions that the patient maintains pertaining to his or her relationships.

Among the prime goals of interpersonal psychotherapy that Klerman and Weissman emphasize are the amelioration of depressive symptomatology and the offering of assistance to the patient in developing more productive strategies for coping with current social and interpersonal problems. Thus, intervention will generally assume the form of reassurance on the part of the therapist, clarification of internal emotional states, enhancement of interpersonal communication, and improvement of reality testing.

The therapist applying interpersonal psychotherapy can rely on this mode of treatment for both the parent and the child. With respect to both such patients, the therapist must first forge a working alliance, according to Rounsaville and Chevron (1982). This working alliance, however, is the overall rubric under which the therapy will operate. Specifically, early intervention with the interpersonal model is designed to obtain a careful history of the depressive symptomatology. Once the symptomatology has been assessed, intervention is premised on the notion that the patient is undergoing a kind of "grieving" process, similar to the actual death or loss of a loved object, and primarily due to a defect in the interpersonal relationship between the patient as a child and the caregiver. As Rounsaville and Chevron stress, the patient's depression may be attributable to an actual, literal loss, or may simply be a response to a dyadic relationship in which a defect resulted in feelings of loss. That is, if the caregiver was severely depressed, if the child was subjected to abuse or neglect, if the caregiver resented the child because he or she was handicapped, or if the child was separated from the caregiver as a consequence of hospitalizations and illness—each of these experiences can create feelings of profound loss which interfere with the child's initial forging of an attachment bond to the caregiver and which linger into subsequent relationships.

The strategies devised by the therapist utilizing interpersonal psychotherapy thus operate on two distinct levels. First the therapist must facilitate the process of mourning, whereby the "damage" the patient has experienced through loss can be ameliorated. In this vein, the therapist can work either with the caregiver and/or child to restructure a more fulfilling relationship. If this is not possible, the therapist must himself or herself serve as a surrogate, reassuring and encouraging the child to overcome early feelings of loss and replace them with competence over the environment. Second, the therapists energies will be devoted to helping the child to reestablish relationships that function in a mutually fulfilling, harmonious manner. Once again, this goal can often be accomplished with the cooperation of the caregiver or, in some cases, the therapist must serve as an object with which the child can resurrect a rewarding relationship. Interpersonal psychotherapy thus offers therapists working with children a flexible tool which can be adapted to a wide variety of situations in which children display psychopathology.

Developmental Guidance and Support

Several strategies are offered by the developmental guidance-support model (Fraiberg, Shapiro, & Cherniss, 1980). This model may be used in two situations. In the first, the parents are assessed as possessing competent nurturing skills, but neonatal complications or infant illness/hospitalization have stressed these capacities. In the second, although both infant and parents manifest severe emotional impairment, the parents' innate capacities may be too limited for them to benefit from the intensive analysis posed by a psycotherapeutic model. Thus such treatment emphasizes providing emotional support to strengthen those capacities that do exist, while at the same time, providing information about the infant's growing needs.

Fraiberg et al. (1980) note that this approach is particularly effective in cases where the interactive problem between infant and caregiver is chronic, such as in the case of a handicapped child or a depressed teenage mother whose child displays symptomatology characteristic of organic failure to thrive. Discussing this mode of treatment, the researchers explain that such therapy is, in essence, a form of reeducating the parent, with the therapist assuming the role of "instructor." Developmental guidance is particularly effective when the infant-caregiver relationship is in danger as a consequence of emotional disturbance, or if the infant or caregiver is under chronic external stress. In this situation, the therapist becomes a "bridge" between infant and parents, gradually striving to promote a nurturing dyadic bond which will facilitate the creation of new child-rearing strategies leading to the optimal development of the infant.

Intervention strategies focusing on educational enhancement may be useful for older children who are encountering difficulties in the school environment. As Morris (1974) notes, the family has in recent years assumed prominence as the primary educator of the child. Thus intervention strategies must involve parents in this key aspect of their child's development. Moreover, shifting attention away from the child, and his or her behavioral problems, and toward the role of learning, creates an atmosphere in which the parent can become an active partner in his or her child's therapy.

In fact, as Chess and Hassibi (1978) have pointed out, numerous children who present with maladaptive behavior may actually harbor an intellectual deficit that has provoked the behavioral disorder. These researchers urge, therefore, that all psychiatric evaluations of children include an assessment of educational status, with accompanying recommendations for remedial skills. Indeed, in some cases, remedial education may result in a dramatic abatement of depression and depressive-like symptomatology. For such children, newly acquired feelings of mastery and self-esteem serve as a bulwark against previously experienced feelings of helplessness. Once such new-found confidence has been achieved, the therapist can devote efforts to engaging in more traditional psychotherapy, designed to help the child confront and resolve inner conflicts.

Skills derived from the educational setting may also be adapted to a form of individualized teaching for a depressed child (Petti, Bornstein, Delamater, & Conners, 1980). Siegel, Siegel, and Siegel (1978), who have written extensively on the symptomatology of loneliness, note that children who express loneliness often have faulty perceptions and fail to interpret correctly the feedback of their playmates. Such children require preparation and tutoring in socialization skills, perhaps because these skills were not provided by the caregiver. Phrased another way, the researchers note that such a child requires training in social perception. The therapist must appreciate that either because of innate deficits or environmental frustrations, the lonely child may not learn communication skills in the way most people do, through a process of indirect imitation and observation. Instead, such children may require direct instruction and interventive practice.

In addition, caregivers play a vital role in reshaping the child's communication skills. Parents in these situations should be instructed to separate their own needs from those of the child, and should be guided by the counsel of the therapist. Over-protectiveness on the part of the parents who have witnessed and empathized with the suffering of such a child must be discouraged and replaced by more effective strategies for overcoming the child's deficit in social skills, according to Siegel et al. (1978). In this respect, the therapist plays a pivotal role in reshaping behavior that can result in reinforcement of feelings of helplessness and their accompanying symptomatology.

Infant-Parent Psychotherapy

As a treatment model, infant–parent psychotherapy, formulated by Fraiberg et al. (1980), may be particularly effective in cases where the patient is an infant under the age of 2 years and hence, incapable of verbalizing complex affective states and areas of cognitive confusion. Within the context of psychotherpy, according to Seligman and Pawl (1983), parents are frequently able, in discussing the infant, to ventilate suppressed feelings they have about themselves, their own histories, and their relationship with the therapist. Indeed, the infant may become a symbol for a figure in the parent's own past or may signify a representation of the parental self that is repudiated or negated. Fraiberg et al. (1980) advocate a system of interpretation similar to that used in traditional psychotherapy, in which the parent's past and present are continually contrasted, but in which the focus always returns to the infant. Moreover, during such treatment, the therapist should attempt to perceive the world from the perspective of the infant and understand the dynamics of the transference between infants and parents (Glenn et al., 1978).

During the process of psychotherapy, the therapist must guard against attributing too great an emphasis to the mother's role as provocateur of the symptomatology. Nevertheless, as Anthony and Benedek (1975) have pointed out, in most cases of depression, ambivalence toward the love object is a pivotal component of the patient's depression. In the case of infants, more often that not, this love object will be the maternal figure. The therapist needs to be attuned to this phenomenon of ambivalence, so that interventions can be oriented both toward resolving the infant's conflicts and toward meeting the parents' specific psychological needs.

Applying a psychotherapeutic model can, however, be problematic and the therapist must advance in treatment with the utmost caution. As traditional psychotherapy reveals, the etiologies of guilt, shame, and inferiority complexes often lie buried deep in the patient's earliest experiences and can only be disclosed gradually by interpreting ambivalent attitudes toward parental figures. Anthony and Benedek (1975) also advise engaging in gradual interpretation of parental attitudes toward the infant, lest too rapid disclosure result in an intensification of depressive symptomatology.

Family Therapy

The techniques offered by family therapy may also supply valuable tools to the therapist dealing with an infant or young child. Since, as Chess and Hassibi (1978) point out, most interventive strategies result in some alteration of the equilibrium and transactional patterns of the family, and since infants and young children are virtually always in the care of an adult figure, the strategies provided by family therapy may be particularly appropriate in these cases.

In therapy of this type, one or both parents' behavior can be modified as an integral part of the treatment, so that parental functioning is optimized. Parental discussion, counseling, reattunement, and reeducation are often useful methods for initiating the ameliorative effects of treatment. When possible, Chess and Hassibi (1978) also encourge home visits, which enable the therapist to experience first-hand the dynamics of interaction in their natural setting. Such visits are especially illuminating for child psychiatrists whose training may have concentrated on the investigation of intrapsychic conflict. Seligman and Pawl (1983) indicate another reason why home visits may be productive: parents often appreciate the increased attention and care suggested by such a visit and, as a consequence, may more readily take the therapist into their confidence.

Finally, family therapy provides the therapist with a new perspective, by conceptualizing the infant or child patient as a component actor within the family structure, rather than as an independent, autonomous unit. The therapist is thus challenged to evaluate the totality of family functioning in terms of a system. As a result, environmental stressors, identifications, alliances, and transitions within the family may all be viewed and interpreted as forms of developmentally age-appropriate behaviors for each family member (Mishne, 1983). Family therapy can, then, provide the therapist with a wealth of new data for devising interactive strategies for intervention.

Psychoanalytic Psychotherapies

Various models of treatment exist even within the category of psychotherapy. Supportive psychotherapy, for example, emphasizes symptom relief, with concomitant enhancement of age-appropriate adaptive behaviors. As Mishne (1983) has explained, such supportive techniques do not explore deeply repressed memories, but allow the patient to ventilate more preconscious material and to seek behaviorial change without attempting resolution of ultimate conflicts. In contrast, psychoanalytic psychotherapy—a less intensive version of adult psychoanalysis—provides a more insight-directed treatment that strives for major change beyond symptom reduction. Chess and Hassibi (1978) have noted that children can benefit from analytic comment, interpretation, and clarification. These researchers particularly advocate the technique in cases of children with circumscribed neuroses based on internalized conflicts, where the external milieu is relatively free of stress. Prime candidates for such psychoanalysis, according to these authors, are children with mild phobic symptoms, mild depression, and mild conduct disorder.

Appropriate candidates for child psychoanalysis, according to Sours (1978), include cases in which the child's future emotional development is threatened or compromised, with the patient exhibiting neurotic symptomatology and/or regression. Analysis may also be of value if object constancy has not been achieved despite chronological passage of this developmental milestone. In addition, if the child displays regulatory instability and appears predisposed to anxiety, frustration intolerance, omnipotence, and pathologic aggression, psychoanalysis may be warranted.

Addressing the specific details of child psychoanalysis, Sours has noted that with children, treatment sessions occur approximately two or at most three times a week. Interestingly, however, Glenn (1978) advocates four patient sessions per week, combined with a weekly session with the parents. The goals of this form of therapy, while including symptom resolution and behavioral modification, also encompass a degree of change in basic personality structure, as well as a return to normal developmental manifestations. Transference and other displacements are as fully explored with the child as they would be with an adult, provided of course that the therapist uses age appropriate interpretations. Therapists engaging in this form of therapy with young children must be aware of the particular hindrances encountered among this young age group.

Several researchers have noted that the transference manifestations in children old enough to verbalize do not differ markedly from adult transference. Anna Freud (1965) wrote that the transference phenomena are implicit in the child's relationship with the therapist who, from the child's vantage point, is viewed as a new object suited to absorbing libidinal and aggressive impulses. Bernstein's (1975) classic definition of transference, which includes affective, cognitive, and behavioral responses oriented toward the therapist and embodies infantile conflicts, appears appropriate for children as well as for adults.

With infants and children, however, the transference may also manifest in nontraditional ways. Glenn (1978), for example, has noted that the arena of play therapy may be one in which the infant or young child is clearly transferring and reenacting episodes of the caregiver-infant interaction. To better understand the dynamics of transference, the therapist must begin to perceive the world from the child's perspective, including the child's attitudes towards parents. Observing caregiver-child interaction first hand can further offer the therapist insight into the dynamics of the transference (Glenn et al., 1978). Moreover, with an infant or child, it is not merely the patient's transference that can be analyzed in detail; the therapist is also given an opportunity—generally not available with adult patients—to explore the parent's transference feelings toward their offspring, as well as to the therapist, and thus to develop a coherent understanding of all the transference phenomena involved in the case (Seligman & Pawl, 1983).

Given this unique abundance of transference information, the therapist working with both infant or child and caregiver has increased leeway for formulating and applying intervention strategies. In essence, he or she can devise strategies and observe their impact in vivo. Although Glenn et al. (1978) caution against interpretations given to parents, this team acknowledges that in extreme situations, the therapist can directly intervene to restructure the debilitating effects of negative transference.

Infant and child treatment offers a unique challenge to the therapist. Armed with the insights of the developmental approach, play therapy, and observed infant-caregiver interaction, the therapist is given a broad array of data from which to derive intervention strategies. Finally, the distinct kinds of transference which the therapist is able to observe in this setting—including transference of the infant or child, transference of the parents, and transference between the parents and child—offer insights into the child or infant's earliest development and clues for enhancing the optimal growth and affective regulation of the young patient.

Sours (1978) comments that children who have experienced deprivations in object relations may pose technical difficulties for the psychoanalyst. Early deprivation often requires a new emotional experience, such as the establishment of a therapeutic relationship, before subsequent interpretation through verbalization and clarification can occur. Sours also stresses that child analysis depends essentially on techniques of interpretation to achieve its ameliorating effects. As in the adult analytic setting, resistances and defenses are interpreted, and the analyst serves as the central figure on whom transference feelings are transposed in order to revive unconscious fantasies and attitudes.

Psychoanalysis can only be attempted, however, if the child is old enough and intelligent enough to engage in the process of interpretation. Sours (1978) suggests a trial analytic session, during which the therapist can evaluate the child's capacity for this form of treatment. Glenn (1978) has noted that children under the age of 3 are rarely analyzed, because of their verbal and cognitive limitations. Nevertheless, according to this researcher, prelatency-age children can benefit from psychoanalysis even if their verbal skills are not that sophisticated. Such children can either directly converse with the therapist or can act out fantasies through games and use of toys, clay, and drawings.

Additionally, the parents' motivation and ability to support the child in this endeavor—both emotionally and financially—need to be considered before embarking on psychoanalysis. Bernstein and Sax (1978) add to this list of considerations the child's endowment, including temperamental predisposition, developmental phase for his or her chronological age, the nature of the symptomatology, the intake diagnosis, the degree of internalization of conflict, and a psychiatric assessment of the parents.

Mishne (1983) has distinguished between child problems appropriately subjected to the rigors of psychoanalysis and those more fittingly dealt with by supportive psychotherapeutic techniques. She writes that if the conflict is predominantly internalized, analysis is the treatment of choice, but adds that even neurotic conflicts can be resolved by psychotherapy, if the conflict doesn't seriously impinge on developmental adaptation. Further, because psychotherapy provides more structure than psychoanalysis, it is often preferable for children with less than neurotic symptomatology and less invasive distortions in object relations.

Discussion

Techniques for each of the models outlined here can be advantageously incorporated into the therapeutic format of virtually any infant or child patient. Although infants under the age of 2 years are precluded from engaging in full-fledged psychoanalysis because of inchoate verbal skill, a preponderance of children over that age and the vast majority of children over age 4 can be involved in at least the preliminary forms of insight provided by psychoanalysis. Moreover, even if the infant is developmentally incapable of participating in the psychoanalytic reenactment, an astute therapist can, by observing cognitive and affective manifestations, infer by conjecture the types of inner turmoil experienced by such a young infant. Additionally, parental behavior, as demonstrated verbally in conversations with the therapist and through observed interaction with the child, can be subjected to the same form of pervasive scrutiny reserved for the adult patient in psychoanalysis. Other techniques may be derived from the models of supportive psychotherapy and family therapy.

The developmental psychopathologist venturing into the realm of infant or child treatment should keep in mind two considerations. First, the patient must be assessed within the context of a developmental framework. In this regard, behavioral response will be evaluated in terms of the patient's "goodness or poorness of fit" with the environment. The ultimate question is whether the patient is regulating in an adaptive or maladaptive fashion. Second, the therapist must be eclectic in borrowing techniques from the variety of treatment models available. He or she must approach treatment with a fierce determination to design creative strategies geared to the individual patient's requirements.

SPECIFIC THERAPEUTIC INTERVENTIONS FOR POPULATIONS AT-RISK

As a guiding principle, the initial evaluation process should be used by the therapist to determine the specific orientation of treatment strategies. The treatment models discussed earlier will, at this juncture, be reassessed in terms of each of the high-risk populations isolated in previous chapters.

Psychotherapeutic Guidance and Support

This therapeutic mode essentially seeks to foster competent nurturing skills, by providing emotional support, counseling, and guidance for caregivers trapped in a mutually frustrating and stifling dyadic exchange. As Minde and Minde (1981) have described this form of treatment, the therapist's main goal is to retrain the mother, enabling her to engage in effective interaction within the dyad. This form of treatment is premised on the notion that the flaw lies neither with the infant nor with the caregiver. Rather, the defect is one that manifests itself during sequences of interaction; for this reason the interactive episodes must be restructured. During the process of instilling guidance and support techniques, the therapist will, in effect, be coaching the mother in the skills of nurturance. As maternal skills are honed, the therapist's influence is felt vicariously by the mother and infant, until eventually the mother is capable of assuming the caregiving role on her own.

Such therapy has been particularly effective in cases of handicapped infant-caregiver dyads. Marfo and Kysela (1984), discussing treatment techniques in handicapped child populations, first note that the diversity within the population of mentally handicapped children alone precludes rigid adherence to any specific therapeutic modality. Thus these researchers advocate development of unique programs for each patient dyad. Nevertheless, they have reported success in relying on the guidance-support model.

Marfo and Kysela (1984) refer to this form of treatment as the "parent therapy model," stressing that the goal is to foster competent parenting techniques and to assist parents in resolving the residue of negative or ambivalent feelings that, in varying degrees, generally follow the birth of a handicapped child. The approach taken may be characterized as didactic, in the sense that parents are taught specific behavioral strategies for enhancing their child's skills and competencies.

Since a shared, gratifying communication system between caregiver and infant is an essential precursor for the infant's optimal development, energy is devoted to enhancing dyadic exchange by instructing the caregiver in sensitive responses to his or her infant's precise developmental impairment. But in addition to enlarging maternal awareness of her infant's handicap, such therapy also strives to incorporate methods for developing the infant's capacities to their fullest extent.

Marfo and Kysela (1984) have articulated several goals in such therapy. First, parental guilt, confusion, anxiety, anger, and the host of other unproductive emotional conflicts that attend the birth of a handicapped child need to be addressed and resolved. Second, specific skill training must be given to the caregivers in a manner supportive of their efforts. Third, the therapist needs to focus the manifestation of these skills within the arena of the infant-caregiver exchange, for it is ultimately in this domain that maternal guidance will exert its greatest impact on the child's development. Fourth, the therapeutic team must assure that the family is provided adquate social support and access to all relevant community support services. A prerequisite to this type of therapy is that the parents need to understand the full ramifications of the handicap and to accept responsibility for their feelings about the child.

Guidance and supportive therapy may also be valuable in instances of parental psychopathology and parental abuse or neglect. In these cases, if the caregiver is developmentally incapable of or emotionally too immature to engage in fullfledged psychotherapy, guidance and supportive techniques may serve to ameliorate a highly conflicted situation. Or, if the child has been removed from his or her biological parents and placed with either adoptive or foster parents, these new caregivers may benefit from the skills derived from this therapy. In addition, even if the therapist has adopted a more intensive treatment mode as the primary vehicle for therapy, the techniques derived from the guidance and supportive model may serve as useful adjuncts that can be integrated into more sophisticated treatment strategies.

Infant-Parent Psychotherapy

This treatment model is applicable to virtually any dyad in which the parent makes the voluntary commitment necessary for the treatment. On some occasions, individual sessions with parent or child may augment mutual therapy. Since parental resistance may be encountered when the techniques of psychotherapy are employed, therapists are cautioned that a full parental evaluation is essential prior to instituting this form of treatment. Even if parental consent is given during the early phases of treatment, as the therapy progresses, latent conflicts may surface involving the parent's guilt about the fact that the child requires psychiatric attention or ambivalence about the child's improvement. Indeed, in many instances, the child's symptomatology is actually the overt manifestation of the parent's own psychopathology and the parent may feel threatened that the child's recovery will focus attention on the real source of disorder.

Infant-parent psychotherapy can be particularly effective in cases of parental psychopathology such as depression. Indeed, the child's therapy may provide the caregiver with a necessary rationale or "excuse" for entering therapy himself or herself. In this context, the therapist can deal with the parent as he or she would with another individual patient, with the significant exception that the infant and the caregiver-infant interaction become further variables for interpretation and modification within the therapeutic setting. Eventually, the parent should be alerted to the fact that his or her own psychopathology is no longer an individual problem; of all known risk factors, the existence of parental psychopathology is the one most closely associated with infant and childhood depression.

Parents of handicapped children can also benefit from psychotherapy. Here, the therapist's efforts should be devoted to uncovering areas of ambivalence and conflict with respect to having a handicapped child that parents may have repressed. The advantages of psychotherapy in restructuring and forging an enhanced self-esteem will also be of benefit in such dyads. Parents with an increased sense of self-esteem will eventually transmit these feelings to their offspring, which will, in turn, facilitate the child's own development of an intact and adaptive sense of self.

Psychotherapy in dyads where the infant or child has been abused or neglected may be more problematic. Although such parents are often prime candidates for the personality restructuring that can only be accomplished by intensive disclosure, interpretation, and resolution of unconscious conflict, resistance and denial is frequently encountered by therapists dealing with such caregivers. If, however, a modest commitment can be obtained from the parent, psychotherapy—while a long and ardous process—may represent hope for breaking the cycle of abuse, which is commonly passed from generation to generation.

When the abused or handicapped patient is an infant, the therapist's first efforts should be devoted to assessing the extent of damage the infant has suffered developmentally. Subsequent strategies should be devised for creating an adaptive sense of self, with particular emphasis on sufficient contingency experiences promoted within the context of a nurturing dyadic exchange.

Sours (1978) has written that children who present with neurotic symptomatology, structural ego defects, preverbal disturbances, and failures in separation-individuation frequently require the structure offered by psychotherapy and the relationship with the therapist. This advice is particularly true in cases of child abuse/neglect, maternal depression, and infant or child handicaps. The therapist must, however, use caution in the extent of his or her intervention, since, as Bernstein and Sax (1978) have cautioned, unstable parents who provide a threatening, excessively stimulating, or depriving environment constitute a contraindication to some specific therapeutic interventions (e.g., child psychoanalysis).

Child Psychoanalysis

The techniques of child psychoanalysis can be applied to virtually any population at risk for depression. In these cases, the child has been brought to treatment either voluntarily or involuntarily. Provided the child has sufficient development of cognitive capacities, most cases can benefit from the techniques of analysis.

In cases of parental psychopathology or abuse/neglect, the therapist must exert intensive effort toward analyzing the child's resistances and defenses before meaningful interpretation can occur. Similar warnings apply for handicapped and hospitalized children. In each of these at-risk populations, the child may have come to perceive himself or herself as the incipient cause of the problem. That is, abused children may believe that they deserve to be abused. Their self-esteem is notoriously poor and extensive therapy often reveals an external locus of control, coupled with feelings of helplessness and debilitation in confronting a hostile, unresponsive universe. For such children, analysis must be geared toward restructuring self-representations and establishing a trusting affective rapport with the therapist.

With handicapped children, a similar cycle of self-blame and guilt may be present. Once again, the therapist's efforts should be geared toward revealing poor self-concepts and constructing the foundation on which more rewarding self-images can be built.

Therapy Designed for Hospitalized Children

Lyth (1985) has specifically addressed the issue of developmental problems encountered in children who have been hospitalized for physical illness or institutionalized for psychiatric disturbances. She notes that many children's facilities do not handle authority in a manner conducive to enhancing child development. Thus institutions tend to be authoritarian and rigid, rather than authoritative and responsible.

Significantly, since hospitals often impose maternal separation on children as a consequence of medical treatment, these institutions must be educated to the now well-documented association between caregiver deprivation and infant or child depression. Indeed, in the institutional setting, the child can experience a loss of control over his or her own boundaries, and this loss of control can contaminate the development of identity. To counteract such debilitating emotions, hospitals need to institute regimens that permit greater caregiver-child interaction, and, when the caregiver must be absent for medical reasons, a surrogate must be assigned the special care of the child. This surrogate system can ameliorate some of the effects of separation.

Lyth (1985) notes that the staff in children's wards should be specially trained to control their own personal sense of boundaries, so as to avoid a negative transference from the patient to the staff, which would replicate repetitive maladaptive interactions between them. By serving as role models, the staff can thus transmit feelings of adaptiveness to the child, helping him or her to control projections and introjections and to strengthen the development of a secure sense of self. Above all, caregiving by staff must not be done in an indiscriminate fashion. Either a special surrogate, in the form of a nurse, can be assigned to the child, or the staff should be composed of a firmly–bound unit, enabling the child to form subsidiary attachments to other adults.

By instituting these techniques for effective boundary control, the infant or child is given a more entrenched sense of belonging, a sense that there is something to identify with, of having "a place" where "I" belong. To achieve this sense of identification in the child, hospitals should avoid multiple indiscriminate caregiving and move closer to the family model. One suggestion by Lyth (1985) is to divide the ward into small units, each with its own staff and accompanying sense of family proximity, privacy, and intimate interaction.

Therapy Designed for Puerperal Depression

Treatment of puerperal depression is often a disarmingly complex task for the therapist working with both the mother and infant. According to Scott (1984), puerperal depression requires an analysis of four distinct phenomena occuring simultaneously for the caregiver. Thus, puerperal depression is generally a function of biochemical, intrapsychic, interpersonal, and social factors, each of which contributes to the maternal symptomatology and each of which plays a unique role depending on the individual.

With respect to specific investigating techniques, Scott emphasizes investigating how the mother perceives of the infant. Therapists should formulate basic questions and answers for themselves, such as "What does *this* baby mean to *this* mother?" and what the actual words "mother," "father," and "baby" mean to the mother. In addition, the mother's destructive impulses toward both herself and her infant need to be evaluated.

Moreover, puerperal depression generally presents with a distinctive symptom, such as feeding difficulty, which the therapist should be alert to, since this symptom may have a symbolic significance for the mother. A thorough psychosocial history of the maternal, familial, and marital relationship needs to be documented, with particular queries concerning the mother's response to her pregnancy.

Once these diagnostic steps have been performed, the therapist can devise an interventive protocol relying on physical treatment of symptoms, supportive psychotherapy, marital therapy, and mobilization of social support networks. None of these areas should be ignored. Throughout the duration of the treatment process, the therapist must function as a supportive bulwark for the mother in her efforts to construct an optimal relationship with her infant.

Therapy Designed for Seasonal Affective Disorder

One form of psychopathology that has recently come to the attention of researchers is seasonal affective disorder. This disorder, which is characterized by a form of depression that surfaces during the fall and winter months, appears to be triggered by the degree of sunlight to which the patient is exposed. The symptomatology of the disorder has been catalogued by several research teams and includes a repetitive cycle of winter-fall depression and summer-spring hypomania, hypersomnia, anergia, fatigue, carbohydrate craving, and weight gain (Hellekson et al., 1986; Wehr et al., 1986). Significantly, the syndrome occurs predominantly in women, often beginning in early childhood.

Unlike other forms of affective disturbance, therapists have reported a high degree of success when treating these patients with phototherapy. Hellekson et al. (1986) reported that six patients displayed significant amelioration of depressive symptomatology after three 2-hour exposures to bright artificial light. Relapse occurred when the treatment was withdrawn.

For therapists involved in the treatment of young children, seasonal affective disorder needs to be considered when arriving at an initial differential diagnosis. Not only is the disorder known to affect children, but equally significant, since the disorder primarily strikes young women and since a preponderance of young children are cared for by their mothers, a woman affected by this condition may keep transferring her periodic depressed affect to the child. Thus, in keeping with the notion that infants and young children seen for therapy are generally involved in a strong dyadic relationship with their caregivers, all caregivers should be queried with respect to the possible presence of seasonal affective disorder during the initial intake process. If it appears that the caregiver is in fact afflicted with this condition, two positive aspects should be emphasized. First, seasonal affective disorder responds favorably to phototherapy treatment. Second, parents are often guilt-ridden and anxious if their young children manifest disturbed symptomatology. If this symptomatology is caused by seasonal affective disorder, the caregiver may be reassured in discovering that the prognosis, both for herself and her child, is positive.

DRUG TREATMENT OF PREADOLESCENT DEPRESSION

During the past 10 years, the psychopharmacologic treatment of children has become much more accepted and effective than in previous decades

(Wiener, 1984). However, there persists a natural reticence to alter a child's affective state with an exogenous agent.

Furthermore, it can be difficult to gauge the synergistic effects of maturation and drug handling in prepubescent pharmacotherapy. (Maturation may influence drug response in a variety of ways; for example, the relatively larger size of the liver and the great quantity of body water and extracellular fluid in younger children combine to make them, proportionate to their size, generally less sensitive to drugs than adults [Pearce, 1980/81]). These treatment difficulties have resulted in a serious lack of adequate research on child psychopharmacology that is only now beginning to be reversed.

Nevertheless, despite these concerns, more and more psychotropic agents are being applied in child populations. Investigators in one study found that 42 percent of children with symptoms of depression had been given a psychopharmacologic agent prior to being seen in a child psychiatric clinic for the first time (Stack, 1972). This dramatic change in treatment mode is no doubt partly due to an increase in the number and quality of psychopharmacologic treatments available and partly to increased recognition that depressive disorders do occur in childhood, presenting with much the same symptomatology as in adult populations (Weller et al., 1983b; Wiener, 1984).

Historical Perspective

It is significant that the use of psychoactive drugs in children has always been preceded by their use in adults. The one exception to this rule is the use of stimulants (Wiener, 1984). In 1942, Bender and Cottingham observed noticeable improvement in hyperactivity, attention span, and organization of activity with benzedrine (Bender & Cottingham, 1942).

The 1960s saw the the introduction of antidepressant medications and lithium into the field of childhood depression (Wiener & Jaffe, 1977). This development occurred even though the definition of childhood depression was much more nebulous than it is today. Over the past 20 years, a marked refinement in the classification of depression has occurred, resulting in the acceptance of the notion that major depressive disorders occur in children and that they have signs and symptoms similar and often identical to those seen in depressed adults (Petti, 1983; Puig-Antich, 1984; Weller, 1983a). In light of this consensus, the success of antidepressant therapy in adults has fostered the use of antidepressants in children.

Pretreatment Considerations: Advantages and Disadvantages

Two of the most difficult therapeutic considerations associated with the pharmacologic treatment of prepubescent depression are the role of physical maturation, which may be of critical importance in defining the drug response, and the specific indications for treatment. However, as Pearce (1980/81) points out, aside from the simple pharmacologic action, there are a number of advantages in administering drug treatment to a child. Any guilt the parents may feel is reduced when the focus of treatment is shifted from their behavior to their child's organic condition and to drug therapy. A child who is classified as being "sick" enough to warrant use of medicine can be seen as needing extra care and tolerance, and this favorable shift in parental attitude may be enhanced by the fact that antidepressants work rapidly to produce their effect. The child also benefits from this rapid action because a prolonged period of poor performance at school may adversely affect expectations and attitudes for an extended period of time.

While these considerations are all to the good, there is one dangerous potential consequence of antidepressant drug therapy. The patient and family may eventually come to think that any problems that may arise in the future will be solvable and reversible with drug therapy. This faulty inference may preempt the search for underlying causes and alternate methods of dealing with the situation.

Indications. Determining the indications for antidepressant treatment in a specific case is made difficult because of the lack of precise methods for assessing psychiatric symptoms in terms of degree, duration, and severity (Puig-Antich, 1984). In an attempt to deal with this problem, the National Institute of Mental Health has called for definition and clarification of the operational criteria for diagnosing childhood depression, and assessment of age-related factors that might influence treatment response (Schulterbrandt & Raskin, 1977).

If criteria for children similar to the criteria for adults are used, roughly 7 percent of pediatric patients, and 30 to 60 percent of child psychiatric outpatients can be diagnosed as having had a major depressive episode (Preskorn et al., 1982). Among these cases, significantly, positive outcomes have been documented as a result of drug therapy. For example, response rates of 40 to 90 percent have been reported in children taking tricyclic antidepressants (Puig-Antich et al., 1979; Weinberg et al., 1973).

Children with endogenous depression may respond best to a multi-dimensional treatment plan, including psychotherapeutic interventions and, where appropriate, pharmacological agents. In the absence of more refined systems of symptom assessment, drug treatment of childhood depression may be indicated in situations where psychosocial stress factors cannot be eliminated and where the depression is generating secondary effects, such as negative feelings in parents and others. Also, psychophar-macologic treatment may be advisable when a dramatic and rapid therapeutic response is needed, such as in cases of severe depression with suicidal thoughts. However, medication is often contraindicated if the child's living situation is so chaotic that proper supervision of the drug regimen cannot be assured (Pearce, 1980/81).

Therapy with Specific Antidepressant Agents

The Tricyclics—Imipramine. Several studies have shown a strong relationship in depressed adults between therapeutic response and plasma concentrations of the tricyclic antidepressants, primarily imipramine and nortriptyline (APA, 1985; Preskorn, Weller, & Weller, 1982). The importance of plasma concentrations, rather than dosages, cannot be overemphasized.

In addition to clearing the liver rapidly, the tricyclic antidepressants are highly lipid soluble and bond extensively to tissues and plasma protein. These pharmacodynamic properties result in a large volume of distribution and the production of plasma elimination half-lives that are of intermediate duration. Such properties account for the fact that there are dramatic interindividual differences in steady-state plasma concentrations and response to this class of agent (APA, 1985). As an example, investigators in one study observed a 36-fold difference in plasma concentrations of desmethylimipramine between two patients given a standard dose (Sjoqvist & Bertilsson, 1984).

Studies in children are rapidly increasing in number, but many more are needed before definitive conclusions can be drawn. Nevertheless, it is not difficult to recognize the added importance of monitoring tricyclic plasma blood levels in children, who have even more physiologic factors influencing drug handling than do adults.

In one study, the results of which were typical of child treatment with tricyclics, the imipramine steady-state plasma levels of 20 children aged 6 to 12 years diagnosed with major depressive disorder were monitored (Weller et al., 1983b). Concentrations of desmethylimipramine, the major active metabolite of imipramine were also monitored. Two weeks of initial in-hospital observation and counseling with no pharmacologic treatment were followed by 3 weeks of administration of 75 milligrams of imipramine before going to bed for those patients who did not remit after the first 2 weeks. At the end of the fifth week, treatment was continued for 3 more weeks with imipramine at an adjusted dose for children who did not respond to the 75 milligram treatment.

Of the 20 patients, none responded at the end of the 2-week nondrug treatment period. However, after 3 weeks of therapy with imipramine at 75 milligrams per day, there was a remission rate of 80 percent for children whose plasma drug levels were within the range of 125 to 225 nanograms per milliliter. For children outside this range, the remission rate was zero. At the end of the second 3-week phase, there was a 93 percent response within the 125 to 225 nanograms per milliliter range and a 25 percent response in children outside this range.

These results were very similar to those obtained by Preskorn et al. (1982) in 20 seriously depressed hospitalized children, aged 7 to 12 years. The paradigm of Preskorn et al. was the same three-phase design employed by Weller et al. (1983b), and the effective plasma concentrations found in this study also fell between 125 and 225 nanograms per milliliter of imipramine. The authors point out that the minimum effective concentration for children (125 nanograms per milliliter) is very close to that for adults (120 nanograms per milliliter). This finding further underscores the importance of monitoring plasma concentrations of the drug in child populations.

On a more subjective level, it is interesting to note Petti's (1983) description of his overall clinical experience with imipramine after treating 60 depressed inpatient children. Petti observes that children, as a rule, rapidly regain contact with their feelings, experience a decrease in anxiety, and make impressive strides in sustaining feelings of well-being after psychopharmacologic treatment. Once well-being is experienced, a transient feeling of depression may recur, which indicates the child is in touch with his or her feelings, perhaps for the first time. As this familiarity with affective state continues, an ability to describe articulately a sense of powerlessness and hopelessness emerges. Thus, interaction and integration with the environment can begin and genuine therapeutic progress can ensue.

The Tricyclics—Nortriptyline. Nortriptyline, another tricyclic anti-depressive, has been evaluated in children with much less frequency than imipramine. In one preliminary study, 9 prepubertal and 11 postpubertal children with DSM-III criteria for major depressive disorder were given single doses of nortriptyline (25 milligrams for children under 10, 50 milligrams for older subjects) and had plasma samples taken every 12 hours for 2 days (Geller, 1984). While patients were not tested for effect on affective state, a variance was discovered between the two age groups, pointing to the importance of monitoring plasma concentrations of nortriptyline in these groups as well as in adult groups.

The Tricyclics—Toxicity. Due to the wide variation in plasma concentrations of the tricyclic antidepressants, the possibility of toxicity due to accumulation is perhaps just as important as maintaining therapeutic plasma drug levels. In adults, imipramine and the other tricyclics can cause serious adverse effects such as intracardiac conduction problems and impaired memory. Indications are that this class of drug can produce side effects in children similar to those seen in adults (Wiener, 1984). Therefore, blood monitoring and caution are mandated while using tricyclics in prepubescent children.

Monoamine Oxidase (MAO) Inhibitors. There are even fewer reports of treatment of depressed children with MAO inhibitors than with tricyclics. Frommer (1967) first reported on MAO inhibitor treatment of depressed children. In her original double-blind crossover study, she found that phenelzine with chlordiazepoxide was more effective than phenobarbitol and placebo. While it is difficult to draw any conclusions from this study, in a subsequent trial with MAO inhibitors, which included 50 children having phobias and depression, an 81 percent improvement rate in phobic ratings and a 66 percent improvement in depression were recorded.

Summary

The fact that antidepressant medication, particularly the tricyclics, appear to be an effective means of treating depression in childhood lends support to the contention that there is a similarity in the nature of depression between the adult and child states. However, it is dangerous to draw too close a parallel between the adult and childhood affective disorders, since maturational considerations affect not only drug handling but etiology as well.

Many more studies are needed to delineate the parameters of drug treatment in children. However, it seems safe to say that, as is true in adulthood, the more typical the symptoms of depression in childhood, and the less overlap with other disorders (e.g., anxiety), the better the chances of recovery.

CONCLUDING REMARKS

The task of the infant and child therapist is a formidable one. The final aim of treatment with such patients remains the achievement of an optimally functioning, mutually regulated dyadic exchange (in the case of infants) and the instilling of a sense of mastery, competence and high self-esteem (in older children). However, these goals are often elusive.

The therapist may use the developmental perspective to provide a comprehensive vision of maturation—plugging in data pertaining to such parameters as infant temperament, attachment, and self—and may rely on techniques culled from the treatment models discussed. In instances where an infant or child is in a specific high-risk group for depression, the therapist should design a special regimen to ameliorate the impact of the risk factor. Additionally, for cases exhibiting specific endogenous symptomatology, pharmacologic agents may alleviate overt signs of disorder and, hence, permit a more thorough delving into the inner conflict through such techniques as psychotherapy. It should be remembered that even patients who are treated successfully with medication alone may benefit from psychotherapeutic support and exploration. The implications of the experience of being depressed must always be explored, independent of the psychotherapeutic or psychopharmacologic intervention for depression per se.

The treatment suggestions offered here should serve merely as a blueprint. In the final analysis, each individual therapist must bring to bear his or her unique talents and creativity, approaching each infant or child as both an embodiment of development and a singular entity. It is only by adding the extra ingredients of therapist and patient individuality that the goals of treatment can come to fruition. In meeting this challenge, the hope that infant and child psychopathology can be conquered may be transformed into a bold reality.

References

Aber, J. L., III, & Zigler, E. (1981). Developmental considerations in the definition of child maltreatment. *New Directions for Child Development, 11,* 1–29.

Abraham, K. (1912). Notes on the psychoanalytic investigation and treatment of manic-depressive insanity and allied conditions. In K. Abraham (Ed.), *Selected papers* (pp. 137–156). London: Hogarth.

Abramson, L. Y., Seligman, M. E. P., & Teasdale, J. D. (1978). Learned helplessness in humans: Critique and reformulation. *Journal of Abnormal Psychology, 87,* 49–74.

Achenbach, T. M., & Edelbrock, C. S. (1978). The classification of child psychopathology: A review and analysis of empirical efforts. *Psychological Bulletin, 85,* 1275–1280.

Achenbach, T. M., & Edelbrock, C. S. (1981). Behavioral problems and competencies reported by parents of normal and disturbed children age four through sixteen. *Monographs of the Society for Child Development, 46* (1, Serial No. 188). 1–82.

Ackerly, W. C. (1967). Latency-age children who threaten or attempt to kill themselves. *Journal of the American Academy of Child Psychiatry, 6,* 242–261.

Adam, K. S. (1982). Loss, suicide, and attachment. In C. M. Parkes & J. Stevenson-Hinde (Eds.), *The place of attachment in human behavior* (pp. 269–294). New York: Basic Books.

Adler, R., & Raphael, B. (1983). Review of children of alcoholics. *Australian and New Zealand Journal of Psychiatry, 17,* 3–8.

Agle, D. P. (1964). Psychiatric studies of patients with hemophilia and related states. *Archives of Internal Medicine, 114,* 76–82.

Agren, J., & Terenius, L. (1983). Depression and CSF endorphin fraction I: Seasonal variation and higher levels in unipolar than bipolar patients. *Psychiatry Research, 10,* 303–311.

Ainsworth, M. D. S. (1962). The effects of maternal deprivation: A review of findings and controversy in the context of research strategy. *WHO Public Health Papers, 14,* 97–165.

Ainsworth, M. D. S. (1967). *Infancy in Uganda: Infant care and the growth of love.* Baltimore: Johns Hopkins University Press.

Ainsworth, M. D. S. (1973). The development of infant-mother attachment. In B. M. Caldwell & H. R. Ricciuti (Eds.), *Review of Child Development Research* (pp. 1–94). Chicago: University of Chicago Press.

Ainsworth, M. D. S. (1979, April). *Attachment: Retrospect and prospect.* Presidential address at the meeting of the Society for Research in Child Development, San Francisco.

Ainsworth, M. D. S., Bell, S. M. V., & Stayton, D. J. (1971). Individual differences in strange-situation behaviour of 1-year-olds. In H. R. Schaffer (Ed.), *The origins of human social relations* (pp. 17–57). London: Academic. Ainsworth, M. D. S., Blehar, M. C., Waters, E., & Wall, S. (1978). *Patterns of attachment: A psychological study of the strange situation.* Hillsdale, NJ: Erlbaum.

Ainsworth, M. D. S., & Wittig, B. A. (1969). Attachment and exploration behavior of one-year-olds in a strange-situation. In B. M. Foss (Ed.), *Determinants of infant behavior* (Vol. 4, pp. 113–136). London: Methuen.

Akiskal, H. S., Rosenthal, T. L., Haykal, R. F., Lemni, H., Rosenthal, R. H., & Scott, S. A. (1980). Characterological depressions: Clinical and sleep EEG findings separating 'subaffective dysthymias' from 'character spectrum disorders.' *Archives of General Psychiatry, 37,* 777–783.

Albert, N., & Beck, A. T. (1975). Incidence of depression in early adolescence. A preliminary study. *Journal of Youth and Adolescence, 4,* 301–307.

Alexander, I.E., & Alderstein, A.M. (1958). Affective Responses to the Concept of Death in a Population of Children and Early Adolescents. *Journal of Genetic Psychology, 93,* 167–177.

Allen, M. G. (1976). Twin studies of affective illness. *Archives of General Psychiatry, 33,* 1467–1478.

Alloy, L. B., Abramson, L. Y., & Viscusi, D. (1981). Induced mood and the illusion of control. *Journal of Personality and Social Psychology, 41,* 1129–1140.

Alloy, L. B., Peterson, C., Abramson, L. Y., & Seligman, M. E. (1984). Attributional style and the generality of learned helplessness. *Journal of Personality and Social Psychology, 46,* 681–687.

Allport, G. W. (1937). *Personality: A psychosocial interpretation.* New York: Holt.

Als, H. (1981). *Infant individuality: Assessing patterns of very early development.* New York: Basic Books.

Als, H., Tronick, E., & Brazelton, T. B. (1980). Affective reciprocity and the development of autonomy: The study of a blind infant. *Journal of the American Academy of Child Psychiatry, 19,* 22–44.

Altemeier, W. A., III, Vietze, P. M., Sherrod, K. B., Sandler, H. M., Falsey, S., & O'Connor, S.(1979). Prediction of child maltreament during pregnancy. *Journal of Child Psychiatry, 18,* 205–218.

Alvy, K. (1975). Preventing child abuse. *American Journal of Psychology, 30,* 921–928.

American Humane Association: Annual Report (1985). *Highlights of Official Child Neglect and Abuse Reporting.* Denver: American Humane Association.

American Psychiatric Association. (1980). *Diagnostic and statistical manual of mental disorders (DSM-III)* (3rd Ed.). Washington, DC.

American Psychiatric Association (1985). Tricyclic antidepressants—Blood level measurements and clinical outcome: An APA task force report. *American Journal of Psychiatry, 142,* 155–162.

Anders, T. F., Sachar, E. J., Kream, J., Rolfwarg, H. P., & Hellman, L. (1970). Behavioral state and plasma cortisol response in the human newborn. *Pediatrics, 46,* 532–537.

Antell, S. E., & Keating, D. P. (1983). Perception of numerical invariance in neonates. *Child Development, 54,* 695–701.

Anthony, E. J. (1978). A mind that lost itself: A prospective study of mental decompensation from birth to breakdown. *Connecticut Medicine, 42,* 591–593.

Anthony, E. J. (1983). An overview of the effects of maternal depression on the infant and child. In H. L. Morrison (Ed.), *Children of depressed parents: Risk, identification and intervention* (pp. 1–16). New York: Grune & Stratton.

Anthony, E. J., & Benedek, T. (1975). Introductory comment to Treatment chapter. In E. J. Anthony & T. Benedek (Eds.), *Depression and human existence (pp. 426–430).* Boston: Little, Brown.

Arai, K., Yanaihara, T., & Okinaga, S. (1976). Adrenocorticotropic hormone in human fetal blood at delivery. *American Journal of Obstetrics and Gynecology, 125,* 1136–1140.

Arajarvi, T., & Huttunen, M. (1972). Encopresis and enuresis as symptoms of depression. In A. L. Annell (Ed.), *Depressive states in childhood and adolescence* (pp. 212–217). Stockholm: Almquist & Wiksell.

Arend, R., Gove, F., & Sroufe, L.A. (1979). Continuity of individual adaptation from infancy to kindergarten: A reductive study of ego resilience and curiosity in pre-schoolers. *Child Development, 50,* 950–959.

Baechler, J. (1979). *Suicides* (B. Cooper, Trans.). New York: Basic Books.

Bakan, D. (1971). *Slaughter of the innocents: Study of the battered child phenomenon.* San Francisco: Jossey-Bass.

Bakwin, H. (1942). Loneliness in infants. *American Journal of Disabled Children, 63,* 30–40.

Bakwin, H. (1949). Emotional deprivation in infants, *Journal of Pediatrics, 35,* 512–521.

Bakwin, H. (1957). Suicide in children and adolescents. *Journal of Pediatrics, 50,* 749–769.

Bandura, A. (1978). The self system in reciprocal determinism. *American Psychologist, 33,* 344–357.

Bane, M. J. (1986). Household composition and poverty. In S. H. Danzinger & D. H. Weinberg (Eds.), *Fighting poverty: What works and what doesn't* (pp. 209–231). Cambridge, MA: Harvard University Press.

Barbero, G. J. (1984). Children with recurrent hospitalizations: A problem of disabled children, parents, and physicians. *Developmental Behavioral Pediatrics, 5,* 319–324.

Baron, M., Klotz, J., Mendlewicz, J., & Rainer, J. (1981). Multiple-threshold transmission of affective disorders. *Archives of General Psychiatry, 38,* 79–84.

Barrera, M. E., & Maurer, D. (1981). Discrimination of strangers by the three-month-old. *Child Development, 52,* 558–563.

Bates, J. E., Maslin, C. A., & Frankel, K. A. (1985). Attachment and security, mother-child interaction, and temperament as predictors of behavior-problem ratings at age three years. In I. Bretherton & E. Waters (Eds.), *Growing points of attachment theory and research. Monographs of the Society for Research in Child Development, 50,* 167–193.

Bayley, N. (1969). *Bayley scales of infant depression.* Cleveland, OH: Psychological Corporation.

Beck, A. T., Sethin, B. B., & Tuthill, R. W. (1963). Childhood bereavement and adult depression. *Archives of General Psychiatry, 9,* 295–302.

Beck, A. T., & Beck, R. (1972). Screening Depressed Patients in Family Practice. A Rapid Technic. *Postgraduate Medicine, 52,* 81–85.

Beckman, P. J. (1983). Influence of selected child characteristics on stress in families of handicapped infants. *American Journal of Mental Deficiency, 88,* 150-156.

Beckwith, L. (1972). Relationships between infants' social behavior and their mothers' behavior. *Child Development, 43,* 397–411.

Beckwith, L. (1979). The influence of caregiver–infant interaction on development. In E. J. Sell (Ed.), *Follow-up of high-risk newborn: A practical approach.* Springfield, IL: Thomas.

Bedi, A. R., & Halikas, J. A. (1985). Alcoholism and affective disorder. *Alcoholism, 9,* 133–134.

Bell, R. Q., & Harper, L. V. (1977). *Child effects on adults.* Hillsdale, NJ: Erlbaum.

Bell, S. M., (1970). The development of the concept of object as related to infant–mother attachment. *Child Development, 11,* 291–311.

Bell, S. M., & Ainsworth, M. (1972). Infant crying and maternal responsiveness. *Child Development, 43,* 1171–1190.

Belsky, J. (1980). Child maltreatment: An ecological integration. *American Journal of Psychology, 35,* 320–335.

Belsky, J. (1985). Experimenting with the family in the newborn period. *Child Development, 56,* 407–414.

Belsky, J., & Benn, J. (1982). Beyond bonding: A family-centered approach to enhancing early parent-infant relations. In L. A. Bond & J. M. Joffe (Eds.), *Facilitating infant and early childhood development* (pp. 281–308). Hanover, NH: University Press of New England.

Belsky, J., Rovine, M., & Taylor, D. (1984). The Pennsylvanian infant and family development project, III: The origins of individual differences in infant-mother attachment and infant contributions. *Child Development, 55,* 718–728.

Bemesderfer, S., & Cohler, B. J. (1983). Depressive reactions during separation period: individuation and self among children of psychotic depressed mothers. In H.L. Morrison (Ed.), *Children of depressed parents: risk, identification, and intervention* (pp. 159–188). New York: Grune & Stratton.

Bender, L., & Cottingham, F. (1942). The use of amphetamine sulfate (Benzedrine) in child psychiatry. *American Journal of Psychiatry, 99,* 116–121.

Bengston, V. L., & Treas, J. (1980). The changing family context of mental health and aging. In J. E. Birren & R. B. Sloane (Eds.), *Handbook of mental health and aging* (pp. 400–428). Englewood Cliffs, NJ: Prentice-Hall.

Berbaum, M. L., & Moreland, R. L. (1980). Intellectual development within the family: A new application of the confluence model. *Developmental Psychology, 16,* 506–515.

Berbaum, M. L., & Moreland, R. L. (1985). Intellectual development within transracial adoptive families: Retesting the confluence model. *Child Development, 56,* 207–216.

Berkman, L. F., & Syme, S. L. (1979). Social networks, host resistance, and mortality: A nine-year follow-up study of Alameda County residents. *American Journal of Epidemiology, 109,* 186–204.

Bernheimer, L. P., Young, M. S., & Winton, P. J. (1983). Stress over time: Parents with young handicapped children. *Developmental and Behavioral Pediatrics, 4,* 177–181.

Bernstein, G., & Garfinkel, B. (1986). School phobia: the overlap of affective and anxiety disorders. *Journal of the American Academy of Child Psychiatry, 25,* 235–241.

Bernstein, I. (1975). On the Technique of Child and Adolescent Analysis. *Journal of the American Psychoanalytic Association, 23,* 190–232.

Bernstein, I., & Sax, A. M. (1978). Indications and contraindications for child analysis. In J. Glenn (Ed.), *Child analysis and therapy* (pp. 67–108). New York: Jason Aronson.

Berry, P., Gunn, P., & Andrews, R. (1980). Behavior of Down Syndrome Infants in a Strange Situation. *American Journal of Mental Deficiency, 85,* 213–218.

Bertelsen, A., Harvald, B., & Hauge, M. (1977). A Danish twin study of manic-depressive disorders. *British Journal of Psychiatry, 130,* 330–351.

Bertenthal, B. I., & Fischer, K. W. (1978). The development of self-recognition in the infant. *Developmental Psychology, 14,* 44–50.

Beverly, B. I. (1936). The effect of illness upon emotional development. *Journal of Pediatrics, 8,* 533–543.

Bible, C., & French, A. P. (1979). Depression in the child abuse syndrome. In A. P. French & I. N. Berlin (Eds.), *Depression in children and adolescents* (pp. 184–209). New York: Human Sciences Press.

Bibring, E. (1953). The mechanism of depression. In P. Greenacre (Ed.), *Affective disorders: Psychoanalytic contribution to their study* (pp. 13–48). New York: International Universities Press.

Blacher, J. (1984a). Attachment and severely handicapped children: Implications for intervention. *Developmental and Behavioral Pediatrics, 5,* 178–183.

Blacher, J. (1984b). Sequential stages of parental adjustment to the birth of a child with handicaps: Fact or artifact? *Mental Retardation, 22,* 55–68.

Blacher, J., & Meyers, C. E. (1983). A review of attachment formation and disorder of handicapped children. *American Journal of Mental Deficiency, 87,* 359–371.

Blanchard, M., & Main, M. (1979). Avoidance of the attachment figure and social-emotional adjustment in day-care infants. *Developmental Psychology, 15,* 445–446.

Blass, E. M., Ganchrow, J. R., & Steiner, J. E. (1984). Classical conditioning in newborn humans 2-48 hours of age. *Infant Behavior and Development, 7,* 223–235.

Blazer, D. G. (1982). Social support and mortality in an elderly community population. *American Journal of Epidemiology, 115,* 684-694.

Bliss, E. L., Migeon, C. H., Branch, C. H., & Samuels, L. T. (1956). Reaction of the adrenal cortex to emotional stress. *Psychosomatic Medicine, 18,* 56–76.

Blom, G. E. (1958). The reactions of hospitalized children to illness. *Pediatrics, 22,* 590–600.

Blumberg, M. L. (1974). Psychopathology of the abusing parent. *American Journal of Psychotherapy, 28,* 21–29.

Blumberg, M. L. (1977). Depression in children on a general pediatric service. *American Journal of Psychotherapy, 32,* 20.

Blumberg, M.L. (1977). Treatment of the Abused Child and the Child Abuser. *American Journal of Psychotherapy, 31*, 204–215.

Blumberg, M. L. (1981). Depression in abused and neglected children. *American Journal of Psychotherapy, 35*, 342–355.

Bond, L. A. (1982). From prevention to promotion: Optimizing infant development. In L. A. Bond & J. M. Joffe (Eds.), *Facilitating infant and early childhood development* (pp. 5–39). Hanover, NH: University Press of New England.

Bornstein, M. H., & Sigman, M. D. (1986). Continuity in mental development from infancy. *Child Development, 57*, 251–274.

Bousha, D. M., & Twentyman, C. T. (1984). Mother–child interactional style in abuse, neglect, and control groups: Naturalistic observations in the home. *Journal of Abnormal Psychology, 93*, 106–114.

Bower, T. G. R., Broughton, J., & Moore, M. K. (1970). Demonstration of intention in the reaching behavior of neonate humans. *Nature, 14*, 679–681.

Bowlby, J. (1944). Forty-four juvenile thieves: Their characters and home life. *International Journal of Psychoanalysis, 25*, 163–171.

Bowlby, J. (1951). Maternal Love and Mental Health. *W.H.O. Monogram, No. 2*. London: H.M.S.O.

Bowlby, J. (1958). The nature of the child's tie to its mother. *International Journal of Psychoanalysis, 39*, 350–373.

Bowlby, J. (1960). Grief and mourning in infancy and early childhood. *Psychoanalytic Study of the Child, 15*, 9–52.

Bowlby, J. (1969). *Attachment and loss: Vol. 1. Attachment.* London, Hogarth Press.

Bowlby, J. (1973). *Attachment and loss: Vol. 2. Separation anxiety and anger.* London: Hogarth.

Bowlby, J. (1977). The making and breaking of affectional bonds: II. Some principles of psychotherapy. *British Journal of Psychiatry, 130*, 421–431.

Bowlby, J. (1980). *Attachment and loss: Vol. 3. Loss.* New York: Basic Books.

Bowlby, J. (1982). *Attachment and loss: Vol. 1. Attachment* (2nd ed.). New York: Basic Books.

Bowlby, J., Ainsworth, M., Boston, M., & Rosenbluth, D. (1956). The effects of mother–child separation: A follow-up study. *British Journal of Medicine and Psychology, 29*, 211–247.

Bowlby, J., Robertson, J., & Rosenbluth, D. (1952). A two-year-old goes to the hospital. *Psychoanalytic Study of the Child, 7*, 82–94.

Boyd, J. H., & Weissman, M. M. (1981). Epidemiology of affective disorders. *Archives of General Psychiatry, 38*, 1039–1046.

Bradley, R. H., & Caldwell, B. H. (1979). Home observation for measurement of the environment: A revision of the preschool scale. *American Journal of Mental Deficiency, 84*, 235–244. Philadelphia: Lippincott.

Brazelton, T. B. (1973). Neonatal behavioral assessment scale. *Clinics in Developmental Medicine, 50*, 1–66.

Brazelton, T. B., & Als, H. (1979). Four early stages in the development of mother-infant interaction. *The Psychoanalytic Study of the Child, 34*, 349–369.

Brazelton, T. B., Koslowski, B., & Main, M. (1974). The origins of reciprocity: The early mother-infant interaction. In M. Lewis & L. A. Rosenblum (Eds.), *The effect of the infant on its caregiver* (pp. 49–76). New York: Wiley.

Breier, A., Charney, D. S., & Heninger, G. R. (1984). Major depression in patients with agoraphobia and panic disorder. *Archives of General Psychiatry, 41*, 1129–1135.

Brennemann, J. (1932). The infant ward. *American Journal of Diseases of Children, 43*, 577–584.

Breslau, N. (1985). Psychiatric disorder in children with physical disabilities. *Journal of the American Academy of Child Psychiatry, 24,* 87–94.

Breslau, N., & Davis, G. C. (1985). Refining DSM-III criteria in major depression: an assessment of the descriptive validity of criterion symptoms. *Journal of Affective Disorders, 9,* 199–206.

Breslau, N., & Davis, G. C. (1986). Chronic Stress and Major Depression. *Archives of General Psychiatry, 43,* 309–314.

Bridges, F. A., & Cicchetti, D. (1982). Mothers' ratings of the temperament characteristics of Down's Syndrome infants. *Developmental Psychology, 18,* 238–244.

Bridges, K. M. B. (1933). Emotional development in early infancy. *Child Development, 3,* 324–341.

Brim, O. G., Jr. (1976). Life-span development of the theory of oneself: Implications for child development. *Advances in Child Development and Behavior, 11,* 241–251.

Brim, O. G., Jr., White, K. L., & Zill, N. (1979). *Child trends international: A plan for organization to improve the quality, scope and use of information about children.* Unpublished manuscript.

Brodie, B. (1974). Views of healthy children toward illness. *American Journal of Public Health, 64,* 1156–1159.

Bromet, E. J., & Cornely, P. J. (1984). Correlates of depression in mothers of young children. *Journal of American Academy of Child Psychiatry, 23,* 335–342.

Bromet, E. J., Schulberg, H. C., & Dunn, L. (1982). Reactions of psychiatric patients to the Three Mile Island nuclear accident. *Archives of General Psychiatry, 39,* 725–730.

Bronfenbrenner, U. (1977). Toward an experimental ecology of human development. *American Journal of Psychology, 32,* 513–529.

Bronfenbrenner, U. (1979). *The ecology of human development: Experiments by nature and design.* Cambridge, MA: Harvard University Press.

Brooks-Gunn, J., & Lewis, M. (1984). Maternal responsivity in interactions with handicapped infants. *Child Development, 55,* 782–793.

Broucek, F. (1979). Efficacy in infancy: A review of some experimental studies and their possible implications for clinical theory. *International Journal of Psychoanalysis, 60,* 311–316.

Broughton, J. (1978) Development of concepts of self, mind, reality and knowledge. *New Directions for Child Development, 1,* 75–100.

Broussard, E. R. (1976). Neonatal prediction and outcome at 10/11 years. *Child Psychiatry and Human Development, 7,* 85–93.

Broussard, E. R. (1982). Primary prevention of psychosocial disorders: Assessment of outcome. In L. A. Bond & J. M. Joffe (Eds.), *Facilitating infant and early childhood development* (pp. 180–196). Hanover, NH: University Press of New England.

Broussard, E. R., & Cornes, C. C. (1981). Identification of mother-infant systems in distress: What can we do? *Journal of Preventative Psychiatry, 1,* 119–132.

Brown, G. W., Bhrolchain, M. N., & Harris, T. (1975). Social class and psychiatric disturbance among women in an urban population. *Sociology, 9,* 225–254.

Brown, G., & Harris, T. (1978). *Social origins of depression: A study of psychiatric disorders in women.* New York: Free Press.

Brown, R. D., & Semple, L. (1970). Effects of unfamiliarity on the overt verbalization and preconceptual motor behavior of nursery school children. *British Journal of Educational Psychology, 40,* 291–298.

Brumbeck, R. A., Dietz-Schmidt, S., & Weinberg, W. A. (1977). Depression in children referred to an educational diagnosis center—Diagnosis and treatment and analysis of criteria and literature review. *Diseases of the Nervous System, 38,* 529–535.

Bryant, B. K. (1985). The neighborhood walk: Sources of support in middle childhood. *Monographs of the Society for Research in Child Development, 50* (3, Serial No. 210), 1–122.

Bryant, H. D., Billingsley, A., & Kerry, G. (1963). Physical abuse of children: An agency study. *Child Welfare, 42,* 125–130.

Burden, R. L. (1980). Measuring the effects of stress on mothers of handicapped infants: Must depression always follow? *Child Care Health Development, 6,* 111–125.

Burgess, R.L., & Conger, R. D. (1977). Family interaction patterns related to child abuse and neglect: Some preliminary findings. *Child Abuse & Neglect: The International Journal, 1,* 269–277.

Burgess, R.L., & Conger, R. D. (1978). Family interaction in abusive, neglectful, and normal families. *Child Development, 49,* 1163–1173.

Burgner, M., & Edgcumbe, R. (1972). Some problems in the conceptualization of early object relationships. *The Psychoanalytic Study of the Child, 27,* 313–332.

Burland, J. A. (1986). The vicissitudes of maternal deprivation. In R. F. Lax, S. Bach, & J. A. Burland (Eds.). *Self and object constancy: Clinical and theoretical perspectives* (pp. 324–347). New York: Guilford.

Burnard, E. D., Todd, D. A., John, E., & Hindmarsh, K. W. (1982). Beta-endorphin levels in newborn cerebrospinal fluid. *Australian Pediatric Journal, 18,* 258–263.

Burstein, S., & Meichenbaum, D. (1979). The work of worrying in children undergoing surgery. *Journal of Abnormal Psychology, 7,* 121–132.

Buss, A. H., & Plomin, R. (1975). *A temperament theory of personality.* New York: Wiley.

Byrd, D. E. (1979, March). *Intersexual assault: A review of empirical findings.* Paper presented at the annual meeting of the Eastern Sociological Society, New York.

Cacciari, E., Cicognani, A., Pirazoli, P., Dallacasa, P., Mazzaracchio, M. A., Tassoni, P., Bernardi, F., Salardi, S., & Zappulla, F. (1976). GH, ACTH, LH and FSH behaviour in the first seven days of life. *Acta Paediatrica Scandinavica, 65,* 337–341.

Cadoret, R. J., O'Gorman, T. W., Heywood, E., & Troughton, E. (1985). Genetic and environmental factors in major depression. *Journal of Affective Disorders, 9,* 155–164.

Call, J. D. (1974). Helping infants cope with change. *Early Child Development and Care, 3,* 229–247.

Cameron, J.M., Johnson, H.R.M., & Camps, R. E. (1966). The Battered child syndrome. *Medicine, Science, and the Law, 6,* 2–21.

Campos, J. J., Barrett, K., Lamb, M. E., Goldsmith, M. E., & Stenberg, C. (1983). Socioemotional development. In M. M. Haith & J. J. Campos (Eds.), *Handbook of child psychology: Vol. 2. Infancy and developmental psychobiology* (pp. 783–916). New York: Wiley.

Cantwell, D. P. (1983a). Depression in childhood: clinical picture and diagnostic criteria. In D. P. Cantwell, & G. A. Carlson (Eds.), *Affective disorders in childhood and adolescence: An update* (pp. 3–18). New York: Spectrum Publishers, Inc.

Cantwell, D. P. (1983b). Childhood depression what do we know, where do we go. In J. B. Guze, F. J. Earls, & J. E. Barrett (Eds.), *Childhood Psychopathology and development* (pp. 67–85). New York: Raven Press.

Cantwell, D. P. (1983c). Assessment of childhood depression: an overview. In D. P. Cantwell & G. A. Carlson (Eds.), *Affective disorders in childhood and adolescence: An update* (pp. 3–18). New York: SP Medical and Scientific Books.

Cantwell, D. P. (1983d). Overview of etiologic factors. In D. P. Cantwell & G. A. Carlson (Eds.), *Affective disorders in childhood and adolescence: An update* (pp. 206–219). New York: SP Medical and Scientific Books.

Caplan, G. (1974). *Social systems and community mental health.* New York: Behavioral Publications.

Caplan, R. D. (1979). Social support, person–environment fit, and coping. In L. A. Ferman & J. P. Gordus (Eds.), *Mental health and the economy* (pp. 89–138). Kalamazoo, Michigan: Upjohn Institute for Employment Research.

Carey, W. B. (1970). A simplified method for measuring infant temperament. *Journal of Pediatrics, 77,* 188–194.

Carey, W. B. (1983). Intervention strategies using temperament data. In T. B. Brazelton & B. M. Lester (Eds.), *New approaches to developmental screening of infants* (pp. 245–258). New York: Elsevier.

Carey, W. B., & McDevitt, S. C. (1978). Stability and change in individual temperament diagnoses from infancy to early childhood. *Journal of American Academy of Child Psychiatry, 17,* 331–337.

Carlson, G. A. (1979). *Lithium carbonate use in adolescents: clinical indications and management.* Chicago, IL: University of Chicago Press.

Carlson, G. A. (1983). Bipolar affective disorders in childhood and adolescence. In D. P. Cantwell, & G. A. Carlson (Eds.). *Affective disorders in childhood and adolescence: An Update* (pp. 61–83). New York: Spectrum Publishers, Inc.

Carlson, G. A., & Cantwell, D. P. (1980). Unmasking masked depression in children and adolescents. *American Journal of Psychiatry, 137,* 445–449.

Carlson, G. A., & Cantwell, D. P. (1982). Diagnosis of childhood depression: A comparison of the Weinberg and DSM-III criteria. *Journal of the American Academy of Child Psychiatry, 21,* 247–250.

Carlson, G. A., Davenport, Y. B., & Jamison, K. (1977). A comparison of outcome in adolescent and late onset bipolar manic depressive illness. *American Journal of Psychiatry, 134,* 919–922.

Carlson, G. A., & Garber, J. (1986). Developmental issues in the classification of depression in children. In M. Rutter, C. E. Izard, & P. B. Read (Eds.), *Depression in young people* (pp. 399–434). New York: The Guilford Press.

Carroll, B. J. (1982). The dexamethasone suppression test for melancholia. *British Journal of Psychiatry, 140,* 292–304.

Carroll, B. J. (1983). Biologic markers and treatment response. *Journal of Clinical Psychology, 44,* 30–40.

Carroll, B. J., Curtis, G. C., & Mendels, J. (1976). Neuroeondocrine regulation in depression: i. limbic system adrenocortical dysfunction. *Archives of General Psychiatry, 33,* 1039–1044.

Carroll, B. J., Feinberg, M.,& Greden, J. F. (1981). A specific laboratory test for the diagnosis of melancholia. *Archives of General Psychiatry, 38,* 15–22.

Casler, L. (1961). Maternal deprivation: a critical review of the literature. *Monographs of the Society for Research in Child Development, 26* (2, Serial No. 80).

Cassell, J. (1974). An epidemiological perspective of psychosocial factors in disease etiology. *American Journal of Public Health, 64,* 1040–1043.

Cassens, B.J. (1985). Social consequences of the acquired immunodeficiency syndrome. *Annals of Internal Medicine, 103,* 768–771.

Cavenar, J. O., & Butts, N. T. (1977). Fatherhood and emotional illness. *American Journal of Psychiatry, 134,* 429–431.

Ceroni, G. B., Neri, C., & Pezzuli, H. (1984). Chronicity in major depression: A naturalistic prospective study. *Journal of Affective Disorders, 7,* 123–132.

Chambers, W. J., Puig-Antich, J., & Tabrizi, M. A. (1978). The ongoing development of the Kiddie-SADS (schedule of affective disorders and schizophrenia for school-age children). Read before the *American Academy of Child Psychiatry,* Annual meeting. San Diego, October 27, 1978.

Chance, M. R. A. (1962). An interpretation of some agonistic postures: The role of "cut-off" acts and postures. *Symposia of the Zoological Society of London, 8,* 71–89.

Chapin, H. D. (1915). Are institutions for infants necessary? *Journal of the American Medical Association, 64,* 1.

Cherniss, D. S., Pawl, J., & Fraiberg, S. (1980). Nina: Developmental, guidance and supportive treatment for a failure to thrive infant and her adolescent mother. In S. Fraiberg (Ed.), *Clinical studies in infant mental health* (pp. 103–120). New York: Basic Books.

Chess, S. (1970). Temperament and children at risk. In E. J. Anthony & C. Koupernik (Eds.), *The child in his family* (pp. 121–130). New York: Wiley-Interscience.

Chess, S. (1978). The plasticity of human development: Alternative pathways. *Journal of the American Academy of Child Psychiatry, 17,* 80–91.

Chess, S., & Fernandez, P. (1980). Do deaf children have a typical personality? *Journal of the American Academy of Child Psychiatry, 19,* 654–664.

Chess, S., & Hassibi, M. (1978). *Principles and practice of child psychiatry.* New York: Plenum.

Chess, S., & Thomas, A. (1982). Infant bonding: mystique and reality. *American Journal of Orthopsychiatry, 52,* 213–222.

Chess, S., & Thomas, A. (1984). *Origins and evolution of behavior disorders: From infancy to early adult life.* New York: Brunner/Mazel.

Chess, S., Thomas, A., Birch, H. G., Hertzig, M. E., & Korn, S. (1963). Practical implications. *Behavioral individuality in early childhood.* New York: New York University Press.

Chess, S., Thomas, A., & Hassibi, M. (1983). Depression in childhood and adolescence: A prospective study of six cases. *Journal of Nervous and Mental Disease, 171,* 411–420.

Chess, S., Thomas, A., Korn, S., Mittelman, D., & Cohen, J. (1983). Early parental attitudes, divorce and separation, and young adult outcome: Findings of a longitudinal study. *Journal of the American Academy of Child Psychiatry, 22,* 47–51.

Church, Joseph A., Allen, James R., & Stiehm, E. Richard (1985). New scarlet letter(s), pediatric AIDS. *Pediatrics, 77,* 423–427.

Cicchetti, D. (1984). The emergence of developmental psychopathology. *Child Development, 55,* 1–7.

Cicchetti, D. V., & Prusoff, B. A. (1983). Reliability of depression. *Archives of General Psychiatry, 40,* 987–990.

Cicchetti, D., & Rizley, R. (1981). Developmental perspectives on the etiology, intergenerational transmission, and sequelae of child maltreatment. *New Directions for Child Development, 11,* 31–55.

Cicchetti, D., & Schneider-Rosen, K. (1984a). Theoretical and empirical considerations in the investigation of the relationship between affect and cognition in atypical populations of infants. In C. E. Izard, J. Kagan, & R. B. Zajonc (Eds.), *Emotions, cognition, and behavior* (pp. 366–406). Cambridge, England: Cambridge University Press.

Cicchetti, D., & Schneider-Rosen, K. (1984b). Toward a transactional model of childhood depression. *New Directions for Child Development, 26,* 5–27.

Cicchetti, D., & Schneider-Rosen, K. (1986). An organizational approach to childhood depression. In M. Rutter, C. E. Izard & P. B. Read (Eds.), *Depression in young people—developmental and clinical perspectives* (pp. 71–134). New York: The Guilford Press.

Cicchetti, D., & Serafica, F. C. (1981). Interplay among behavioral systems: Illustrations from the study of attachment, affiliation, and wariness in young children with Down's Syndrome. *Developmental Psychology, 17,* 36–49.

Cicchetti, D., & Sroufe, L.A. (1976). The Relationship between affective and cognitive development in Down's Syndrome infants. *Child Development, 47,* 920–929.

Cicchetti, D., & Sroufe, L.S. (1978). An Organizational view of affect: Illustration from the study of Down's Syndrome infants. In M. Lewis & L. Rosenblum (Eds.) *The Development of Affect*. New York: Plenum.

Clancy, H., & McBride, G. (1975). The isolation syndrome in childhood. *Developmental Medicine and Child Neurology, 17,* 198–219.

Clarke-Stewart, K. A. (1973). Interactions between mothers and their young children: Characteristics and consequences. *Monographs of the Society for Research in Child Development, 38,* (Serial No. 153), 6–7.

Cleary, P. D., & Mechanic, D. (1982). Sex differences in psychological distress among married women. *Journal of Health Services, 24,* 111–121.

Cobb, S. (1976). Social support as a moderator of life stress. *Psychosomatic Medicine, 38,* 300–314.

Cohen, M. I., Raphling, D. L., & Green, P. E. (1966). Psychological aspects of the maltreatment syndrome in childhood. *Journal of Pediatrics, 69,* 279–284.

Cohen, M. R., Pickar, D., Extein, I., Gold, M. S., & Sweeney, D. R. (1984). Plasma cortisol and beta-endorphin immunoreactivity in nonmajor and major depression. *American Journal of Psychiatry, 141,* 628–632.

Cohen, M. R., Pickar, D., & Dubois, M. (1981). Surgical stress and endorphins. *Lancet, 1,* 213–214.

Cohen, S., & Wills, T. A. (1985). Stress, social support, and the buffering hypothesis. *Psychological Bulletin, 98,* 310–357.

Cohen-Sandler, R., & Berman, A. L. (1980). Diagnosis and treatment of childhood depression and self-destructive behavior. *Journal of Family Practice, 11,* 51–58.

Cohen-Sandler, R., Berman, A. L., & King, R. A. (1982a). A follow-up study of hospitalized suicidal children. *Journal of American Academy of Child Psychiatry, 21,* 398–403.

Cohen-Sandler, R., Berman, A. L., & King, R. A. (1982b). Life stress and symptomology: Determinants of suicidal behavior in children. *Journal of American Academy of Child Psychiatry, 21,* 178–186.

Cohler, B. J., Grunebaum, H. U., Weiss, J. L., Gamer, E., & Gallant, D. H. (1977). Disturbance of attention among schizophrenic, depressed and well mothers and their young children. *Journal of Child Psychology and Psychiatry, 18,* 115–135.

Colbert, P., Newman, B., Ney, P., & Young, J. (1982). Learning disabilities as a symptom of depression in children. *Journal of Learning Disabilities, 15,* 333–336.

Committee on Child Psychiatry. (1982). *The process of child therapy*. New York: Brunner/Mazel.

Conger, J. C., & Farrell, A. D. (1981). Behavioral components of heterosocial skills. *Behavioral Therapy, 12,* 41–55.

Conger, J. J. (1981). Freedom and commitment: Families, youth, and social change. *American Psychologist, 36,* 1475–1484.

Connell, J. P., & Furman, W. (1984). The study of transitions: Conceptual and methodological issues. In R. N. Emde & R. J. Harmon, *Continuities and discontinuities in development* (pp. 153–173). New York: Plenum.

Conners, C. K. (1964). Visual and verbal approach motives as a function of discrepancy from expectancy level. *Perceptual and Motor Skills, 18,* 457–464.

Conners, C. K., Himmelhock, J., Goyette, C. H., Ulrich, R., & Neil, J. F. (1979). Children of parents with affective illness. *Journal of the American Academy of Child Psychiatry, 18,* 600–607.

Cotterell, J. L. (1986). Work and community influence on the quality of child rearing. *Child Development, 57,* 362–374.

Crittenden, P. M. (1985a). Maltreated infants: Vulnerability and resilience. *Journal of Child Psychology and Psychiatry, 26,* 85–96.

Crittenden, P. M. (1985b). Social networks, quality of child rearing, and child development. *Child Development, 56,* 1299–1313.

Crittenden, P.M., & Bonvillian, J. D. (1984). The Relationship between maternal risk status and maternal sensitivity. *American Journal of Orthopsychiatry, 54,* 250–262.

Crockenberg, S. B. (1981). Infant irritability, mother responsiveness, and social support influences on the security of infant–mother attachment. *Child Development, 52,* 857–865.

Crook, T., Raskin, A., & Eliot, J. (1981). Parent–child relationships and adult depressions. *Child Development, 52,* 950–957.

Crowe, R. R., Noyes, R., Pauls, D. L., & Slymen, D. (1983). A family study of panic disorder. *Archives of General Psychiatry, 40,* 1065–1069.

Cummings, S. T. (1976). The impact of the child's deficiency on the father: A study of fathers of mentally retarded and of chronically ill children. *American Journal of Orthopsychiatry, 46,* 246–255.

Cummings, S. T., Bayley, H.C., & Rie, H.E. (1966). Effects of the child's deficiency on the mother: A study of mothers of mentally retarded and of chronically ill children. *American Journal of Orthopsychiatry, 36,* 595–608.

Curran, B. E. (1979). Suicide. *Pediatric Clinics of North America, 26,* 737–746.

Curtis, G. (1963). Violence Breeds Violence. *American Journal of Psychiatry, 120,* 386–387.

Cytryn, L., McKnew, D. H., Jr., Bartko, J. J., Lamour, M., & Hamovitt, J. (1982). Offspring of patients with affective disorders: II. *Journal of American Academy of Child Psychiatry, 21,* 389–391.

Cytryn, L., McKnew, D. H., & Bunney, W. E., Jr. (1980). Diagnosis of depression in children: A reassessment. *American Journal of Psychiatry, 137,* 22–25.

Cytryn, L., McKnew, D. H., Zahn-Waxler, C., & Gershon, E. S. (1986). Developmental issues in risk research: The offspring of affectively ill parents. In M. Rutter, C. E. Izard, & P. B. Read (Eds.), *Depression in Young People,* New York: The Guilford Press.

Cytryn, L., & McKnew, T. (1974). Factors influencing the changing clinical expression of the depressive process in children. *American Journal of Psychiatry, 131,* 879–881.

Dackis, C. A., Gold, M. S., Pottash, A. L. C., & Sweeney, D. R. (1986). Evaluating depression in alcoholics. *Psychiatry Research, 17,* 105–109.

Dackis, C. A., Pottash, A. L. C., Annito, W., & Gold, M. S. (1985). *Dexamethasone suppresion test specificity for depression in opiate addicts.* New York: American Psychiatric Association meeting, May, New York.

Damon, W., & Hart, D. (1982). The development of self-understanding from infancy through adolescence. *Child Development, 53,* 841–864.

Darwin, C. (1877). A biographical sketch of an infant. *Mind—A Quarterly Review of Psychology and Philosophy, 2,* 285–294.

Davenport, Y. B., Zahn-Waxler, C., Adland, M. L., & Mayfield, A. (1984). Early child-rearing practices in families with a manic-depressive parent. *American Journal of Psychiatry, 141,* 230–235.

David, M. (1983). Early treatment of infants at risk in disturbed families. In J. D. Call, E. Galenson, & R. L. Tyson (Eds.), *Frontiers of infant psychiatry* (pp. 110–114). New York: Basic Books.

Davidson, J. (1968). Infantile depression in a "normal" child. *Journal of the American Academy of Child Psychiatry, 37,* 67–94.

Davis, J. M., & Rovee-Collier, C. K. (1983). Alleviated forgetting of a learned contingency in an 8-week-old infant. *Developmental Psychology, 19,* 353–365.

Davis, K., & Schoen, C. (1978). *Health and war on poverty: A ten-year appraisal.* Washington, DC: Brookings Institute.

Daws, D. (1985). Two papers on work in a baby clinic: Standing next to the weighing scales. *Journal of Child Psychotherapy, 11,* 77–85.

Day, R. H., & McKenzie, B. E. (1977). Constancies in the perceptual world of the infant. In W. Epstein (Ed.), *Stability and constancy in visual perception: Mechanism and processes* (pp. 285–321). New York: Wiley.

Dayton, G. O., Jones, M. H., Aiu, P., Rowson, R. A., Steele, B., & Rose, M. (1964). Developmental study of coordinated eye movements in the human infant: 1. Visual acuity in the newborn human: A study based on induced optokinetic nystagmus recorded by electro-oculography. *Archives of Ophthalmology, 71,* 865–870.

Dean, A. (1986). Social support in epidemiological perspective. In N. Lin, A. Dean, & W. Ensel (Eds.), *Social support, life events, and depression* (pp. 3–15). Orlando, FL: Academic.

Dean, A., & Lin, N. (1977). The stress buffering role of social support. *Journal of Nervous and Mental Disease, 165,* 403–413.

DeCasper, A. J., & Carstens, A. A. (1981). Contingencies of stimulation: Effects on learning and emotion in neonates. *Infant Behavior and Development, 4,* 19–35.

DeCasper, A. J., & Fifer, W. P. (1980). Of human bonding: Newborns prefer their mothers' voices. *Science, 208,* 1174–1176.

Decina, P., Kestenbaum, C. J., Farber, S., Kron, L., Gargan, M., Sackeim, H. A., & Fieve, R. R. (1983). Clinical and psychological assessment of children of bipolar probands. *American Journal of Psychiatry, 140,* 548–553.

DeFrain, J., & Eirick, R. (1981). Coping as divorced single parents: A comparative study of fathers and mothers. *Family Relations, 30,* 265–274.

DeJons, R., Rubinow, D. R., Roy-Byrne, P., Hoban, M. C., & Grover, G. N. (1985). Premenstrual mood disorder and psychiatric illness. *American Journal of Psychiatry, 142,* 1359–1361.

DeLozier, P. P. (1982). Attachment theory and child abuse. In C. M. Parkes & J. Stevenson-Hinde (Eds.), *The place of attachment in human behavior* (pp. 95–117). New York: Basic Books.

Delsordo, J.D. (1963). Protective case work for abused children. *Children, 10,* 213–218.

Derryberry, D., & Rothbart, M. K. (1984). Emotion, attention and temperament. In C. E. Izard, J. Kagan, & R. B. Zajonc (Eds.), *Emotion, cognition and behavior* (pp. 132–166). Cambridge, England: Cambridge University Press.

Deutsch, H. (1942). Some psychoanalytic observations in surgery. *Psychosomatic Medicine, 4,* 105–115.

Dietrich, K. N., Starr, R. H., & Weisfeld, G. E. (1983). Infant maltreatment: Caretaker–infant interaction and developmental consequences at different levels of parenting failure. *Pediatrics, 72,* 532–540.

Dilley, J.W., Ochtill, H.N., Perl, M., & Volberding, P.A. (1985). Findings in psychiatric consultations with patients with Acquired Immune Deficiency Syndrome. *American Journal of Psychiatry, 142,* 82–86.

Dolgoff, R., & Feldstein, D. (1984). *Understanding social welfare.* New York: Longman.

Donovan, W. L., & Leavitt, L. A. (1985). Simulating conditions of learned helplessness: The effects of interventions and attributions. *Child Development, 56,* 594–603.

Dosen, A. (1984). Depressive conditions in mentally handicapped children. *Acta Paedopsychiatrica, 50,* 29–40.

Douglas, G. (1956). Psychotic mothers. *Lancet, 1,* 124–125.

Douglas, J. W. B. (1975). Early hospital admissions and later disturbances of behaviour and learning. *Developmental Medicine and Child Neurology, 17,* 456–480.

Duncan, G. J., Coe, R. D., Corcoran, M. E., Hill, M. S., Hoffman, S. D., & Morgan, J. H. (1986). An overview of family economic mobility. In A. S. Skolnick & J. H. Skolnick (Eds.), *Family in transition* (pp. 104–120). Boston: Little, Brown.

Durkheim, E. (1951). *Suicide.* (J. A. Spaulding & G. Simpson, trans.). Glenco, IL: Free Press. (Original work published in 1897).

Earle, E. M. (1979). The psychological effects of mutilating surgery in children and adolescents. *Psychoanalytic Study of the Child, 34,* 527–546.

Earls, F. (1982). Application of DSM-III in an epidemiological study of preschool children. *American Journal of Psychiatry, 139,* 242–243.

Earls, F. (1984). The epidemiology of depression in children and adolescents. *Pediatric Annals, 13,* 23–31.

Ebeling, N. B., & Hill, D. A. (1975). *Child abuse: Intervention and treatment.* Acton, MA: Publishing Sciences Group.

Edelstein, C. K., Ray-Byrne, R., Fawzy, A. I., & Domfield, L. (1983). *Effects of weight loss on the dexamethasone suppresion test.* New York: American Psychiatric Association.

Egeland, B. (1979). Preliminary results of a prospective study of the antecedents of child abuse. *Child Abuse & Neglect, 3,* 269–278.

Egeland, B., Breitenbucher, M., & Rosenberg, D. (1980). Prospective study of the significance of life stress in the etiology of child abuse. *Journal of Consulting and Clinical Psychology, 48,* 195–205.

Egeland, B., Cicchetti, D., & Taraldson, B. (1976, April). Child abuse: A family affair. In *Proceedings of the NP Masse Research Seminar on Child Abuse* (pp. 28–52). Paris, France.

Egeland, B., & Farber, E. A. (1984). Infant–mother attachment: Factors related to its development and changes over time. *Child Development, 55,* 753–771.

Egeland, B., & Sroufe, L. A. (1981a). Attachment and early maltreatment. *Child Development, 52,* 44–52.

Egeland, B., & Sroufe, L. A. (1981b). Developmental sequelae of maltreatment in infancy. *New Directions for Child Development, 11,* 77–92.

Egeland, B., & Vaughn, B. (1981). Failure of "bond formation" as a cause of abuse, neglect, and maltreatment. *American Journal of Orthopsychiatry, 51,* 78-84.

Eiser, C., Patterson, D., & Tripp, J. H. (1984). Illness experience and children's concepts of health and illness. *Child Care Health Development, 10,* 157–162.

Elmer, E. (1967). *Children in jeopardy: A study of abused minors and their families.* Pittsburgh, PA: University of Pittsburgh Press.

Elmer, E., & Gregg, C. S. (1967). Developmental characteristics of abused children. *Pediatrics, 40,* 596–602.

Elmer, E., Gregg, G., Wright, B., Reinhart, J. B., McHenry, T., Girdony, B., Geisel, P., & Wittenberg, C. (1977). Studies of child abuse and infant accidents. In J. L. Schwartz & L. H. Schwartz (Eds.), *Vulnerable Infants.* New York: McGraw-Hill.

Emde, R. N. (1983). The prerepresentational self and its affective core. In *The psychoanalytic study of the child.* (Vol. 38, pp. 165–192). New Haven, CT: Yale University Press.

Emde, R. N., & Brown, C. (1978). Adaptation to the birth of a Down's Syndrome infant: Grieving and maternal attachment. *Journal of the American Academy of Child Psychiatry, 17,* 299–323.

Emde, R. N., Gaensbauer, T., & Harmon, R. J. (1981). Using our emotions: Some principles for appraising emotional development and intervention. In M. Lewis & L. T. Taft (Eds.),

Developmental disabilities: Theory, assessment, and intervention (pp. 409-424). New York: SP Medical & Scientific Books.

Emde, R. N., Katz, E. L., & Thorpe, J. K. (1978). Emotional expression in infancy: II. Early deviations in Down's Syndrome. In M. Lewis & L. A. Rosenblum (Eds.), *The development of affect* (pp. 351–360). New York: Plenum.

Emde, R. N., Polak, P. R., & Spitz, R. A. (1965). Analytic depression in an infant raised in an institution. *Journal of the American Academy of Child Psychiatry, 4*, 545–553.

Emde, R. N., & Sorce, J. F. (1983). The rewards of infancy: Emotional availability and maternal referencing. In J. D. Call, E. Galenson, & R. L. Tyson (Eds.), *Frontiers of infant psychiatry* (pp. 17–30). New York: Basic Books.

Engel, G. L. (1962). Anxiety and depressive–withdrawal: The primary effects of unpleasure. *The International Journal of Psychoanalysis, 43*, 89–97.

Engel, G. L., & Reichsman, F. (1956). Spontaneous and experimentally induced depressions in an infant with gastric fistula: A contribution to the problem of depression. *Journal of the American Psychiatric Association, 4*, 428–452.

Engel, G. L., Reichsman, F., Harway, V. T., & Hess, D. W. (1985). Monica: infant-feeding behavior of a mother gastric fistula-fed as an infant: a 30-year longitudinal study of enduring effects. In E. J. Anthony, & G. H. Pollock (Eds.), *Parental influences in health and disease*. Boston: Little, Brown.

Engel, G., & Schmale, A. H. (1973). Conservation–withdrawal. A primary regulatory process for organismic homeostasis. *Physiology, emotion and psychosomatic illness*. CIBA Foundation Symposium 8. Amsterdam: Excerpta Medica, 57–85.

Erickson, M. F., Sroufe, L. A., & Egeland, B. (1985). The relationship between quality of attachment and behavior problems in preschool in a high-risk sample. In I. *Monographs of the Society for Research in Child Development, 50*, 147–166.

Estroff, T. W., Herrera, C., Gaines, R., Shaffer, D., Gould, M., & Green, A. H. (1984). Maternal psychopathology and perception of child behavior in psychiatrically referred and child maltreatment families. *Journal of the American Academy of Child Psychiatry, 23*, 649–652.

Evans, S. L., Reinhart, J. B., & Succip, R. A. (1972). Failure to thrive: A study of 45 children and their families. *Journal of the American Academy of Child Psychiatry, 11*, 440–457.

Eysenck, H. J., & Eysenck, S. B. (1969). *Personality structure and measurement*. London: Routledge & Kegan Paul.

Facchinetti, F., Bagnoli, F., Bracci, R., & Genazzani, R. (1982). Plasma opioids in the first hours of life. *Pediatric Research, 16*, 95–98.

Fagen, J. W., & Ohr, P. S. (1985). Temperament and crying in response to the violation of a learned expectancy in early infancy. *Infant Behavior and Development, 8*, 157–166.

Fagen, J. W., & Rovee-Collier, C. K., (1976). Effects of quantitative shifts in a visual reinforcer on the instrumental response in infants. *Journal of Experimental Child Psychology, 21*, 349–360.

Fagen, J. W., Morrongiello, B. A., Rovee-Collier, C., & Gekowski, M. J. (1984). Expectancies and memory retrieval in three-month-old infants. *Child Development, 55*, 936–943.

Fantz, R. L., & Miranda, S. B. (1975). Newborn infant attention to form of contour. *Child Development, 46*, 224–228.

Faris, R. E., & Dunham, H. W. (1939). *Mental disorders in urban areas*. Chicago: University of Chicago Press.

Feighner, J. P., Robins, E., Guze, S. B., Woodruff, R. A., Winokur, G., & Munoz, R. (1972). Diagnostic criteria for use in psychiatric research. *Archives of General Psychiatry, 26*, 57–63.

Feinberg, M., & Carroll, B. J. (1984). 'Biological markers' for endogenous depression. *Archives of General Psychiatry, 41*, 1080–1085.

Ferguson, B. F. (1979). Preparing young children for hospitalization; a comparison of two methods. *Pediatrics, 64,* 656–664.

Fergusson, D. M., Horwood, L. J., & Shannon, F. T. (1984). Relationship of family life events, maternal depression and child-rearing problems. *Pediatrics, 73,* 773.

Fetters, L. (1981). Object permanence development in infants with motor handicaps. *Journal of Physical Therapy, 61,* 327–333.

Field, T. M. (1977). Effect of early separation, interactive deficits, and experimental manipulations on infant–mother face-to-face interaction. *Child Development, 48,* 763–771.

Field, T. M. (1984a). Early interactions between infants and their postpartum depressed mothers. *Infant Behavior and Development, 7,* 517–522.

Field, T. M. (1984b). Perinatal risk factors for infant depression. In J. D. Call, E. Galenson, & R.L. Tyson (Eds.), *Frontiers in psychiatry* (Vol. 2, pp. 152–159). New York: Basic Books.

Field, T. M., & Miller, S. (1969). Admission of children to hospital. *Ulster Medical Journal, 38,* 172–175.

Field, T. M., Vega-Lahr, N., & Jagadish, S. (1984). Separation stress of nursery school infants and toddlers graduating to new classes. *Infant Behavior and Development, 7,* 277–284.

Field, T., & Reite, M. (1984). Children's responses to separation from mother during the birth of another child. *Child Development, 55.* 1308–1316.

Field, T., Sandberg, D., Garcia, R., Vega-Lahr, N., Goldstein, S., & Guy, L. (1985). Pregnancy problems, postpartum depression and early mother–infant interactions. *Developmental Psychology, 21,* 1152–1156.

Fieve, R. R., Mendlewicz, J., & Fleiss, J. L. (1973). Manic–depressive illness: Linkage with the Xg blood group. *American Journal of Psychiatry, 130,* 1355–1359.

Fine, M. A., Moreland, J. R., & Schwebel, A. I. (1983). Long-term effects of divorce on parent-child relationships. *Developmental Psychology, 19,* 703–713.

Fineman, J. B., & Boris, M. (1983). Outcomes of early intervention: A summary of an ongoing follow-up study. In J. D. Call, E. Galenson, & R. L. Tyson (Eds.), *Frontiers of infant psychiatry* (pp. 231–234). New York: Basic Books.

Finkelstein, N. W., & Ramey, C. T. (1977). Learning to control the environment in infancy. *Child Development, 48,* 806–819.

Fischer, J., & Gochros, H. L. (1975). *Planned behavior changes.* London: Free Press.

Fischer, M., & Gottesman, I. (1980). A study of parents both hospitalized for psychiatric disorders. In L. N. Robbins, P. J. Clayton, & J. K. Wing (Eds.), *The social consequences of psychiatric illness* (pp. 77–90). New York: Brunner/Mazel.

Fisher, L., Harder, D. W., & Kokes, R. F. (1980). Child competence and psychiatric risk. III. Comparisons based on diagnosis of hospitalized parent. *Journal of Nervous and Mental Disease, 168,* 338–342.

Fisher, S.H. (1958). Skeletal manifestations of parent-induced trauma in infants and children. *Southern Medical Journal, 51,* 956–960.

Flynn, J. P. (1975). *Spouse assault: Its dimensions and characteristics in Kalamazoo County, Michigan.* Unpublished manuscript, Kalamazoo; Western Michigan University.

Fontana, V. J. (1973). *Somewhere a child is crying; Maltreatment—Causes and prevention.* New York: Macmillan.

Fontana, V. J. (1985). Child abuse, past, present, and future. *Human Ecology Forum,* 5–7.

Ford, A. B., Rushforth, N. B., & Sudak, H. S. (1984). The causes of suicide: Review and comment. In H. S. Sudak, A. B. Ford, & N. B. Rushforth (Eds.), *Suicide in the young* (pp. 159-182). Boston: John Wright-PSG.

Forsyth, D. (1934). Psychological effects of bodily illness in children. *Lancet, 2,* 15–18.

Fraiberg, S. (1982a). The adolescent mother and her infant. *Adolescent Psychiatry, 10,* 7–23.

Fraiberg, S. (1982b). Pathological defenses in infancy. *Psychoanalytic Quarterly, 51,* 612–635.

Fraiberg, S., Shapiro, V., & Cherniss, D. P. (1980). Treatment modalities. In S. Fraiberg (Ed.), *Clinical studies in infant mental health: The first year of life* (pp. 49-77). New York: Basic Books.

Frangos, E., Athanassenas, G., Tsitourides, S., Psilolignos, P., Robos, A., Katsanous, N., & Bulgaris, C. (1980). Seasonality of the episodes of recurrent affective psychoses: Possible prophylactic interventions. *Journal of Affective Disorders, 2,* 239–247.

Freedman, D. A., & Brown, S. L. (1968). On the role of coenesthetic stimulation in the development of psychic structure. *Psychoanalytic Quarterly, 37,* 418–438.

Freedman, D. A., Montgomery, J. R., Wilson, R., Bealmear, P. M., & South, M. A. (1976). Further observations on the effect of reverse isolation from birth on cognitive and affective development. *Journal of the American Academy of Child Psychiatry, 15,* 593–603.

Freeman, L. N., Poznanski, E. O., Grossman, J. A., Buschbaum, Y. Y., & Banegas, M. D. (1985). Psychotic and depressed children: A new entity. *Journal of the American Academy of Child Psychiatry, 24,* 95–102.

Freud, A. (1952). The role of bodily illness in the mental life of children. *Psychoanalytic Study of the Child, 7,* 69–81.

Freud, A. (1953). A two year-old goes to the hospital; scientific film by James Robertson. *International Journal of Psychoanalysis, 34,* 284–287.

Freud, A. (1965). Normality and pathology in childhood. *The Writings of Anna Freud 6.* New York: International Universities Press.

Freud A. (1971). Indications and contradictions for child analysis. In *Problems of psychoanalytic training, diagnosis, and the technique of therapy: 1966-1970. The writings of Anna Freud* (Vol. 7, pp. 110–123). New York: International Universities Press.

Freud, S. (1925). Instincts and their vicissitudes. *Collected Papers* (Vol. 4, pp. 60–83). London: Hogarth. (Original work published 1915).

Freud, S. (1938). *An outline of psychoanalysis.* London, England: Hogarth.

Friedman, S., Bruno, L. A., & Vietze, P. (1974). Newborn habituation to visual stimuli: A sex difference in novelty detection. *Journal of Experimental Child Psychology, 18,* 242–251.

Friedrich, W. N., & Boriskin, J. A. (1976). The role of the child in abuse: A review of the literature. *American Journal of Psychiatry, 46,* 580–590.

Friedrich, W. N., Tyler, J. D., & Clark, J. A. (1985). Personality and psychophysiological variables in abusive, neglectful, and low-income control mothers. *Journal of Nervous and Mental Disease, 173,* 449–460.

Fritz, G. K. (1980). Attempted suicide in a five-year-old boy. *Clinical Pediatrics, 19,* 448–450.

Frodi, A. M. (1981). Contribution of infant characteristics to child abuse. *American Journal of Mental Deficiency, 85,* 341–349.

Frodi, A., Bridges, L., & Grolnick, W. (1985). Correlates of mastery-related behavior: A short-term longitudinal study of infants in their second year. *Child Development, 56,* 1291–1298.

Frodi, A., & Thompson, N. (1985). Infant's affective responses in the Strange Situation: Effects of prematurity and of quality of attachment. *Child Development, 56,* 1280–1290.

Froman, P. K. (1971). The development of a depression scale for the Personality Inventory for Children (PIC). Unpublished manuscript. University of Minnesota.

Frommer, E. A. (1967). Treatment of childhood depression with antidepressant drugs. *British Medical Journal, 1,* 729–732.

Frommer, E. A., & O'Shea, G. (1973). Antenatal identification of women liable to have problems managing their infants. *British Journal of Psychiatry, 123,* 149–156.

Furman, E. (1957). Treatment of under-fives by way of their parents. *The Psychoanalytic Study of the Child, 12,* 250–262.

Furman, E. (1984). Some difficulties in assessing depression and suicide in childhood. In H. S. Sudak, A. B. Ford, & N. B. Rushforth (Eds.), *Suicide in the young* (pp. 245–258). Boston: J. Wright, PSG.

Furman, R.A. (1964). Death and the young child: Some preliminary considerations. *Psychoanalytic Study of the Child, 19,* 321–333.

Gaensbauer, T. J. (1980). Anaclitic depression in a three-and-one-half month-old child. *American Journal of Psychiatry, 137,* 841–842.

Gaensbauer, T. J. (1982). Regulation of emotional expression in infants from two contrasting caretaker environments. *Journal of the American Academy of Child Psychiatry, 21,* 163–171.

Gaensbauer, T. J., Connell, J. P., & Schultz, L. A. (1983). Emotion and attachment: Interrelationships in a structured laboratory paradigm. *Developmental Psychology, 19,* 815–831.

Gaensbauer, T. J., & Emde, R. N. (1979). *Patterning of emotional expression in a playroom laboratory situation. 2,* 162–178.

Gaensbauer, T. J., Harmon, R. J., Cytryn, L., & McKnew, D. (1984a). Social and affective development in infants with a manic–depressive parent. *American Journal of Psychiatry, 141,* 223–229.

Gaensbauer, T. J., Harmon, R. J., & Mrazek, D. (1980). Affective behaviour patterns in abused and/or neglected infants. In N. Frude (Ed.), *Psychological approaches to child abuse* (pp. 113–136). London: Batesford Academic and Educational.

Gaensbauer, T. J., & Hiatt, S. (1984). Facial communication of emotion in early infancy. In N. A. Fox & R. J. Davidson (Eds.), *The psychobiology of affective development* (pp. 207–209). Hillsdale, NJ: Erlbaum.

Gaensbauer, T.J., Mrazek, D., & Emde, R.N. (1981). Patterning of emotional response in a playroom laboratory situation. *Infant Behavior and Development, 2,* 673–691.

Gaensbauer, T.J., & Sands, K. (1979). Distorted affective communications in abused/neglected infants and their potential impact on caretakers. *Journal of the American Academy of Child Psychiatry, 18,* 236–250.

Galdston, R. (1965). Observations of children who have been physically abused and their parents. *American Journal of Psychiatry, 122,* 440–443.

Galdston, R. (1981). The domestic dimensions of violence: Child abuse. *Psycholanalytic Study of the Child, 36,* 391–414.

Gamer, E., Gallant, D., Grunebaum, H. U., & Bertram, J. C. (1977). Children of psychotic mothers: Performance of three-year-old children on tests of attention. *Archives of General Psychiatry, 34,* 592–597.

Garbarino, J. (1976). A Preliminary study of some ecological correlates of child abuse: The impact of socio-economic stress on mothers. *Child Development, 47,* 178–185.

Garbarino, J. (1977). The human ecology of child maltreatment: A conceptual model for research. *Journal of Marriage and the Family, 39,* 721–735.

Garbarino, J., & Gilliam, G. (1980). *Understanding abusive families.* Lexington, MA: Lexington Books.

Garber, J. (1984). The developmental progression of depression in female children. *New Directions for Child Development, 26,* 29–58.

Garfinkel, B. D., & Golombek, H. (1974). Suicide and depression in childhood and adolescence. *Canadian Medical Association Journal, 110,* 1278–1281.

Garmezy, N. (1985). Stress-resistant children: The search for protective factors. In J. E. Stevenson (Ed.), *Recent research in developmental psychopathology* (pp. 213–233). New York: Pergamon.

Garmezy, N. (1986). Developmental aspects of children's responses to the stress of separation and loss. In M. Rutter, C. E. Izard, & P. B. Read (Eds.), *Depression in young people: Developmental and critical perspectives* (pp. 297–323). New York: Guilford.

Geller, B., Cooper, T. B., Chestnut, E., Abel, H. S., & Anker, J. H. (1984). Nortriptyline Pharmacokinetic Parameters in Depressed Children and Adolescents: Preliminary Data. *Journal of Clinical Pharmacology, 4,* 265–269.

Gelles, R. J. (1973). Child abuse as psychopathology: A sociological critique and reformulation. *American Journal of Orthopsychiatry, 43,* 611–621.

Gelles, R. J., & Straus, M. A. (1979). Determinants of violence in the family: Toward a theoretical integration. In W. R. Burr, R. Hill, F. I. Nye (Eds.), *Contemporary theories about the family* (Vol. 1, pp. 549–581). New York: Free Press.

George, C., & Main, M. (1979). Social interactions of young abused children: Approach, avoidance and aggression. *Child Development, 50,* 306–318.

Gershon, E. S., Bunney, W. E., Jr., Leckman, J. F., Eerdewesh, M., & DeBauche, B. A. (1976). The inheritance of affective disorders: A review of data and hypotheses. *Behavioral Genetics, 6,* 227–261.

Gibson, E. J. (1969). *Principles of perceptual learning and development.* New York: Appelton-Century-Crofts.

Gil, D. G. (1968). Legally reported child abuse: A nationwide survey. In D. G. Gil (Ed.), *Social work practice.* New York: Columbia University Press.

Gil, D. G. (1969). Physical abuse of children: Findings and implications of a nationwide survey. *Pediatrics, 44,* suppl, 857–864.

Gil, D. G. (1970). *Violence against children: Physical child abuse in the United States.* Cambridge, MA: Harvard University Press.

Gilligan, C. (1977). In a different voice: Women's conceptions of self and morality. *Harvard Educational Review, 47,* 481–517.

Giovannoni, J.M., & Becerra, M. (1979). *Defining Child Abuse.* New York: Free Press.

Glaser, H. H., Harrison, G. S., & Lynn, D. B. (1964). Emotional implications of congenital heart disease in children. *Pediatrics, 33,* 367–379.

Glaser, K. (1968). Masked depression in children and adolescents. *Annual Progress in Child Psychiatry and Child Development, 1,* 345–355.

Glenn, J. (1978). The psychoanalysis of prelatency children. In J. Glenn (Ed.), *Child analysis and therapy* (pp. 163–203). New York: Jason Aronson.

Glenn, J., Sabot, L. M., & Bernstein, I. (1978). The role of parents in child analysis. In J. Glenn (Ed.), *Child analysis and therapy* (pp. 393–426). New York: Jason Aronson.

Gochman, D. S. (1971). Some correlates of children's health beliefs and potential health behavior. *Journal of Health and Social Behavior, 12,* 148–154.

Goldsmith, H. H., & Campos, J. J. (1982). Toward a theory of infant temperament. In R. N. Emde & R. J. Harmon (Eds.), *The development of attachment and affiliative systems* (pp. 161–193). New York: Plenum.

Gould, R.E. (1965). Suicide problems in children and adolescents. *American Journal of Psychotherapy, 19,* 228–246.

Graham, F. K. (1979). Distinguishing among orienting, defense and startle responses. In M. D. Kimmel, E. H. Van Olst, & J. F. Orlebeke (Eds.), *The orienting reflex in humans* (pp. 137–167). New York: Erlbaum.

Green, A. H. (1968). Self-destruction in physically abused schizophrenic children: Report of cases. *Archives of General Psychiatry, 19,* 171–197.

Green, A. H. (1976). Psychodynamic approach to the study and treatment of abusive parents. *Journal of the American Academy of Child Psychiatry, 15,* 414–429.

Green, A. H. (1978a). Psychopathology of abused children. *Journal of the American Academy of Child Psychiatry, 17,* 92–104.

Green, A. H. (1978b). Self-destructive behavior in battered children. *American Journal of Psychiatry, 135,* 579–582.

Green, A. H. (1983). Child abuse: Dimensions of psychological trauma in abused children. *Journal of the American Academy of Child Psychiatry, 22,* 231–237.

Green, A. H., Gaines, R., & Sandgrund, A. (1974). Child abuse: Pathological syndrome of family interaction. *American Journal of Psychiatry, 131,* 882–886.

Green, M., & Solnit, A. J. (1964). Reactions to the threatened loss of a child; a vulnerable child syndrome. *Pediatrics, 34,* 58–66.

Green, W. H., Campbell, M., & David, R. (1984). Psychosocial dwarfism: A critical review of the evidence. *Journal of the American Academy of Psychiatry, 23,* 39–48.

Greenberg, M. T. (1980). Social Interaction Between Deaf Preschoolers and Their Mothers: The Effects of Communication Method and Communication Competence. *Developmental Psychology, 16,* 465–474.

Greenberg, M. T., & Marvin, R. S. (1979). Attachment Patterns in Profoundly Deaf Preschool Children. *Merrill-Palmer Quarterly, 25,* 265–279.

Greenberg, N. H. (1970). Atypical behavior during infancy: Infant deviation in relation to behavior and personality of the mother. In E.J. Anthony & C. Coupernik (Eds.), *The child in his family* (Vol. 1, pp. 87–120). New York: Wiley.

Greenberg, R., & Field, T. (1982). Temperament ratings of handicapped infants during classroom, mother, and teacher interactions. *Journal of Pediatric Psychology, 7,* 387–405.

Greenspan, S. I. (1979). *Intellegence and adaptation: An intergeneration of psychoanalytic and Piagetian developmental psychology.* New York: International Universities Press.

Greenspan, S. I. (1981). *Psychopathology and adaptation in infancy and early childhood: Principles of clinical diagnosis and preventive intervention.* New York: International Universities Press.

Greenspan, S.I., & Porges, S.W. (1984). Psychopathology in infancy and early childhood: clinical perspectives on the organization of sensory and affective-thematic experience. *Child Development, 55,* 49–70.

Gregg, G.S., & Elmer, E. (1969). Infant Injuries: Accident or Abuse? *Pediatrics, 44,* 434–439.

Grossmann, K. E., Grossmann, K., Huber, F., & Warner, U. (1981). German children's behavior toward their mothers at 12 months and their fathers at 18 months in Ainsworth's Strange Situation. *International Journal of Behavioral Development, 4,* 157–181.

Group for the Advancement of Psychiatry (1982). The Developmental Stages. *The Process of Child Therapy.* New York: Brunner/Mazel Publishers.

Grunebaum, H., Cohler, B., & Kauffman, C. (1978). Children of depressed and schizophrenic mothers. *Child Psychiatry and Human Development, 8,* 219–228.

Guillemin, R., Vargo, T., Rossier, J., Minick, S., Ling, N., Rivier, C., Vale, W., & Bloom, F. (1977). [B]-endorphin and adrenocorticotropin are secreted concomitantly by the pituitary gland. *Science, 197,* 1367–1369.

Gunn, P., Berry, P., & Andrews, R. J. (1983). The temperament of Down's Syndrome toddlers: A research noted. *Journal of Child Psychology and Psychiatry, 24,* 601–605.

Gunnar, M. R. (1980). Control, warning signals, and distress in infancy. *Developmental Psychology, 16,* 281–289.

Gunnar, M. R., Malone, S., Vance, G., & Fische, R. O. (1985). Coping with aversive stimulation in the neonatal period: Quiet sleep and plasma cortisol levels during recovery from circumcision. *Child Development, 56,* 824–834.

Gunnar, M. R., & Stone, C. (1984). The effects of positive maternal affect on infant responses to pleasant, ambiguous, and fear-provoking toys. *Child Development, 55,* 1231–1236.

Gutai, J., George, R., Koeff, S., & Bacon, G. E. (1972). Adrenal response to physical stress and the effect of adrenocorticotropic hormone in newborn infants. *Journal of Pediatrics, 81,* 719–725.

Haber, R. M. (1958). Discrepancy from adaption level as a source of affect. *Journal of Experimental Psychology, 56,* 370–375.

Haggerty, R. J. (1968). Diagnosis and treatment: Tonsils and adenoids—A problem revisited. *Pediatrics, 41,* 815–817.

Halbreich, U., & Endicott, J. (1985). Relationship of dysphoric premenstrual changes to depressive disorders. *Acta-Psychiatry-Scandinavia, 71,* 331–338.

Hampton, R. L., & Newberger, E. H. (1985). Child abuse incidence and reporting by hospitals: Significance of severity, class, and race. *American Journal of Public Health, 75,* 56–60.

Harmon, R. J., Morgan, G. A., & Glicken, M. S. W. (1984). Continuities and discontinuities in affective and cognitive–motivational development. *Child Abuse & Neglect, 8,* 157–167.

Harmon, R. J., Morgan, G. H., & Klein, R. P. (1977). Determinants of normal variation in infants' negative reactions to unfamiliar adults. *Journal of Child Psychiatry, 16,* 670–683.

Harmon, R. J., Wagonfeld, S., & Emde, R. N. (1982). Anaclitic depression: A follow-up from infancy to puberty. *The Psychoanalytic Study of the Child, 37,* 67–94.

Harris, P., & MacFarlane, A. (1974). The growth of the effective visual field from birth to seven weeks. *Journal of Experimental Child Psychology, 18,* 340–348.

Harter, S. (1974). Pleasure derived by children from cognitive challenge and mastery. *Child Development, 45,* 661–669.

Harter, S. (1977). The effects of social reinforcement and task difficulty level on the pleasure derived by normal and retarded children from cognitive challenge and mastery. *Journal of Experimental Child Psychology, 24,* 476–494.

Harter, S. (1978). Effectance motivation reconsidered: Toward a developmental model. *Human Development, 21,* 34–64.

Harter, S. (1982). The perceived competence scale for children. *Child Development, 53,* 87–97.

Harter, S. (1983). Developmental perspectives on the self-system. In E. M. Hetherington (Ed.), *Handbook of child psychology: Vol. 4. Socialization, personality and social development* (pp. 275–385). New York: Wiley.

Harter, S., & Pike, R. (1984). The pictorial scale of perceived competence and social acceptance for young children. *Child Development, 55,* 1969–1982.

Harvey, D. H. P., & Greenway, A. P. (1982). How parent attitudes and emotional reactions affect their handicapped child's self-concept. *Psychological Medicine, 12,* 357–370.

Harvey, D. H., & Greenway, A. P. (1984). The self-concept of physically handicapped children and their non-handicapped siblings: An empirical investigation. *Journal of Child Psychology and Psychiatry, 25,* 273–284.

Helfer, R. E. (1975). The relationship between lack of bonding and child abuse and neglect. In M. H. Klaus, T. Leger, & M. A. Trause (Eds.), *Maternal attachment and mothering disorders: A round table.* Skillman, N.J.: Johnson & Johnson Baby Products Company.

Helfer, R. E., McKinney, J. P., & Kempe, R. (1976). Arresting or freezing the developmental process. In R. E. Helfer & C. H. Kempe (Eds.), *Child abuse and neglect: The family and the community* (pp. 55–73). Cambridge, MA: Ballinger.

Hellekson, C.J., Kline, J.A., & Rosenthal, N.E. (1986). Phototherapy for seasonal affective disorder in Alaska. *American Journal of Psychiatry, 143,* 1035–1037.

Helzer, J. E., Robins, L. N., Croughan, J. L., & Welner, A. (1981). Renard diagnostic interview: its reliability and procedural validity with physicians and lay interviewers. *Archives of General Psychiatry, 38,* 393–398.

Henderson, N. D. (1982). Human behavior genetics. *Annual Review of Psychology, 33,* 403–440.

Henderson, S. (1981). Social relationships, adversity and neurosis: An analysis of prospective observations. *British Journal of Psychiatry, 138,* 391–398.

Henderson, S., Byrne, D. G., & Duncan-Jones, P. (1981). *Neurosis and the social environment.* New York: Academic.

Herrenkohl, R. C., & Herrenkohl, E. C. (1981). Some antecedents and developmental consequences of child maltreatment. *New Directions for Child Development, 11,* 57–76.

Herrenkohl, R. C., Herrenkohl, E. C., & Egolf, B. (1983a). Circumstances surrounding the occurrence of child maltreatment. *Journal of Consulting and Clinical Psychology, 51,* 424–431.

Herrenkohl, R. C., Herrenkohl, E. C., & Toedter, L. J. (1983b). Perspectives on the intergenerational transmission of abuse. In D. Finkelhor, R. J. Gelles, G. T. Hotaling (Eds.), *The dark side of families* (pp. 305–316). Beverly Hills, CA: Sage.

Herrenkohl, R. C., Herrenkohl, E. C., Toedter, L. J., & Yanushefski, A. M. (1984). Recent studies in child abuse: Parent child interactions in abusive and nonabusive families. *Journal of the American Academy of Child Psychiatry, 23,* 641–648.

Hiatt, S., Campos, J. J., & Emde, R. N. (1979). Facial patterning and infant emotional expression: Happiness, surprise, and fear. *Child Development, 50,* 1020–1035.

Higgins, E. T. R., Klein, R., & Strauman, T. (1985). Self-concept discrepancy theory: a psychological model for distinguishing among different aspects of depression and anxiety. *Social Cognition, 3,* 5176.

Hindeman, M. (1977). Child abuse and neglect: The Alcohol connection. *Alcohol, Health and Research World, 3,* 2–7.

Hirschfeld, R. M. A., Klerman, G. L., Clayton, P. J., & Keller, M. B. (1983). Personality and depression. *Archives of General Psychiatry, 40,* 993–998.

Hoffman, M. L. (1977). Empathy, its development and prosocial implications. *Nebraska Symposium on Motivation, 25,* 169–217.

Hoffman, M. L. (1982a). Development of prosocial motivation: Empathy and guilt. In N. Eisenberg (Ed.), *The development of prosocial behavior* (pp. 281–313). New York: Academic.

Hoffman, M. L. (1982b). The measurement of empathy. In C. E. Izard (Ed.), *Measuring emotions in infants and children* (pp. 279–296). Cambridge, England: Cambridge University Press.

Hoffman, M. L. (1984). Interaction of affect and cognition in empathy. In C. E. Izard, J. Kagan, & R. B. Zajonc (Eds.), *Emotions, cognition and behavior* (pp. 103–131). Cambridge, England: Cambridge University Press.

Holinger, P. C. (1980). Violent deaths as a leading cause of mortality: An epidemiologic study of suicide, homicide and accidents. *American Journal of Psychiatry, 137,* 472–476.

Holland, Jimmie C., & Tross, Susan (1985). The Psychosocial and neuropsychiatric sequelae of the acquired immunodeficiency syndrome and related disorders. *Annals of Internal Medicine, 103,* 760–764.

Hollenbeck, A. R., Susman, E. J., Nannis, E. D., Strope, B. E., Herson, S. P., Levine, A. S., & Pizzo, P. A. (1980). Children with serious illness: Behavioral correlates of separation and isolation. *Child Psychiatry and Human Development, 11,* 3–11.

Hollingshead, A., & Redlich, F. (1958). *Social class and mental illness.* New York: Wiley.

Holmes, S. (1976). The use of control by a hospitalized five-year-old girl. *Maternal-Child Nursing Journal, 5,* 189–197.

Holmes, T., & Masuda, N. (1974). Life change and illness susceptibility. In B. S. Dohrenwend & B. P. Dohrenwend (Eds.), *Stressful life events: Their nature and effects* (pp. 45–78). New York: Wiley.

Holmes, T., & Rahe, R., (1967). The social readjustment rating scale. *Journal of Psychosomatic Research, 11,* 213–218.

Holter, J.C., & Friedman, S.B. (1968). Principles of management in child abuse cases. *American Journal of Orthopsychiatry, 38,* 127–136.

Hopkins, J. R., Zelazo, P. R., Jacobson, S. W., & Kagan, J. (1976). Infant reactivity to stimulus–schema discrepancy. *Genetic Psychology Monographs, 93,* 27–62.

Hourcade, J. J., & Parette, H. P. (1986). Early intervention programming: Correlates of progress. *Perceptual and Motor Skills, 62,* 58.

House, J. S., Robbins, C., & Metzner, H. L. (1982). The association of social relationships and activities with mortality: Prospective evidence from the Tecumseh Community Health Study. *American Journal of Epidemiology, 116,* 123–140.

Howells, J. G. (1956). Day foster-care and the nursery. *Lancet, 1,* 1254–1255.

Howells, J. G. (1963). Child-parent separation as a therapeutic procedure. *American Journal of Psychiatry, 119,* 922–926.

Howells, J. G., & Layng, J. (1955). Separation experiences and mental health: A Statistical study. *Lancet, 2,* 285–288.

Hubert, N. C., Wachs, T. D., Peters-Martin, P., & Gandour, M. J. (1982). The study of early temperament: Measurement and conceptual issues. *Child Development, 53,* 571–600.

Hudson, J. I., Laffer, P. S., & Pope, H. G., Jr. (1982). Bulimia related to affect disorder by family history and response to the dexamethasone suppression test. *American Journal of Psychiatry, 139,* 685–687.

Hug-Hellmuth, H. (1965). The Child's concept of death. Trans. from Das Kind und seine Vorsellung vom Tode in Imago, I:286. 1912 by Kris, A.O. *Psychoanalytic Quarterly, 34,* 499–516.

Hunter, R. S., Kilstron, N., Kraybill, E. N., & Loda, F. (1978). Antecedents of child abuse and neglect in premature infants: A Prospective study in a newborn intensive care unit. *Pediatrics, 61,* 629–635.

Husain, S. A., & Vandiver, T. (1984). *Suicide in children and adolescents.* New York: Spectrum.

Hyson, M. C., & Izard, C. E. (1985). Continuities and changes in emotion expressions during brief separation at 13 and 18 months. *Developmental Psychology, 21,* 1165–1170.

Illingworth, R. S., & Holt, K. S. (1955). Children in hospital; some observations on their reactions with special reference to daily visiting. *Lancet, 2,* 1257–1262.

Izard, C. E. (1977). *Human emotions.* New York: Plenum.

Izard, C. E. (1979). *The maximally discriminative facial movement coding system (MAX).* Newark, Delaware: University of Delaware Instruction Resources Center.

Izard, C. E., & Buechler, S. (1982). Theoretical perspectives on emotions in developmental disabilities. In M. Lewis & L. T. Taft (Eds), *Developmental disabilities: Theory, assessment, and intervention* (pp. 353–369). New York: SP Medical & Scientific Books.

Izard, C. E., Huebner, R. R., Risser, D., McGinnis, G., & Dougherty, L. (1980). The young infant's ability to produce discrete emotion expressions. *Developmental Psychology, 16,* 132–140.

Izard, C. E., & Schwartz, G. M. (1986). Patterns of emotion in depression. In M. Rutter, C.E. Izard, & P.B. Read (Eds.), *Depression in young people: Developmental and critical perspectives.* New York: Guilford.

Jacob, T., Dunn, N. J., & Leonard, K. (1983). Pattern of alcohol abuse and family stability. *Alcoholism: Clinical and Experimental Research, 17,* 105–109.

Jacobs, J. W. (1982). The effect of divorce on fathers: An overview of the literature. *American Journal of Psychiatry, 139,* 1235–1241.

Jacobziner, H. (1965). Attempted suicides in adolescence. *Journal of the American Medical Association, 191,* 7–11.

Jaudes, P. K., & Diamond, L. J. (1985). The Handicapped Child and Child Abuse. *Child Abuse and Neglect: The International Journal, 9,* 341–347.

Jellinek, M. S., & Slovik, L. S. (1981). Divorce: Impact on children. *The New England Journal of Medicine, 305,* 557–560.

Jensen, R. A. (1955). The hospitalized child: Round Table 1954. *American Journal of Orthopsychiatry, 25,* 293–318.

Jessner, L., Blom, G. E., & Waldfogel, S. (1952). Emotional implications of tonsillectomy and adenoidectomy on children. *Psychoanalytic Study of the Child, 7,* 126–169.

Johnson, B., & Morse, H. A. (1968). Injured children and their parents. *Children, 15,* 147–152.

Jordan, M. K., & O'Grady, D. J. (1982). Children's health beliefs and concepts: Implications for child health care. In P. Karoly, J. J. Steffen, & D. J. O'Grady (Eds.), *Child health psychology: Concepts and issues.* New York: Pergamon.

Justice, B., & Duncan, D. F. (1975). Physical abuse of children. *Public Health Reviews, 4,* 183–200.

Kagan, J. (1981). *The second year.* Cambridge: Harvard University Press.

Kagan, J. (1982). Comments on the construct of difficult temperament. *Merrill Palmer Quarterly, 8,* 21–24.

Kagan, J. (1983). Retrieval difficulty in reading disability. *Topics in Learning and Learning Disabilities, 3,* 75–83.

Kagan, J. (1984). Continuity and change in the opening years of life. In R. N. Emde & R. J. Harmon (Eds.), *Continuities and discontinuities in development* (pp. 15-39). London: Plenum.

Kalin, N. H., & Carnes, M. (1984). Biological correlates of attachment bond disruption in human and nonhuman primates. *Progress in Neuropsychopharmacology and Biological Psychiatry, 8,* 459–469.

Kaplan, B. H., Cassel, J. C., & Gore, S. (1977). Social support and health. *Medical Care, 15,* 47–58.

Kaplan, S. J., Pelcovitz, D., Salzinger, S., & Ganeles, D. (1983). Psychopathology of parents of abused and neglected children and adolescents. *Journal of the American Academy of Child Psychiatry, 22,* 238–244.

Kaplan, S. J., & Zitrin, A. (1983a). Psychiatrists and child abuse. I. Case assessment by child protective services. *Journal of the American Academy of Child Psychiatry, 22,* 253–256.

Kaplan, S. J., & Zitrin, A. (1983b). Psychiatrists and child abuse. II. Case assessment by hospitals. *Journal of the American Academy of Child Psychiatry, 22,* 257–261.

Kashani, J., Barbero, G. J., & Bolander, F. (1981a). Depression in hospitalized pediatric patients. *Journal of the American Academy of Child Psychiatry, 20,* 123–134.

Kashani, J. H., Barbero, G. J., & Bolander, F. D. (1981b). Depression in hospitalized pediatric patients. *Journal of the American Academy of Child Psychiatry, 20,* 123–134.

Kashani, J., Burk, J. P., & Reid, J. C. (1985). Depressed children of depressed parents. *Canadian Journal of Psychiatry, 30,* 265–269.

Kashani, J. H., & Cantwell, D. P. (1983). Characteristics of children admitted to inpatient community mental health centers. *Archives of General Psychiatry, 40,* 397–401.

Kashani, J. H., & Carlson, G. A. (1985). Major depressive disorder in a preschooler. *Journal of the American Academy of Child Psychiatry, 24,* 490–494.

Kashani, J. H., Carlson, G. A., Horwitz, E., & Reid, R. C. (1985). Dysphoric mood in young children referred to a child development unit. *Child Psychiatry and Human Development, 15,* 234–242.

Kashani, J., Husain, A., Shekim, W. O., Hodges, K. K., Cytryn, L., & McKnew, D. H. (1981). Current perspectives on childhood depression. *American Journal of Psychiatry, 138,* 143–153.

Katz, J. (1979). Depression in the young child. In J. Nowells (Ed.), *Modern perspectives in the psychiatry of infancy* (pp. 435–449). New York: Brunner/Mazel.

Kauffman, C., Grunebaum, H., Cohler, B., & Gamer, E. (1979). Superkids: Competent children of psychotic mothers. *American Journal of Psychiatry, 136,* 1398–1402.

Kauppila, A., Simila, S., Ylikorkala, O., Koivisto, M., Makela, P., & Haapalahti, J. (1976). ACTH levels in maternal, fetal and neonatal plasma after short-term prenatal dexamethasone therapy. *British Journal of Obstetrics and Gynecology, 84,* 124–128.

Kavanagh, C. (1982). Emotional abuse and mental injury: A critique of the concepts and a recommendation for practice. *Journal of the American Academy of Child Psychiatry, 21,* 171–177.

Kazdin, A. E., Sherick, R. B., Esveldt-Dawson, K., & Rancurello, M. D. (1985). Nonverbal behavior and childhood depression. *Journal of the American Academy of Child Psychiatry, 24,* 303–309.

Keller, A., Ford, L. H., & Meacham, J. A. (1978). Dimensions of self-concept in preschool children. *Developmental Psychology, 14,* 483–489.

Keller, M. B., Lavori, P. W., Rice, J., Coryell, W., & Hirschfeld, R. M. A. (1986). The persistent risk of chronicity in recurrent episodes of nonbipolar major depressive disorder: A prospective follow-up. *American Journal of Psychiatry, 143,* 24–28.

Keller, M. B., & Shapiro, R. W. (1982). 'Double depression': Superimposition of acute depressive episodes on chronic depressive disorders. *American Journal of Psychiatry, 139,* 438–442.

Keller, M. B., Shapiro, R. W., Lavori, P. W., & Wolfe, N. (1982). Relapse in major depressive disorder: analysis with the life table. *Archives of General Psychiatry, 39,* 911–915.

Kelly, J. B., & Wallerstein, J. S. (1976). The effects of parental divorce: Experiences of the child in early latency. *American Journal of Orthopsychiatry, 46,* 20–32.

Kempe, C. H., Silverman, F. N., & Steele, B. F. (1962). The battered child syndrome. *Journal of the American Medical Association, 181,* 17–240.

Kempe, R. S., & Kempe, C. H. (1978). *Child Abuse.* Cambridge, MA: Harvard University Press.

Kendler, K. S., & Eaves, L. J. (1986). Models for the joint effect of genotype and environment on liability to psychiatric illness. *The American Journal of Psychiatry, 143,* 279–289.

Kennerley, H., & Gath, D. (1985). Maternity blues reassessed. *Psychiatric Developments, 1,* 1–17.

Kenny, T. J. (1975). The hospitalized child. *Pediatric Clinics of North America, 22,* 583–593.

Kerkhofs, M., Hoffmann, G., DeMartelaere, V., Linkowski, A., & Mendlewica, J. (1985). Sleep EEG recordings in depressive disorders. *Journal of Affective Disorders, 9,* 47–53.

Kernberg, P. F. (1984). Reflections in the mirror: Mother–child interactions, self-awareness, and self-recognition. In J. D. Call, E. Galenson, & R. Tyson (Eds.), *Frontiers of infant psychiatry* (pp. 101–110). New York: Basic Books.

Kestenberg, J. S., & Buelte, A. (1983). Prevention, infant therapy, and the treatment of adults, III: Periods of vulnerability in transition from stability to mobility and vice versa. In J.D. Call, E. Galenson, & R.L. Tyson (Eds.), *Frontiers of infant psychiatry* (pp. 200–216). New York: Basic Books.

Kim, S. P., & Ferrara, A., (1980). *Comparative temperament profiles of children with chronic diseases.* Presented at the 28th annual meeting of the American Academy of Child Psychiatry.

Kim, S. P., Ferrara, A., & Chess, S. (1980). Temperament in asthmatic children. *Journal of Pediatrics, 97,* 483-486.

Kim, S. P., Ferrara, A., Mattsson, A., & Chess, S. (1981). *Comparative temperament profiles for children with chronic diseases.* Presented at the 28th Annual Meeting of the American Academy of Child Psychiatry.

Kitzinger, M., & Hunt, H. (1985). The effect of residential setting on sleep and behavior patterns of young visually handicapped-children. In J. E. Stevenson (Ed.), *Recent research in developmental psychopathology* (pp. 73–80). New York: Pergamon.

Klaus, M. H., & Kennell, J. L. (1970). Mothers separated from their newborn infants. *Pediatric Clinics of North America, 17,* 1015–1037.

Klaus, M. H., & Kennell, J. H. (1976). *Mother–infant bonding.* St. Louis, MO: Mosby.

Klee, S. H., & Garfinkel, B. D. (1984). Identification of depression in children and adolescents: the role of the dexamethasone suppression test. *Journal of the American Academy of Child Psychiatry, 23,* 410–415.

Klein, D. C., & Seligman, M. E. P. (1976). Reversal of performance deficits in learned helplessness and depression. *Journal of Abnormal Psychology, 85,* 11–26.

Klein, D. F. (1982). Anxiety reconceptualized. In D. F. Klein & J. A. Robkins (Eds.), *Anxiety: New research and current concepts.* New York: Raven.

Klein, D. K., Depue, R. A., & Slater, J. F. (1985). Cyclothymia in the adolescent offspring of parents with bipolar affective disorder. *Journal of Abnormal Psychology, 94,* 115–127.

Klein, M. (1932). *The Psychoanalysis of Children.* New York: Norton.

Klein, M., & Stern, L. (1971). Low birth weight and the battered child syndrome. *American Journal of Diseases of Children, 122,* 15–18.

Klerman, G. L. (1980). Overview of affective disorders. In H. I. Kaplan, A. M. Freedman, & B. J. Saddock (Eds.) *Comprehensive textbook of psychiatry/III* (Vol. 2. pp. 1305-1319). Boston: Williams & Wilkins.

Klermen, G. L., & Weissman, M. M. (1982). Interpersonal psychotherapy: Theory and research. In J. Rush (Ed.) *Short Term Psychotherapies for Depression.* New York: Guilford Press, 86–106.

Kogan, L., Smith, J., & Jenkins, S. (1977). Ecological validity of indicator data as predictors of survey findings. *Journal of Social Service Research, 1,* 117–132.

Kolin, I., Scherzer, A., New, B., & Garfield, M. (1971). Studies of the school age child with meningomyelocele: social and emotional adaption. *Journal of Pediatrics, 78,* 1013–1019.

Koocher, G. P. (1973). Childhood, death and cognitive development. *Developmental Psychology, 9,* 369–375.

Koocher, G. P. (1981). Children's conceptions of death. *New Directions for Child Development, 14,* 85–99.

Kopp, C. B. (1982). Antecedents of self-regulation: A developmental perspective. *Developmental Psychology, 18,* 199–214.

Kosky, R. (1983). Childhood suicidal behavior. *Journal of Child Psychology and Psychiatry, 24,* 457–468.

Kovacs, M. (1978). *Children's depression inventory (CDI).* Unpublished manuscript. University of Pittsburgh.

Kovacs, M., Feinberg, T., Crouse-Novak, M. A., Paulauskas, S., & Finkelstein, R. (1984a). Depressive disorders in childhood: I. a longitudinal prospective study of characteristics and recovery. *Archives of General Psychiatry, 41,* 229–237.

Kovacs, M., Feinberg, T., Crouse-Novak, M. A., Paulauskas, S., Pollock, M., & Finkelstein, R. (1984b). Depressive disorders in childhood: II. a longitudinal study of risk for subsequent major depression. *Archives of General Psychiatry, 41,* 643–649.

Kovacs, M., & Paulauskas, S. L. (1984). Developmental stage and the expression of depressive disorders in children: An empirical analysis. *New Directions for Child Development, 26,* 59–80.

Kraepelin, E. (1921). *Manic-depressive insanity and paranoia.* Edinburgh, Scotland: Livingstone.

Kramer, S., & Byerly, L. J. (1978). Technique of psychoanalysis of the latency child. In J. Glenn (Ed.), *Child analysis and therapy* (pp. 205–236). New York: Jason Aronson.

Kraus, M. A., & Redman, E. S. (1986). Postpartum depression—an interactional view. *Journal of Marital and Family Therapy, 12,* 63–74.

Kroll, P. D., Stock, D. F., & James, M. E. (1985). The Behavior of adult alcoholic men abused as children. *Journal of Nervous and Mental Disease, 173,*] 689–693.

Kun, A. (1977). Development of the magnitude covariation and compensation schemata in ability and effort attributions of performance. *Child Development, 48,* 862–873.

Kurdek, L. A., Blisk, D., & Siesky, A. E. (1981). Correlates of children's long-term adjustment to their parents' divorce. *Developmental Psychology, 17,* 565–579.

Kuyler, P. L., Rosenthal, L., Igel, G., Dunner, D. L., & Fieve, R. R. (1980). Psychopathology among children of manic-depressive patients. *Biological Psychiatry, 15,* 589–597.

Laird, J. D. (1974). Self-attribution of emotion: The effects of expressive behavior on the quality of emotional experience. *Journal of Personality and Social Psychology, 29,* 475–486.

Lamb, M. E., Gaensbauer, T. J., Malkin, C. M., & Schultz, L.A. (1985). The effects of child maltreatment on security of infant-adult attachment. *Infant Behavior and Development, 8,* 35–45.

Lambert, S. A. (1984). Variables that affect the school-age child's reaction to hospitalization and surgery: A review of the literature. *Maternal-Child Nursing Journal, 13,* 1–18.

Lamontagne, L. L. (1984). Children's locus of control beliefs as predictors of preoperative coping behavior. *Nursing Research, 33,* 76–79, 85.

Lang, P. J., Levin, D. N., Miller, G. A., & Kozak, M. J. (1983). Fear behavior, fear imagery, and the psychophysiology of emotion: The problem of affective response integration. *Journal of Abnormal Psychology, 92,* 276–306.

Langer, E. J. (1975). The illusion of control. *Journal of Personality and Social Psychology, 32,* 311–328.

Langer, W. L. (1974). Infanticide: A historical survey. *History of Childhood Quarterly, 2,* 355–365.

Langford, W. S. (1948). Physical illness and convalescence; their meaning to the child. *Journal of Pediatrics, 33,* 242.

Langford, W. S. (1961). The child in the pediatric hospital: Adaptation to illness and hospitalization. *American Journal of Orthopsychiatry, 31,* 667–684.

Langsdorf, P., Izard, C. E., Rayais, M., & Hembree, E. A. (1983). Interest expression, visual fixation, and heart rate changes in 2- to 8-month-old infants. *Development Psychology, 19,* 375–386.

Lansman, M., Farr, S., & Hunt, E. (1984). Expectancy and dual-task interference. *Journal of Experimental Psychology, 10,* 195–204.

Lapouse, R. (1966). The epidemiology of behavior disorders in children. *Journal of Affective Disorders of Children, 3,* 594–599.

Lawler, R. H., Nakielny, W., & Wright, N. A. (1966). Psychological Implications of Cystic Fibrosis. *Canadian Medical Association Journal, 94,* 1043–1046.

Leckman, J. F., Weissman, M. M., Merikangas, K. R., Pauls, D. L., & Prusoff, B. A. (1983). Panic disorder and major depression: increased risk of depression, alcoholism, panic, and phobic disorders in families of depressed probands with panic disorder. *Archives of General Psychiatry, 40,* 1055–1069.

Leifer, A. D., Leiderman, P. H., Barnett, C. R., & Williams, J. (1972). Effects of mother-infant separation on maternal attachment behavior. *Child Development, 43,* 1203–1218.

Leonard, M. F., Rhymes, J. P., & Solnitt, A. J. (1966). Failure to thrive in infants. *American Journal of Diseases of Children, 111,* 600–612.

Leonhard, K. (1957). *Aufteilung der endogenen psychosen [Classification of endogenous psychoses].* Berlin: Akademie-Verlag.

Lerner, J. V., & Galambos, N. L. (1986). Child development and family change: The influences of maternal employment on infants and toddlers. In L. P. Lipsitt & C. Rovee-Collier (Eds.), *Advances in infancy research* (pp. 39–70). Norwood, NJ: ABLEX Publishing.

Lester, B. M., Hoffman, J., & Brazelton, T. B. (1985). The rhythmic structure of mother-infant interaction in term and preterm infants. *Child Development, 56,* 15–27.

Levy, D. M. (1945). Psychic trauma of operations in children and note on combat neurosis. *American Journal of Diseases of Children, 69,* 7–25.

Lewis, D. A., Kathol, R. G., Sherman, B. M., Winokur, G., & Schlesser, M. A. (1983). Differentiation of depressive subtypes by insulin insensitivity in the recovered phase. *Archives of General Psychiatry, 40,* 167–170.

Lewis, M. (1967). Mother-infant interaction and cognitive development: A motivational construct. In V. Vaughan (Ed.), *Issues in human development* (pp. 32–37). Washington, D.C.: U.S. Government Printing Office.

Lewis, M., & Brooks-Gunn, J. (1979). *Social congition and the acquisition of self.* New York: Plenum.

Lewis, M., Brooks-Gunn, J., & Jaskir, J. (1985). Individual differences in visual self-recognition as a function of mother-infant attachment relationship. *Developmental Psychology, 21,* 1181–1187.

Lewis, M., & Goldberg, S. (1969). Perceptual-cognitive development in infancy: A generalized expectancy model as a function of the mother–infant interaction. *Merrill-Palmer Quarterly, 15,* 81–100.

Lewis, M., & Schaeffer, S. (1979). Peer behavior and mother–infant interaction in maltreated children. In M. Lewis & L. Rosenblum (Eds.), *The uncommon child: The genesis of behavior* (Vol. 3). New York: Plenum.

Lewis, M., & Schaeffer, S. (1981). Peer behavior & mother–infant interaction in maltreated children. In M. Lewis & L. A. Rosenblum (Eds.) *The Uncommon Child.* New York: Plenum, 193–224.

Lewis, M., Sullivan, M. W., & Brooks-Gunn, J. (1985). Emotional behaviour during the learning of the contingency in early infancy. *British Journal of Developmental Psychology, 3,* 307–316.

Lezak, M. D. (1978). Living with chracteristically altered brain injured patients. *Journal of Clinical Psychiatry, 39,* 592–598.

Light, R. (1973). Abused and neglected children in America: A study of alternative policies. *Harvard Educational Review, 43,* 556–598.

Lin, N. (1986a). Conceptualizing social support. In N. Lin, A. Dean, & W. Ensel (Eds.), *Social support, life events, and depression* (pp. 17–30). Orlando, FL: Academic.

Lin, N. (1986b). Epilogue: In retrospect and prospect. In N. Lin, A. Dean, & W. Ensel (Eds.), *Social support, life events, and depression* (pp. 333–342). Orlando, FL: Academic.

Lindemann, E. (1941). Observations on psychiatric sequelae to surgical procedures in women. *American Journal of Psychiatry, 98,* 132–139.

Ling, W., Oftedal, G., & Weinberg, W. A. (1970). Depressive illness in children presenting a severe headache. *American Journal of Diseases of Childhood, 120,* 122–124.

Lingjaerde, L. (1983). The biochemistry of depression. *Acta Psychiatrica Scandinavica Supplementum, 302,* 36–51.

Lichtenberg, P. (1971). Social policy: Social work contributions to the economy. In R. Morris, B. Dana, P. Glasser, R. Marks, M. Rein, P. Schreiber, & B. Saunders (Ed.), *Encyclopedia of social work* (Vol. 11, pp. 1426–1432). New York: National Association of Social Workers.

Livingston, R., Reis, C. J., & Ringdahl, I. C. (1984). Abnormal dexamethasone suppression test results in depressed and nondepressed children. *American Journal of Psychiatry, 141,* 106–108.

Lobovits, D. A., & Handal, P. J. (1985). Childhood depression: Prevalence using DSM-III criteria and validity of parent and child depression scales. *Journal of Pediatric Psychology, 10,* 45–54.

Loftus, E. F., & Grober, E. H. (1973). Retrieval from semantic memory by young children. *Developmental Psychology, 8, 310.*

Loosen, P. T., & Prange, A. J. (1982). Serum thyrotropin response to thyrotrypsin-releasing hormone in psychiatric patients: a review. *American Journal of Psychiatry, 139,* 405–416.

Lourie, R. S. (1966). Clinical studies of attempted suicide in childhood. *Clinical Proceedings of the Children's Hospital of the District of Columbia, 22,* 163–173.

Lowe, T. L., & Cohen, D. J. (1980). Mania in childhood and adolescence. In R. H. Belmaker, & H. M. van Praag (Eds.), *Mania: an evolving concept* (pp. 111–117). New York: Spectrum.

Lowrey, L. G. (1940). Personality distortion and early institutional care. *American Journal of Orthopsychiatry, 10,* 576–585.

Lozoff, B., Brittenham, G. M., Trause, M. A., Kennell, J. H., & Klaus, M. H. (1977). The mother–newborn relationship: Limits of adaptability. *Journal of Pediatrics, 91,* 1–12.

Lucas, H. R., Lockett, H. J., & Grimm, F. (1965). Amitriptyline in childhood depressions. *Diseases of the Nervous System, 26,* 105–111.

Lussier, A. (1980). The physical handicap and the body ego. *International Journal of Psycho-analysis, 61,* 179–185.

Lynch, M. A. (1975). Ill-health and child abuse. *Lancet, 2,* 317–319.

Lynch, M. A., & Roberts, J., (1977). Predicting child abuse: Signs of bonding failure in the maternity hospital. *British Medical Journal, 1,* 624–626.

Lyth, I. M. (1985). The development of self in children in institutions. *Journal of Child Psychotherapy, 11,* 49–64.

MacKinnon, C. E., Brody, G. H., & Stoneman, Z. (1982). The effects of divorce and maternal employment on the home environments of preschool children. *Child Development, 53,* 1392–1399.

Mahler, M. (1958). Autism and symbiosis: Two extreme disturbances of identity. *International Journal of Psychoanalysis, 29,* 77–83.

Mahler, M. S. (1966). Notes on the development of basic moods: The depressive affect. *Selected papers of Margaret S. Mahler: Volume II, separation-individuation.* New York: Jason Aronson.

Mahler, M. S. (1972). Rapprochement subphase of the separation individuation process. *Psychoanalytic Quarterly, 41,* 487–506.

Mahler, M., Pine, F., & Bergman, A. (1975). *The psychological birth of the human infant.* New York: Basic Books.

Mahmood, T., Reveley, A. M., & Murray, R. M. (1983). Genetic studies of affective and anxiety disorders. In M. Weller (Ed.), *The scientific basis of psychiatry* (pp. 266–277). London: Bailliere Tindall.

Maier, S. F., & Seligman, M. E. P. (1976). Learned helplessness: Theory and evidence. *Journal of Experimental Psychology, 105,* 3–46.

Maier, S., Seligman, M. E., & Solomon, R. L. (1967). Fear conditioning and learned helplessness. In R. Church & B. Campbell (Eds.), *Punishment and aversive behavior* (p. 34). New York: Appleton-Century-Crofts.

Main, M. (1977). Analysis of a peculiar form of reunion behavior seen in some day-care children: Its history and sequelae in children who are home reared. In R. Webb (Ed.), *Social development in childhood: day-care programs and research* (pp. 33–78). Baltimore, MD: Johns Hopkins University Press.

Main, M. (1983). Exploration, play and cognitive functioning related to infant-mother attachment. *Infant Behavior and Development, 6,* 167–174.

Main, M., & Goldwyn, R. (1984). Predicting rejection of her infant from mother's representation of her own experience: Implications for the abused-abusing intergenerational cycle. *Child Abuse and Neglect, 8,* 203–217.

Main, M., Kaplan, N., & Cassidy, J. (1985). Security in infancy, childhood and adulthood: A move to the level of representation. *Monographs of the Society for Research in Child Development, 50,* 66–104.

Main, M., & Stadtman, J. (1981). Infant response to rejection of physical contact by the mother. *Journal of the American Academy of Child Psychiatry, 20,* 292–307.

Main, M., Tomasini, L., & Tolan, W. (1979). Differences among mothers of infants judged to differ in security. *Developmental Psychology, 15,* 472–477.

Main, M., & Weston, D. R. (1981). The quality of the toddler's relationship to mother and to father: Related to conflict behavior and readiness to establish new relationships. *Child Development, 52,* 932–940.

Main, T. F. (1958). Mothers with children in a psychiatric hospital. *Lancet, 2,* 845–847.

Mans, L., Cicchetti, D., & Sroufe, L. A. (1978). Mirror reactions of Down's Syndrome infants and toddlers: Cognitive underpinnings of self-recognition. *Child Development, 49,* 1247–1250.

Marfo, K., & Kysela, G. M. (1984). Early intervention with mentally handicapped children: A critical appraisal of applied research. *Journal of Pediatric Psychology, 10,* 305–324.

Maris, R.W., & Lazerwitz, B. (1981). *Pathways to suicide: A survery of self-destructive behaviors.* Baltimore, MD: Johns Hopkins University Press.

Martin, H. P., & Beezley, P. (1977). Behavioral observations of abused children. *Developmental Medicine and Child Neurology, 19,* 373–387.

Mason, E. A. (1965). The hospitalized child—His emotional needs. *New England Journal of Medicine, 272,* 406–414.

Masters, J. C., Barden, R.C., & Ford, M. E. (1979). Affective states, expressive behavior and learning in children. *Journal of Personality and Social Psychology, 3,* 380–390.

Masters, J. C., & Furman, W. (1976). Effects of affective states on noncontingent outcome expectancies and beliefs in internal or external control. *Developmental Psychology, 12,* 481–482.

Matas, L., Arend, R. A., & Sroufe, L. A. (1978). Continuity of adaptation in the second year: The relationship between quality of attachment and later competence. *Child Development, 49,* 547–556.

Matheny, A. P., & Dolan, A. B. (1975). Persons, situations, and time: A genetic view of behavioral change in children. *Journal of Personality and Social Psychology, 32,* 1106–1110.

Matthews, J., Akil, H., Greden, J., & Watson, S. (1982). Plasma measures of beta-endorphin-like immunoreactivity in depressives and other psychiatric subjects. *Life Sciences, 31,* 1867–1870.

Mattsson, A. (1972). Long-term physical illness in childhood: A challenge to psychosocial adaptation. *Pediatrics, 50,* 801–811.

Mattsson, A., Seese, L. R., & Hawkins, J. W. (1969). Suicidal behavior as child psychiatric emergency: Clinical characteristics and follow-up results. *Archives of General Psychiatry, 20,* 0–109.

Maziad, M., Cote, R., Boudreault, M., Thivierge, J., & Caperaa, P. (1984). The New York longitudinal studies' model of temperament: gender differences and demographic correlates in a French-speaking population. *Journal of the American Academy of Child Psychiatry, 23,* 582–587.

McCall, R. B. (1970a). IQ pattern over age: Comparisons among siblings and parent-child pairs. *Science, 170,* 644–648.

McCall, R. B. (1970b). The use of multivariate procedures in developmental psychology. In P. Mussen (Ed.), *Carmichael's manual of child psychology* (3rd ed. pp. 1366–1378). New York: Wiley.

McCall, R. B., (1970c). Attention in the infant: avenue to the study of cognitive development. In D. M. Walcher and D. L. Peters (Eds.), *Early childhood: the development of self-regulation* (pp. 107–140). New York: Putnam.

McCall, R. B. (1972). Similarity in IQ profile among related pairs: Infancy and childhood. *Proceedings of the 80th Annual Convention of the American Psychological Association, 7,* 79–80.

McCall, R. B. (1977). Challenges to a science of developmental psychology. *Child Development, 48,* 333–344.

McCall, R. B. (1981). Nature–nurture and the two realms of development: A proposed integration with respect to mental development. *Child Development, 52,* 1–12.

McCall, R. B. (1983). Environmental effects on intelligence: The forgotten realm of discontinuous nonshared within-family factors. *Child Development, 54,* 408–415.

McCall, R. B. (1985). The confluence model and theory. *Child Development, 56,* 217–218.

McCall, R. B., Appelbaum, M. I., & Hogarty, P. S. (1973a). Developmental changes in mental performance. *Monographs of the Society for Research in Child Development, 38,* (3, Serial No. 150), 1–83.

McCall, R. B., Hogarty, P. S., Hamilton, J. S., & Vincent, J. H. (1973b). Habituation rate and the infant's response to visual discrepancies. *Child Development, 44,* 280–287.

McCall, R. B., & Kagan, J. (1967). Stimulus-schema discrepancy and attention in the infant. *Journal of Experimental Child Psychology, 5,* 381–390.

McCall, R. B., & McGhee, P. E. (1977). The discrepancy hypothesis of attention and affect in infants. In I. C. Uzgiris & F. Weizmann (Eds.), *The structuring of experience* (pp. 179–210). New York: Plenum.

McCall, R. B., & Melson, W. H. (1969). Attention in infants as a function of magnitude of discrepancy and habituation rate. *Psychonomic Science, 17,* 317–319.

McCall, R. B., & Kagan, J. (1970). Individual differences in the infant's distribution of attention to stimulus discrepancy. *Developmental Psychology, 2,* 90–98.

McCarthy, E., & Kozak, L. J. (1985). Hospital use by children: United States, 1983. *NCHS Advancedata, 109,* 1–16.

McCollum, A. T., & Gibson, L. E. (1970). Family adaptation to the child with cystic fibrosis. *Journal of Pediatrics, 77,* 571–578.

McConville, B. J., Boag, L. C., & Purchit, A. P. (1973). Three types of childhood depression. *Canadian Psychiatric Association Journal, 18,* 133–138.

McDevitt, J. B. (1975). Separation-individuation and object constancy. *Journal of the American Psychoanalytic Association, 23,* 713–742.

McGuire, D. J. (1982). The problem of children's suicide: Ages 5-14. *Internal Journal of Offender Therapy and Comparative Criminology, 26,* 10–17.

McGuire, L. L., & Meyers, C. E. (1971). Early Personality in the Congenitally Blind Child. *New Outlook, 65,* 137–143.

McIntire, M. S., Angle, C. R., & Schlicht, M. L. (1977). Suicide and self-poisoning in pediatrics. *Advances in Pediatrics, 24,* 291–309.

McKnew, D. H., & Cytryn, L. (1973). Historical background in children with affective disorders. *American Journal of Psychiatry, 130,* 178–180.

McKnew, D. H., & Cytryn, L. (1979). Urinary metabolites in chronically depressed children. *Journal of the American Academy of Child Psychiatry, 18,* 608–615.

McKnew, D. H., Cytryn, L., Efron, M. A., Gershon, E. S., & Bunney, W. E. (1979). Offspring of parents with affective disorders. *British Journal of Psychiatry, 134,* 148–152.

Meadow, K. P., Greenberg, M. T., & Erting, C. (1983). Attachment behavior of dcaf parents. *Journal of American Academy of Child Psychiatry, 22,* 23–28.

Melnick, B., & Hurley, J. R. (1969). Distinctive personality attributes of child-abusing mothers. *Journal of Consulting and Clinical Psychology, 33,* 746–749.

Menahem, S. (1984). Possible conservation-withdrawal in two infants. *Developmental and Behavioral Pediatrics, 5,* 361–363.

Mendlewicz, J., & Rainer, J. D. (1977). Adoption study supporting genetic transmission in manic-depressive illness. *Nature, 268,* 327–329.

Menninger, K. A. (1938). *Man against himself.* New York: Harcourt Brace.

Merikangas, K. R., Leckman, J. F., Prusoff, B. A., Pauls, D. L., & Weissman, M. M. (1985). Familial transmission of depression and alcoholism. *Archives of General Psychiatry, 42,* 367–372.

Merril, E. J. (1962). Physical Abuse of Children: an agency study. In V. de Francis (Ed.), Protecting the Battered Child. Denver: American Humane Association.

Meyendorf, R. (1971). Infant depression due to separation from siblings syndrome or depression retardation starvation and neurological symptoms: a reevaluation of the concept of maternal deprivation. *Psychiatric Clinics, 4,* 321–335.

Meyers, C. E., Zetlin, A., & Blacher-Dixon, J. (1981). The family as affected by schooling for severely retarded children: An invitation to research. *Journal of Community Psychology, 9,* 306–315.

Michaels, J. J. (1943). Psychiatric implications of surgery. *Family, 23,* 363–369.

Milowe, I. D., & Lourie, R. S. (1964). The child's role in the battered child syndrome. *Journal of Pediatrics, 65,* 1079–1081.

Minde, K. K., Marton, P., Manning, D., & Hines, B. (1980). Some determinants of mother–infant interaction in the premature nursery. *Journal of the American Academy of Child Psychiatry, 19,* 1–21.

Minde, K. K., & Minde, R. (1981). Psychiatric intervention in infancy. *Journal of the American Academy of Child Psychiatry, 20,* 217–238.

Minde, K. K., Whitelaw, A., Brown, J., Brown, J., & Fitzhardinge, P. (1983). Effect of neonatal complications in premature infants on early parent–infant interactions. *Developmental Medicine and Child Neurology, 25,* 763–777.

Mintzer, D., Als, H., Tronick, E.Z., & Brazelton, T. B. (1984). Parenting an infant with a birth defect. *Psychoanalytic Study of the Child, 39,* 561–589.

Mishne, J. M. (1983). *Clinical work with children.* New York: Free Press.

Mitchell, R. E., Billings, A. G., & Moos, R. H. (1982). Social support and well-being: Implications for prevention programs. *Journal of Primary Prevention, 3,* 77–98.

Mittelmann, B. (1954). Motility in infants, children, and adults: Patterning and psychodynamics. *Psychoanalytic Study of the Child, 9,* 142–177.

Miyake, K., Chen, S. J., & Campos, J. J. (1985). Infant temperament, mother's mode of interaction, and attachment in Japan: An interim report. *Monographs of the Society for Research in Child Development, 50,* 276–297.

Molla, P. M. (1981). Self-concept in children with and without physical disabilities. *Journal of Psychiatric Nursing and Mental Health Services, 19,* 22–27.

Monane, M., Leitcher, D., & Lewis, D. O. (1984). Physical abuse in psychiatrically hospitalized children and adolescents. *Journal of the American Academy of Child Psychiatry, 23,* 653–658.

Money, J. (1977). The syndrome of abuse dwarfism (psychosocial dwarfism or reversible hyposomatotropism). *American Journal of Diseases of Children, 131,* 508–513.

Moos, R. H., & Billings, A. G. (1982). Children of alcoholics during the recovery period. *Addictive Behaviors, 7,* 155–163.

Mordock, J. B. (1979). The separation–individuation process and developmental disabilities. *Exceptional Children, 46,* 176–184.

Morris, A. G. (1973). Parent education for child education being carried out in a pediatric clinic playroom. *Clinical Pediatrics, 12,* 235–239.

Morris, A. G. (1974). Conducting a parent education program in a pediatric clinic playroom. *Children Today, 3,* 11–14.

Morris, M. G., & Gould, R. W. (1963). Neglected children. Role reversal: A necessary concept in dealing with the "battered child syndrome." *American Journal of Orthopsychiatry, 33,* 298–299.

Morrison, G. C., & Collier, J. G. (1969). Family treatment approaches to suicidal children and adolescents. *Journal of the American Academy of Child Psychiatry, 8,* 140–153.

Morse, W., Sahler, O. J., & Friedman, S. B. (1970). A three-year follow-up study of abused and neglected children. *American Journal of Diseases of Children, 120,* 439–446.

Moynihan, D. P. (1986). *Family and nation.* New York: Harcourt, Brace and Jovanovich.

Mrazek, D. A. (1984). Effects of hospitalization on early child development. In R. N. Emde & R. J. Harmon (Eds.), *Continuities and Discontinuities in Development* (pp. 211–228). New York: Plenum.

Mrazek, David A. (1986). Annotation childhood asthma: Two central questions for child psychiatry. *Journal of Child Psychiatry, 27,* 1–5.

Murphy, J. M., Sobol, A. M., & Neff, R. K. (1984). Stability of prevalence: Depression and anxiety disorders. *Archives of General Psychiatry, 41,* 990–997.

Murphy, M. A. (1982). The family with a handicapped child: A review of the literature. *Developmental and Behavioral Pediatrics, 3,* 73–82.

Myers, J. K., Lindenthal, J. J., & Pepper, M. P. (1971). Life events and psychiatric impairments. *Journal of Nervous and Mental Diseases, 52,* 149–157.

Myers, J. K., & Pepper, M. P. (1972). Life events and mental status: A longitudinal study. *Journal of Health and Social Behavior, 13,* 398–406.

Myers, J. K., Lindenthal, J. J., & Pepper, M.P. (1975). Life events, social integration, and psychiatric symptomatology. *Journal of Health and Social Behavior, 16,* 421–429.

Myers, J. K., Weissman, M. M., Tischler, G. L., Holzer, C. E., Leaf, P. J., Orvaschel, H., Anthory, J. C., Boyd, J. H., Burke, J. D., Kramer, M., & Stoltzman, R. (1984). Six-month prevalence of psychiatric disorders in three communities: 1980-1982. *Archives of General Psychiatry, 41,* 959–967.

Nachman, P. A., & Stern, D. N. (1984). Affect retrieval: A form of recall memory in pre-linguistic infants. In J. D. Call, E. Galenson, & R. L. Tyson (Eds.), *Frontiers of infant psychiatry* (Vol. 2 pp. 95–100). New York: Basic Books.

Nagy, M. (1948). The child's theories concerning death. *Journal of Genetic Psychology, 73,* 3–27.

Naslund, B., Persson-Blennow, I., McNeil, T. F., Kaij, L., & Malmquist-Larsson, A. (1984). Deviations on exploration, attachment, and fear of strangers in high-risk and control infants at one year of age. *American Journal of Orthopsychiatry, 54,* 569–577.

Natapoff, J. N. (1978). Children's views of health: A developmental study. *American Journal of Public Health, 68,* 995–1000.

Newberger, C. M., & Cook, S. J. (1983). Parental awareness and child Abuse: A cognitive developmental analysis of urban and rural samples. *American Journal of Orthopsychiatry, 53,* 512–524.

Newberger, E. (1977). *Statement Printed in Senate hearings on Extension of the Child Abuse Prevention and Treatment Act.* (April 6-7), 44.

Newberger, E. H., Newberger, C. M., & Hampton, R. C. (1983). Child abuse: The current theory base and future research needs. *Journal of the American Academy of Child Psychiatry, 22,* 262–268.

Newson, J. (1974). Towards a theory of infant understanding. *Bulletin of the British Psychological Society, 27,* 251–257.

Nicholls, J. G. (1978). The development of the concepts of effort and ability, perception of academic attainment, and the understanding that difficult tasks require more ability. *Child Development, 49,* 800–814.

Nicholls, J. G., & Miller, A. T. (1985). Differentiation of the concepts of luck and skill. *Developmental Psychology, 21,* 76–82.

Nichols, S. E. (1985). Psychosocial reactions of persons with the acquired immunodeficiency syndrome. *Annals of Internal Medicine, 103,* 765–767.

Nowicki, S., Jr., & Strickland, B. (1973). A Locus of control scale for children. *Journal of Consulting and Clinical Psychology, 40,* 148–154.

NIMH (1977). Depression in children: Diagnosis, treatment, and conceptual models. Edited by J. G. Schulterbrandt & A. Raskin. U. S. Dept. of Health, Education, and Welfare, Public Health Service, Alcohol, Drug Abuse, and Mental Health Administration, National Institute of Mental Health; Washington, D. C.

Okuno, A., Nishimura, Y., & Kawarzaki, T. (1972). Changes in plasma 11-hydroxycorticosteroids after ATCH, insulin and dexamethasone in neonatal infants. *Journal of Clinical Endocrinology, 34,* 516–520.

Oleske, J. M., Minnefor, A., Cooper, R., Jr., Thomas, K., Dela Cruz, A., Ahdieh, H., Guerrero, I., Toshi, V. V., & Desposito, F. (1983). Immunodeficiency in children. *Journal of American Medical Association, 249,* 2345–2349.

Orbach, I., & Glaubman, H. (1978). Suicidal, aggressive, and normal children's perception of personal and impersonal death. *Journal of Clinical Psychology, 34,* 850–857.

Orme, T. C., & Rimmer, J. (1981). Alcoholism and child abuse: A review. *Journal of Studies on Alcohol, 42,* 273–287.

Ossofsky, H. J. (1974). Endogenous depression in infancy and childhood. *Comprehensive Psychiatry, 15,* 19–25.

Oswald, P. F., & Peltzman, P. (1974). The Cry of the Human Infant. *Scientific American, 230,* 84–90.

Papousek, H., & Papousek, M. (1975). Cognitive aspects of preverbal social interaction between human infants and adults. In M. O'Connor (Ed.), *Parent–infant interaction* (pp. 241–269). Amsterdam: Elsevier.

Papousek, H., & Papousek, M. (1979). Early ontogeny of human social interaction: Its biological roots and social dimensions. In M. von Cranach, K. Foppa, W. Lepenies, & D. Ploog (Eds.), *Human ethology: Claims and limits of a new Discipline. Contributions to the colloquium by the Werner-Reimers Stiftung* (pp. 456–490). Cambridge, England: Cambridge University Press.

Papousek, H., & Papousek, M. (1983). Interactional failures: their origins and significance in infant psychiatry. In J. D. Call, E. Galenson, & R. L. Tyson (Eds.), *Frontiers of infant psychiatry* (pp. 31–37). New York: Basic Books.

Papousek, H., & Papousek, M. (1984). The evolution of parent–infant attachment: New psychobiological perspectives. In J. D. Call, E. Galenson, & R. L. Tyson (Eds.), *Frontiers of infant psychiatry* (Vol. 2 pp. 276–283). New York: Basic Books.

Paradise, E. B., & Curcio, F. (1974). Relationship of cognitive and affective behaviors to fear of strangers in male infants. *Developmental Psychology, 10,* 476–483.

Parke, R. D., & Collmer, C. W. (1975). Child abuse: An interdisciplinary analysis. *Review of Child Development Research 9,* 509–590.

Parmelee, A. H. (1986). Children's illnesses: Their beneficial effects on behavioral development. *Child Development, 57,* 1–10.

Parmelee, A. H., Beckwith, L., Cohen, S. E., & Sigman, M. (1983). Social influences on infants at medical risk for behavioral difficulties. In J.D. Call, E. Galenson, & R. L. Tyson (Eds.), *Frontiers of infant psychiatry* (pp. 247–255). New York: Basic Books.

Parrot, M. (1922). Cited by Czerny, A, *Der Arzt als Erzeiher des Kindes* (6th ed.). Leipsig: Franz Deuticke, p. 5.

Parry, G. (1982, April). Paid employment mental health working class mothers. Paper read at British Psychological Society, University of York.

Parry, M. H. (1973). Infant wariness and stimulus discrepancy. *Journal of Experimental Child Psychology, 16,* 377–387.

Patton, R. G., & Gardner, L. I. (1975). Deprivation dwarfism (psychosocial deprivation): Disordered family environment as cause of so-called idiopathic hypopituitarism. In L. I. Gardner (Ed.), *Endocrine and genetic diseases of childhood and adolescence* (2nd ed., pp. 85–98). Philadelphia: Saunders.

Paulsen, M. G. (1974). The law and abused children. In R. E. Helfer & C. H. Kemp, (Eds.), *The battered child* (2nd ed. pp. 153–178). Chicago: University of Chicago Press.

Paulson, M. J., Schwemer, F. T., & Bendel, R. B. (1976). Clinical application of the Pd, Ma, and (OH) Experimental MMPI Scales to further understanding of abusive parents. *Journal of Clinical Psychology, 32,* 558–564.

Paulson, M. J., Stone, D., & Sposto, R. (1978). Suicidal potential and behavior in children ages 4 to 12. *Suicide and Life-Threatening Behavior, 8,* 225–242.

Paykel, E. S. (1974). Life stress and psychiatric disorder: Applications of the clinical approach. In B. S. Dohrenwend & B. P. Dohrenwend (Eds.), *Stressful life events: The nature and effects* (pp. 135–141). New York: Wiley.

Paykel, E. S., Emms, E. M., Fletcher, J., & Rassagy, E. S. (1980). Life events and social support in prepubertal depression. *British Journal of Psychology, 136,* 339–346.

Paykel, E. S., Prusoff, B. A., & Tanner, J. (1976). Temporal stability of symptom patterns in depression. *British Journal of Psychiatry, 128,* 369–374.

Pearce, J. B. (1977). Depressive disorder in childhood. *Journal of Child Psychology and Psychiatry, 18,* 79–82.

Pearce, J. B. (1978). The recognition of depressive disorders in children. *Journal of the Royal Society of Medicine, 71,* 494–500.

Pearce, J. B. (1980/81). Drug treatment of depression in children. *Acta paedopsychiatrica, 46,* 317–328.

Pearson, G. H. J. (1941). Effect of operative procedures on the emotional life of the child. *American Journal of Diseases of Children, 62,* 716–729.

Pederson, F. A., Zaslow, M., Cain, R. L., Anderson, B. J., & Thomas, M. (1979). *Methodology for Assessing Parent Perceptions of Baby Temperament.* Bethesda: Child and Family Research Branch, National Institute of Child Health and Human Development, National Institute of Health.

Pelton, L. H. (1978). Child abuse and neglect: The myth of classlessness. *American Journal of Orthopsychiatry, 48,* 608–617.

Perris, C. (1966). A study of bipolar (manic depressive) and unipolar recurrent depressive psychoses. *Acta Psychiatrica Scandinavica, 42,* Supplement 194, 1–188.

Pervin, L. A. (1963). The need to predict and control under conditions of threat. *Journal of Personality, 31,* 570–587.

Peterson, C., & Seligman, M. E. (1984). Causal explanations as a risk factor for depression: Theory and evidence. *Psychological Review, 91,* 347–374.

Petti, T. A. (1978). Depression in hospitalized child psychiatry patients. *Journal of the American Academy of Child Psychiatry, 17,* 49–59.

Petti, T. A. (1983). Imipramine in the treatment of depressed children. In D. P. Cantwell & G. A. Carlson (Eds.) *Affective disorders in childhood and adolescence—An update* (pp. 375–415). New York: Spectrum.

Petti, T. A., Bornstein, M., Delamater, A., & Conners, C. K. (1980). Evaluation and multimodality treatment of a depressed girl. *Journal of the American Academy of Child Psychiatry, 19,* 690–702.

Petty, L. K., Asarnow, J. R., Carlson, G. A., & Lesser, L. (1985). The dexamethasone suppression test in depressed, dysthymic, and nondepressed children. *American Journal of Psychiatry, 142,* 631–633.

Pfeffer, C. R. (1977). Psychiatric hospital treatment of suicidal children. *Suicide and Life-Threatening Behavior, 8,* 150–160.

Pfeffer, C. R. (1978). Clinical observations of play of suicidal latency age children. *Suicide and Life-Threatening Behavior, 9,* 235–244.

Pfeffer, C. R. (1981). The family system of suicidal children. *American Journal of Psychotherapy, 35,* 330–341.

Pfeffer, C. R., Conte, H. R., & Plutchik, R. (1980). Suicidal behavior in latency-age children: An outpatient population. *Journal of the American Academy of Child Psychiatry, 19,* 703–710.

Pfeffer, C. R., Solomon, G., Plutchik, R., Muzruchi, M. S., & Weiner, A. (1982). Suicidal behavior in latency-age psychiatric inpatients: A replication and cross validation. *Journal of the American Academy of Child Psychiatry, 21,* 564–569.

Philips, I. (1979). Childhood depression: Interpersonal interactions and depressive phenomena. *American Journal of Psychiatry, 136,* 511–515.

Piaget, J. (1930). *The child's conception of physical casuality.* London: Routledge & Kegan Paul.

Piaget, J. (1932). *The moral judgment of the child.* New York: Harcourt Brace.

Piaget, J. (1952). *The origin of intelligence in children.* New York: International Universities Press.

Piaget, J. (1954). *The construction of reality in the child.* New York: Basic Books. (Original work published 1937)

Piaget, J., & Inhelder, B. (1969). *The psychology of the child.* (1969) New York: Basic Books.

Piers, E. V., & Harris, D. (1969). Manual for the Piers Harris Children's Self-Concept Scale. Counsellor Recordings and Tests. Nashville, Tennessee.

Pilowsky, I., Bassett, D. L., Begg, M. W., & Thomas, P. G. (1982). Childhood hospitalization and chronic intractable pain in adults: A controlled retrospective study. *International Journal of Psychiatry and Medicine, 12,* 75–84.

Pine, F. (1982). The experience of self: Aspects of its formulation, expansion, and vulnerability. *The Psychoanalytic Study of the Child, 36,* 143–167.

Plomin, R. (1983). Childhood temperament. *Advances in Clinical Child Psychology, 6,* 45–92.

Plomin, R., & Rowe, D. C. (1979). Genetic and environmental etiology of social behavior in infancy. *Developmental Psychology, 15,* 62–71.

Pohjavuori, M., Rovamo, L., & Laatikainen, T. (1985). Plasma immunoreactive beta-endorphin and cortisol in the newborn infant after elective caesarean section and after spontaneous labour. *European Journal of Obstetrics, Gynecology, and Reproductive Biology, 19,* 67–74.

Polan, H. J., Hellerstein, D., & Amchin, J. (1985). Impact of AIDS-related cases on an inpatient therapeutic milieu. *Hospital Community Psychiatry, 36,* 173–176.

Polansky, N. (1976). Analysis of research on child neglect: The social work viewpoint. In Herner and Company (Eds.), *Four perspectives on the status of child abuse and neglect research* (pp. 202–278). Washington, DC: National Center on Child Abuse and Neglect.

Pollitt, E., & Eichler, A. (1976). Behavioral disturbances among failure to thrive children. *American Journal of Diseases of Children, 130,* 24–29.

Pollitt, E., Eichler, A. W., & Chon, C. (1975). Psychosocial development and behavior of mothers of failure to thrive children. *American Journal of Orthopsychiatry, 45,* 525–537.

Pollock, D., & Steele, B. A. (1972). A Therapeutic approach to the parents. In C. H. Kempe & R. E. Helfer (Eds.), *Helping the Battered Child and His Family.* Philadelphia: Lippincott.

Powell, G. F., Brasel, J. A., & Blizzard, R. M., (1967a). Emotional deprivation and growth retardation simulating idiopathic hypopituitarism. *New England Journal of Medicine, 276,* 1271.

Powell, G. F., Brasel, J. A., Riati, S., & Blizzard, R. M. (1967b). Emotional deprivation and growth retardation simulating idiopathic hypopituitarism. *New England Journal of Medicine, 276,* 1279.

Poznanski, E., Mokdros, H. B., Grossman, J., & Freeman, L. N. (1985). Diagnostic criteria in childhood depression. *American Journal of Psychiatry, 142,* 1168–1173.

Poznanski, E., & Zrull, J. P. (1970). Childhood depression. *Archives of General Psychiatry, 23,* 8–15.

Poznanski, E. O., Grossman, J. A., Buchsbaum, Y., Banegas, M. C., Freeman, L. N., & Gibbons, R. (1984). Preliminary studies of the reliability and validity of the childrens' depression rating scale. *Journal of the American Academy of Child Psychiatry, 23,* 191–197.

Prange, A. J., & Wilson, L. C. (1984). Thyrotropin releasing hormone (TRH) in depression: a preliminary report. *Journal of Psychiartic Research (Oxford), 10,* 155–156.

Preskorn, S. H., Weller, E. B., & Weller, R. A. (1982). Depression in children: Relationship between plasma imipramine levels and response. *Journal of Clinical Psychiatry, 43,* 450–453.

Price, G. G., Walsh, D. J., & Vilberg, W. R. (1984). The confluence model's good predictions of mental age beg the question. *Psychological Bulletin, 96,* 195–200.

Price, L. H., Nelson, J. C., Charney, D. S., & Quinlan, D. M. (1984). The clinical utility of family history for the diagnosis of melancholia. *Journal of Nervous and Mental Disease, 172,* 5–11.

Provence, S. (1978). A clinician's view of affect development in infancy. In M. Lewis & L. A. Rosenblum (Eds), *The Development of Affect* (pp. 293–307). New York: Plenum.

Provence, S. (1983). Case vignettes. *Zero to Three, 3,* 46.

Provence, S., & Lipton, R. C. (1962). *Infants in institutions.* New York: International Universities Press.

Provence, S., & Ritvo, S. (1961). Effects of deprivation on institutionalized infants: Disturbances in development of relationship to inanimate objects. *Psychoanalytic Study of the Child, 16,* 189–205.

Prugh, D. G. (1983). *The Psychosocial Aspects of Pediatrics.* Philadelphia: Lea & Febiger.

Prugh, D. G., Staub, E. M., Sands, H. H., Kirschbaum, R. M., & Lenihan, E. A. (1953). A study of the emotional reactions of children and families to hospitalization and illness. *American Journal of Orthopsychiatry, 23,* 70–106.

Puig-Antich, J. (1982). Major depression and conduct disorder in prepuberty. *Journal of the American Academy of Child Psychiatry, 21,* 118–128.

Puig-Antich, J. (1984). Clinical and treatment aspects of depression in childhood and adolescence. *Pediatric Annals, 13,* 37–45.

Puig-Antich, J. (1986). Psychobiological markers: Effects of age and puberty. In M. Rutter, C. E. Izard, P. B. Read (Eds.), *Depression in young people* (pp. 341–382). New York: Guilford.

Puig-Antich, J., Chambers, W., Halpern, F., Hallon, C., & Sachar, E. J. (1979). Cortisol hypersecretion in prepubertal depressive illness: A preliminary report. *Psychoneuroendocrinology, 4*, 191–197.

Puig-Antich, J., Goetz, R., Hanlon, C., Davies, M., Thompson, J., Chambers, W. J., Tabrizi, M. A., & Weitzman, E. D. (1982). Sleep architecture and REM sleep measures in prepubertal children with major depression. *Archives of General Psychiatry, 39*, 932–939.

Puig-Antich, J., Lukens, E., Davies, M., Goetz, D., Quattrock, J. B., & Todak, G. (1985). Psychosocial functioning in prepubertal major depressive disorders. *Archives of General Psychiatry, 42*, 500–507.

Puig-Antich, J., Novacenko, M. S., Davies, M., Chambers, W. J., Tabrizi, M. A., Krawiec, V., Ambrosini, P. J., & Sachar, E. J. (1984a). Growth hormone secretion in prepubertal children with major depression. *Archives of General Psychiatry, 39*, 932–939.

Puig-Antich, J., Novacenko, H., Goetz, R., Corser, J., Davies, M., & Ryan, N. (1984b). Cortisol and prolactin responses to insulin-induced hypoglycemia in prepubertal major depressives during episode and after recovery. *Journal of the American Academy of Child Psychiatry, 23*, 49–57.

Puig-Antich, J., Perel, J. M., Lupatkin, W., Chambers, W. J., Shea, C., Tabrizi, M. A., & Stiller, R. L. (1979). Plasma levels of imipramine (IMI) and desmethylimipramine (DMI) and clinical response in prepubertal major depressive disorder: A preliminary report. *Journal of the American Academy of Child Psychiatry, 18*, 616–627.

Puig-Antich, J., Tabrizi, M. A., Davies, M., Goetz, R., Chambers, W., Halpern, F., & Sachar, E. J. (1981). Prepubertal endogenous major depressives hyposecrete growth hormone in response to insulin-induced hypoglycemia. *Biological Psychiatry, 16*, 801–818.

Purcell, K., Brady, K., & Chai, H. (1969). The effect on asthma in children on experimental separation from the family. *Psychosomatic Medicine, 31*, 144–164.

Purcell, K., & Weiss, J. H. (1970). Asthma. In C. G. Costello (Ed.), *Symptoms of psychopathology: A handbook* (pp. 597–623). New York: Wiley.

Quinton, D., & Rutter, M. (1976). Early hospital admissions and later disturbances of behavior: An attempted replication of Douglas' findings. *Developmental Medicine and Child Neurology, 18*, 447–459.

Radke-Yarrow, M., Cummings, E. M., Kuczynski, L., & Chapman, M. (1985). Patterns of attachment in two- and three-year-olds in normal families and families with parental depression. *Child Development, 56*, 884–893.

Radke-Yarrow, M., Zahn-Waxler, C., & Chapman, M. (1983). Children's prosocial dispositions and behavior. In P. H. Musson (Ed.), *Handbook of child psychology: Vol. 4. Socialization, personality, and social development* (4th Ed.) New York: Wiley.

Rado, S. (1928). The problem of melancholia. *International Journal of Psychoanalysis, 9*.

Ramey, C. T., & Gowen, J. (1984). A general systems approach to modifying risk for retarded development. *Early Child Development and Care, 16*, 9–26.

Rau, J. H., & Kaye, N. (1977). Joint hospitalization of mother and child: Evaluation in vivo. *Bulletin of the Menninger Clinic, 41*, 385–394.

Reichelderfer, T. E., & Rockland, L. (1963). Maternal deprivation and the effect of loving care. *Clinical Pediatrics, 2*, 449–452.

Reid, A. H. (1980). Psychiatric Disorders in Mentally Handicapped children: A clinical and follow-up study. *Journal of Mental Deficiency Research, 24*, 287–298.

Reite, M., Short, R., Seiler, C., & Pauley, M. (1981). Attachment loss and depression. *Journal of Child Psychology and Psychiatry, 22*, 141–169.

Reynolds, C. R., & Richmond, B. O. (1978). What I think and feel: A revised measure of children's manifest anxiety. *Journal of Abnormal Child Psychiatry, 6,* 271–280.

Renshaw, D. C. (1974). Suicide and depression in children. *Journal of School Health, 44,* 487–489.

Ribble, M. A. (1944). Infantile experience in relation to personality development. In J. McV. Hunt (Ed.), *Personality and the Behavior Disorders* (Vol. 2 pp. 621–651). New York: Ronald.

Richman, J., & Flaherty, J. (1985). Coping and depression: The relative contribution of internal and external resources during a life-cycle transition. *The Journal of Nervous and Mental Disease, 173,* 590–595.

Richman, N., & Graham, P. (1971). A behavioral screening questionnaire for use with three year old children. *Journal of Child Psychology and Psychiatry, 12,* 5–33.

Ricks, M. H. (1985). The social transmission of parental bahavior: Attachment across generations. *Monographs of the Society for Research in Child Development, 50,* 211–227.

Rie, H. E. (1966). Depression in childhood: A survey of some pertinent contributions. *Journal of the American Academy of Child Psychiatry, 5,* 653–685.

Risch, S. C. (1982). Beta-endorphin hypersecretion in depression: Possible cholinergic mechanisms. *Biological Psychiatry, 17,* 1071–1079.

Risch, S. C., Janowsky, D. S., Judd, L. L., Gillin, J. C., & McClure, S. F. (1983). The role of endogenous opioid systems in neuroendocrine regulation. *Psychiatric Clinics of North America, 6,* 429–441.

Robertson, J. (1953). Some responses of young children to loss of maternal care. *Nursing Times, 49,* 382–386.

Robertson, J. (1956). Mother's observations on tonsillectomy of her four-year-old daughter. *Psychoanalytic Study of the Child, 11,* 410–427.

Robertson, J. (1970). *Young Children in Hospital.* London: Tavistock Publications.

Robertson, J., & Bowlby, J. (1952). Responses of young children to separation from their mothers. *Courrier du Centre International de l'Enfance, 2,* 131–142.

Robertson, J., & Robertson J. (1971). Young children in brief separation. *Psychoanalytic Study of the Child, 26,* 264–325.

Robins, L. N., Helzer, J. E., & Weissman, M. M. (1984). Lifetime prevalence of specific psychiatric disorders in three sites. *Archives of General Psychiatry, 41,* 949–958.

Robison, E., & Solomon, F. (1979). Some further findings on the treatment of the mother-child dyad in child abuse. *Child Abuse Neglect, 3,* 247–251.

Rochlin, G. (1959). The loss complex. *Journal of the American Psychoanalytic Association, 7,* 299–316.

Rode, S. S., Chang, P. N., Fisch, R. O., & Sroufe, L. A. (1981). Attachment patterns of infants separated at birth. *Developmental Psychology, 17,* 188–191.

Rose, R. M. (1985). Psychoendocrinology. In J. D. Wilson & D. W. Foster (Eds.). *Williams Textbook of Endocrinology* (7th Ed, 653–681). Philadelphia, PA: W. B. Saunders.

Rosenthal, N. E., Carpenter, C. J., James, S. P., Parry, B. L., Rogers, S., & Wehr, T. (1986). Seasonal affective disorder in children and adolescents. *American Journal of Psychiatry, 143,* 356–358.

Rosenthal, N. E., Sack, D. A., Gillin, J. C., Lewy, A. J., Goodwin, F. K., Davenport, Y., & Mueller, P. S. (1984). Seasonal affective disorder: A description of the syndrome and preliminary findings with light therapy. *Archives of General Psychiatry, 41,* 72–80.

Rosenthal, P. A. (1983), Suicide among preschoolers: Fact or fallacy? *Children Today, 12,* 21–24.

Rosenthal, P. A., & Rosenthal, S. (1984). Suicidal behavior by preschool children. *American Journal of Psychiatry, 141,* 520–525.

Rothbart, M. K. (1981). Measurement of temperament in infancy. *Child Development, 52,* 569–578.

Rothbart, M. K., & Derryberry, D. (1981). Development of individual differences in temperament. In M. E. Lamb & A. L. Brown (Eds.), *Advances in Developmental Psychology* (Vol. 1. pp. 17–86). Hillsdale; Erlbaum.

Rothbart, M. K., & Derryberry, D. (1982). Theoretical issues in temperament. In M. Lewis & L. T. Taft (Eds.), *Developmental disabilities: theory, assessment, and intervention* (pp. 383–400). New York: SP Medical and Scientific Books.

Rothbart, M. K., & Derryberry, D. (1984). Emotion, attention, temperament. In C. E. Izard, J. Kagan, & R. B. Zajonc (Eds.). *Emotions, cognition, behavior.* Cambridge, England: Cambridge University Press.

Rothbart, M. K., & Hanson, M. J. (1983). A caregiver report comparison of temperamental characteristics of Down's Syndrome and normal infants. *Developmental Psychology, 19,* 766–769.

Rotter, J.B. (1966). Generalized expectancies for internal external locus of control of reinforcement. *Psychological Monographs, 80* (1, Whole No. 609).

Rounsaville, B. J., & Chevron, Eve (1982). Interpersonal psychotherapy: Clinical applications. In J. Rush (Ed.) *Short Term Psychotherapies for Depression.* New York: Guilford Press, 86–106.

Rowe, D. C., & Plomin, R. (1981). The importance of shared (E1) environmental influences in behavioral development. *Developmental Psychology, 17,* 517–531.

Rutter, M. (1979). Maternal deprivation, 1972-1978: New findings, new concepts, new approaches. *Child Development, 50,* 283–305.

Rutter, M. (1986). The developmental psychopathology of depression: Issues and perspectives. In M. Rutter, C. E. Izard, & P. B. Read (Eds.), *Depression in young people* (pp. 3–30). New York: Guildford.

Rutter, M., & Garmezy, N. (1983). Developmental psychopathology. In P. H. Mussen (Ed.). *Handbook of child psychology: Vol. 4. Socialization, personality, & social development* (4th Ed, pp. 776–911). New York: Wiley.

Rutter, M., Graham, P., & Yule, W. (1970a). *A Neuropsychiatric Study in Childhood, Clinics in Developmental Medicine 35/36.* London: Spastics International Medical Publishing.

Rutter, M., Tizard, J., & Whitmore, K. (Eds.) (1970b). *Education, Health and Behavior.* London: Longmans.

Ryan, K. M. (1981). Developmental differences in reactions to the physically disabled. *Human Development, 24,* 240–256.

Sabbath, J. C. (1969). The suicidal adolescent—the expendable child. *Journal of the American Academy of Child Psychiatry, 8,* 272–289.

Sameroff, A. J., & Chandler, M. J. (1975). Perinatal risk and the continuum of caretaking causality. In F. D. Harowitz, E. M. Heterington, & S. Scarr-Salapatek (Eds.), *Review of child development research* (Vol. 4. pp. 187-245). Chicago: University of Chicago Press.

Sander, L. W. (1983). A twenty-five-year follow-up of the Pavenstedt Longitudinal Research Project, its relation to early intervention. In J. D. Call, E. Galenson, & R. L.Tyson (Eds.), *Frontiers of infant psychiatry* (pp. 225–230). New York: Basic Books.

Sandgrund, A., Gaines, R., & Green, A. (1974). Child abuse and mental retardation: A Problem of cause and effect. *American Journal of Mental Deficiency, 79,* 327–330.

Scarr, S., & Salapetek, P. (1970). Patterns of fear development during infancy. *Merrill-Palmer Quarterly, 16,* 53–90.

Schachter, R. S. (1984). Kinetic psychotherapy in the treatment of depression in latency age children. *International Journal of Group Psychotherapy, 34,* 83–91.

Schaffer, H. R. (1958). Objective observations on personality development in early infancy. *British Journal of Medical Psychology, 31,* 174–183.

Schaffer, H. R., & Callender, W. M. (1959). Psychologic effects of hospitalization in infancy. *Pediatrics, 25,* 528–539.

Schaffer, H. R., & Emerson, P. E. (1964). The development of social attachments in infancy. *Monographs in Social Research and Child Development, 29,* 3.

Schecter, M. D. (1961). The orthopedically handicapped child; emotional responses. *Archives of General Psychiatry, 4,* 247–253.

Schildkraut, J. J. (1965). The catecholamine hypothesis of affective disorders: A review of supporting evidence. *American Journal of Psychiatry, 122,* 509–522.

Schmale, A. H. (1972). Giving up as a final common pathway to changes in health. *Advances in Psychosomatic Medicine, 8,* 20–40.

Schmitt, B., & Kempe, C. (1975). Neglect and abuse of children. In V. Vaughn & R. Mckay *Nelson Textbook of Pediatrics* (10th ed.). Philadelphia: W. B. Saunders.

Schneider-Rosen, K., & Cicchetti, D. (1984). The relationship between affect and cognition in maltreated infants: Quality of attachment and the development of visual self-recognition. *Child Development, 55,* 648–658.

Schowalter, J. E. (1970). The child's reaction to his own terminal illness. In B. Schoenberg, A. C. Carr, & D. Peretz (Eds.), *Loss and grief: Psychological management in medical practice* (pp. 51–69). New York: Columbia University Press.

Schrut, A. (1964). Suicidal adolescents and children. *Journal of the American Medical Association, 188,* 1103–1107.

Schuckit, M. A. (1986). Genetic and clinical implications of alcoholism and affective disorder. *American Journal of Psychiatry, 143,* 140–147.

Schulterbrandt, M. S., & Raskin, A. (Eds.) (1977). *Depression in childhood: Diagnosis, treatment and conceptual models.* New York: Raven.

Schwab, J. J., & Schwab, M. D. (1978). *Sociocultural roots of mental illness: An epidemiological survey.* New York: Plenum.

Scott, D. (1984). Nursing the impaired mother–infant relationship in puerperal depression. *Australian Journal of Advanced Nursing, 1,* 50–56.

Seidel, U. P., Chadwick, O. F. D., & Rutter, M. (1975). Psychological disorders in crippled children. A comparative study of children with and without brain damage. *Developmental Medicine and Child Neurology (London), 17,* 563–573.

Seligman, M. E. P. (1975). *Helplessness: On depression, development and death.* San Francisco: Freeman.

Seligman, M. E. P., & Maier, S. F. (1967). Failure to escape traumatic shock. *Journal of Experimental Psychology, 74,* 1–9.

Seligman, M. E. P., & Peterson, C. (1986). A learned helplessness perspective on childhood depression: Theory and research. In M. Rutter, C. E. Izard, & P. B. Read (Eds.). *Depression in young people* (pp. 223–249). New York: Guilford.

Seligman, M. E., Peterson, C., Kaslow, N. J., Tanenbaum, R. L., Alloy, L. B., & Abramson, L. Y. (1984). Attributional style and depressive symptoms among children. *Journal of Abnormal Psychology, 93,* 235–238.

Seligman, P. S., & Pawl, H. J. (1983). Impediments to the formation of the working alliance in infant–parent psychotherapy. In J. D. Call, E. Galenson & R. L. Tyson (Eds.), *Frontiers of infant psychiatry* (Vol. 2. pp. 232–237). New York: Basic Books.

Selman, R. (1980). *The Growth of Interpersonal Understanding.* New York: Adademic Press.

Selye, H. (1956). *The stress of life.* New York:McGraw-Hill.

Serafica, F., & Cicchetti, D. (1976). Down's Syndrome children in a strange situation: Attachment and exploration behaviors. *Merrill-Palmer Quarterly, 22,* 137–150.

Shaffer, D., & Fisher, P. (1981a). The epidemiology of suicide in children and young adolescents. *Journal of the American Academy of Child Psychiatry, 20,* 545–565.

Shaffer, D., & Fisher, P. (1981b). Suicide in childhood and early adolescence. In C. F. Wells & I. R. Stuart (Eds.), *Self destructive behavior in children and adolescents* (pp. 75–104). New York: Van Nostrand Reinhold.

Shaw, C. R., & Schelkun, R. F. (1965). Suicidal behavior in children. *Psychiatry, 28,* 157–168.

Shereshefsky, P. M., & Yarrow, L. J. (1973). *Psychological aspects of a first pregnancy and early post-natal adaptation.* New York: Raven.

Sherrod, K. B., O'Connor, S., & Vietze, P. M. (1984). Child health and maltreatment. *Child Development, 55, 1174–1183.*

Shiller, V. M., Izard, C. E., & Hembree, E. A. (1986). Patterns of emotion expression during separation in the strange situation procedure. Developmental Psychology, 22, 378–382.

Shindi, J. (1981). Emotional adjustment of physically handicapped children: A comparison of children with congenital and acquired orthopaedic disabilities. *International Journal of Social Psychiatry, 29,* 292–298.

Siegel, E., Siegel, R., & Siegel, T. (1978). *Help for the lonely child: Strengthening social perception.* New York: Dutton.

Siever, J. L., & Davis, K. L. (1985). Overview: Toward a dysregulation hypothesis of depression. *American Journal of Psychiatry, 142,* 1017–1031.

Sigman, M. (1982). Plasticity in development: Implications for intervention. In L. A.Bond & J. M. Joffe (Eds.), *Facilitating infant and early childhood development* (pp. 98–116). Hanover, NH: University Press of New England.

Silver, A. A. (1984). Children in classes for the severely emotionally handicapped. *Developmental and Behavioral Pediatrics, 5,* 49–54.

Silver, L. B., Dublin, C. C., & Lourie, R. S. (1969). Does violence breed violence? Contributions from a study of the child abuse syndrome. *American Journal of Psychiatry, 126,* 404–407.

Simeonson, R. J., Buckley, L., & Monson, L. (1979). Conceptions of illness causality in hospitalized children. *Journal of Pediatrics and Psychology, 4,* 77–84.

Simoneau, K., & Decarie, T. G. (1979). Cognition and perception in the object concept. *Canadian Journal of Psychology, 33,* 396–407.

Simons, C., Kohle, K., Genscher, U., & Dietrich, M. (1973). The impact of reverse isolation on early childhood development: Two and a half years of treatment in plastic isolations systems. *Psychotherapy and Psychosomatics, 22,* 300–309.

Simpson, K. (1967). The battered baby problem. *Royal Society of Health Journal, 87,* 168–170.

Simpson, K. (1968). The battered baby problem. *South African Medical Journal, 42,* 661–663.

Sjoqvist, F., & Bertilsson, L. (1984). Clinical pharmacology of antidepressant drugs: Pharmogenetics. *Advanced Biochemical Psychopharmacology, 39,* 359–372.

Smith, C. R., Selz, L. J., Bingham, E. Z., Aschenbrenner, B., Standbury, K., & Leiderman, P. H. (1985). Mother's perception of handicapped and normal children. In J. E. Stevenson (Ed.), *Recent research in developmental psychopathology* (pp. 111–124). New York: Pergamon.

Smith, S. M., & Hanson, R. (1975). Interpersonal relationships and child-rearing practices in 214 parents of battered children. *British Journal of Psychiatry, 127,* 513–525.

Smith, S. M., Hanson, R., & Noble, S. (1973). Parents of battered babies: A controlled study. *British Medical Journal, 4,* 388–391.

Solnit, A. J. (1960). Hospitalization: An Aid to physical and psychological health in childhood. *American Journal of Diseases in Children, 99,* 155–163.

Solnit, A. J. (1982). Developmental perspective on self and object constancy. *Psychoanalytic Study of the Child, 32,* 201–217.

Solnit, A. J., & Neubauer, P. B. (1986). Object constancy and early triadic relationship. *Journal of the American Academy of Child Psychiatry, 25,* 23–29.

Solnit, A. J., & Stark, M. H. (1961). Mourning and the birth of a defective child. *Psychoanalytic Study of the Child, 16,* 523–538.

Sorce, J. F., & Emde, R. N. (1982). The meaning of infant emotional expressions: Regularities in caregiving responses in normal and Down's Syndrome infants. *Journal of Child Psychology and Psychiatry, 23,* 145–158.

Sorce, J. F., Emde, R. N., Campos, J., & Klinnert, M. D. (1985). Maternal emotional signaling: Its effect on the visual cliff behavior of 1-year-olds. *Developmental Psychology, 21,* 195–200.

Sours, J. A. (1978). The application of child analytic principles to forms of child psychotherapy. In J. Glenn (Ed.), *Child analysis and therapy* (pp. 615–646). New York: Jason Aronson.

Sovner, R., & Hurley, A. D. (1983). The subjective experience of mentally retarded persons. *Psychiatric Aspects of Mental Retardation Newsletter, 2,* 41–42.

Speece, M. W., & Brent, S. B. (1984). Children's understanding of death: A Review of three components of a death concept. *Child Development, 55,* 1671–1686.

Spence, J. C. (1947). The care of children in hospital. *British Medical Journal, 1,* 125–130.

Spinetta, J., & Rigler, D. (1972). The child-abusing parent: A psychological review. *Psychological Bulletin, 77,* 296–304.

Spitz, R. A. (1945). Hospitalism. An inquiry into the genesis of psychiatric conditions in early childhood. *Psychoanalytic Study of the Child, 1,* 53–74.

Spitz, R. A. (1954). Infantile depression and the general adaptation syndrome—On the relation between physiologic model and psychoanalytic conceptualization. In P. H. Hoch & J. A. Zubin (Eds.), *Depression* (pp. 93–108). New York: Grune & Stratton.

Spitz, R. A. (1965). *The first year of life.* New York: International Universities Press.

Spitz, R. A., & Wolf, K. M. (1946). Anaclitic depression. *Psychoanalytical Study of the Child, 2,* 313–342.

Spitz, R. A., & Wolf, K. M. (1949). Autoerotism: Some empirical findings and hypotheses on three of its manifestations in the first year of life. *Psychoanalytic Study of the Child, 314,* 85–119.

Spitzer, R. L., Endicott, J., & Robbins, E. (1978). Research diagnostic criteria: Rationale and reliability. *Archives of General Psychiatry, 35,* 773–782.

Sroufe, L. A. (1979). The coherence of individual development. *American Psychologist, 34,* 834–841.

Sroufe, L. A. (1983). Infant–caregiver attachment and patterns of adaptation in preschool: The roots of maladaptation and competence. *The Minnesota Symposia On Child Psychology, 16,* 14–83.

Sroufe, L. A. (1985). Attachment classification from the perspective of infant–caregiver relationships and infant temperament. *Child Development, 56,* 1–14.

Sroufe, L. A., & Rutter, M. (1984). The domain of developmental psychology. *Child Development, 55,* 17–29.

Sroufe, L. A., & Waters, E. (1977). Attachment as an original construct. *Child Development, 48,* 1184–1199.

Sroufe, L. A., & Waters, E. (1982). Issues of temperament and attachment: Letter to the editor. *American Journal of Orthopsychiatry, 52,* 743–747.

Sroufe, L. A., Waters, E., & Matas, L. (1974). Contextual determinants of infant affective response. In L. M. Rosenblum (Ed.), *The origins of behavior: Vol. 2 Fear* (pp. 49–72). New York: Wiley.

Stack, J. J. (1972). Chemotherapy in childhood depression. In A. L. Annell (Ed.), *Depressive states in childhood and adolescents* (pp. 460–466). New York: Wiley.

Stahlecker, J. E., & Cohen, M. C. (1985). Application of the strange situation attachment paradigm to a neurologically impaired population. *Child Development, 56,* 502–507.

Standbury, K., & Leiderman, P. H. (1985). Mothers' perceptions of handicapped and normal children. In J. E. Stevenson (Ed.), *Recent research in developmental psychopathology* (pp. 111–124). New York: Plenum.

Starr, R., Ceresnie, S., & Rossi, J. (1976). What child abuse researchers don't tell about child abuse research. *Pediatric Psychology, 1,* 50–53.

Starr, P. (1986). Health care for the poor: The past twenty years. In S. H. Danzinger & D. H. Weinberg (Eds.), *Fighting poverty: What works and what doesn't* (pp. 106–132). Cambridge, MA: Harvard University Press.

Steele, B. F. (1976). Violence within the family. In R. E. Helfer & C. H. Kempe (Eds.), *Child abuse and neglect: The family and the community* (pp. 3–23). Cambridge, MA: Ballinger.

Steele, B. F. (1983). The effect of abuse and neglect on psychological development. In J. D. Call, E. Galenson, & R. L. Tyson (Eds.), *Frontiers of infant psychiatry* (pp. 235–244). New York: Basic Books.

Steele, B. F., & Pollock, C. B. (1968). A psychiatric study of parents who abuse infants and small children. In R. Helfer (Ed.), *The battered child* (pp. 103–147). Chicago: University of Chicago Press.

Steele, B. F., & Pollock, C. B. (1974). A Psychiatric study of parents who abuse infants and small children. In R. E. Heffer & C. H. Kempe (Eds.) *The Battered Child* (2nd ed.). Chicago: University of Chicago Press.

Steinglass, P. (1981a). The alcoholic family at home. *Archives of General Psychiatry, 38,* 578–584.

Steinglass, P. (1981b). The alcoholic family: Patterns of interaction in dry, wet, and transitional stages of alcoholism. *Archives of General Psychiatry, 38,* 578–584.

Steinhausen, H. C. (1981). Chronically ill and handicapped children and adolescents: Personality studies in relation to disease. *Journal of Abnormal Child Psychology, 9,* 291–297.

Steinhausen, H. C., Gobel, D., & Nestler, V. (1984). Psychopathology in the offspring of alcoholic parents. *Journal of the American Academy of Child Psychiatry, 23,* 465–471.

Stern, D. N. (1974). Mother and infant at play: The dyadic interaction involving facial, vocal, and gaze behaviors. In M. Lewis & L. A. Rosenblum (Eds.), *The effects of the infant on its caregiver* (pp. 187–213). New York: Wiley.

Stern, D. N. (1984). Affect attunement. In J. D. Call, E. Galenson, & R. L. Tyson (Eds.), *Frontiers of infant Psychiatry* (Vol. 2, pp. 3–14). New York: Basic Books.

Stern, D. N. (1985). *The interpersonal worlds of the infant.* New York: Basic Books.

Stern, D. N., & Gibbon, J. (1979). Temporal expectancies of social behaviors in mother–infant play. In E. B. Thoman (Ed.), *Origins of the infant's social responsiveness* (pp. 409–429). Hillsdale, N.J.: Erlbaum.

Stern, D. N., Hofer, L., Haft, W., & Dore, J. (1985). Affect attunement: The sharing of feeling states between mother and infant by means of inter-modal fluency. In T. Field & N. A. Fox (Eds.), *Social perception in infants.* Norwood, NJ: Ablex.

Stern, G., & Kruckman, L. (1983). Multi-disciplinary perspectives on postpartum depression: An anthropological critique. *Social Science and Medicine, 17,* 1027–1041.

Stocking, M., Rothney, D., Grosser, G., & Goodwin, R. (1970). Psychopathology in the pediatric hospital: Implications for the pediatrician. *Psychiatry in Medicine, 1,* 329–338.

Stoddard, F. J., & O'Connell, K. G. (1983). Dysphoria in children with severe burns. *Journal of Children in Contemporary Society, 15,* 41–50.

Stone, N. W., & Chesney, B. H. (1978). Attachment behaviors in handicapped infants. *Mental Retardation, 16,* 8–12.

Streissguth, A. P. (1983). Alcohol and pregnancy: An overview and update. *Substance and Alcohol Actions/Misuse, 4,* 149–173.

Strober, M. (1984). Familial aspects of depressive disorder in early adolescence. In E. Weller (Ed.), *An update on Childhood Depression.* Washington, DC: American Psychiatric Press.

Susman, R. N., Trickett, P. K., Iannotti, R. J., Hollenbeck, B. S., & Zahn-Waxler, C. (1985). Child-rearing patterns in depressed, abusive, and normal mothers. *American Journal of Orthopsychiatry, 55,* 237–251.

Swartz, C. M., & Dunner, F. J. (1982). Dexamethasone suppression testing of alcoholics. *Archives of General Psychistry, 39,* 1309–1312.

Tarter, R. E., Hegedus, A. M., Winsten, N. E., & Alterman, A. I. (1984). Neuropsychological, personality, and familial characteristics of physically abused delinquents. *Journal of the American Academy of Child Psychiatry, 23,* 668–674.

Taylor, R. W. (1973). Depression and recovery at nine weeks of age. *Journal of American Academy of Child Psychiatry, 12,* 506–510.

Telzrow, R. W., Snyder, D. M., Tronick, E., Als, H., & Brazelton, T. B. (1980). The behavior of jaundiced infants undergoing phototherapyy. *Developmental Medicine and Child Neurology, 22,* 317–326.

Tennes, K., & Carter, D. (1973). Plasma cortisol levels and behavioral states in early infancy. *Psychosomatic Medicine, 35,* 121–128.

Tennes, K., Downey, K., & Vernaakis, A. (1977). Urinary cortisol excretion rates and anxiety in normal 1-year-old infants. *Psychosomatic Medicine, 39,* 178–187.

Tennes, K. H., & Mason, J. W. (1982). Developmental psychoendocrinology: An approach to the study of emotions. In C. E. Izard (Ed.). *Measuring emotions in infants and children* (pp. 21–38). Cambridge, England: Cambridge University Press.

Thomas, A., & Chess, S. (1977). *Temperament and development.* New York: Bruner/Mazel.

Thomas, A., & Chess, S. (1980). *The dynamics of psychological development.* New York: Bruner/Mazel.

Thomas, A., & Chess, S. (1984). Genesis and evolution of behavior disorders: From infancy to early adult life. *American Journal of Psychiatry, 141,* 1–9.

Thomas, A., Chess, S., & Birch, H. G. (1968). *Temperament and behavior disorders in children.* New York: New York University Press.

Thomas, A., Chess, S., & Birch, H. G. (1970). The origin of personality. *Scientific American, 223,* 102–109.

Thomas, A., Chess, S., Birch, H. G., Hertzig, M. E., & Korn, S. (1963). *Behavioral individuality in early childhood.* New York: New York University Press.

Thompson, R. A., & Cicchetti, D. (1985). Emotional responses of Down Syndrome and normal infants in the strange situation: The organization of affective behavior in infants. *Developmental Psychology, 21,* 828–841.

Thompson, R. A., & Lamb, M. E. (1983). Security of attachment and stranger sociability in infancy. *Developmental Psychology, 19,* 184–191.

Tinbergen, N., & Moynihan, M. (1952). Head flagging in the black-headed gull: Its function and origin. *British Birds, 45,* 19–22.

Tishler, C. L., & McHenry, P. C. (1982). Parental negative self and adolescent suicide attempts. *Journal of the American Academy of Child Psychiatry, 21,* 404–408.

Toolan, J. M. (1962a). Depression in children and adolescents. *American Journal of Orthopsychiatry, 32,* 404–414.

Toolan, J. M. (1962b). Suicide and suicidal attempts in children and adolescents. *American Journal of Psychiatry, 118,* 719–724.

Trad, P. V. (1986). *Infant depression, paradigms and paradoxes.* New York: Springer-Verlag.

Tracy, R. L., & Ainsworth, M. D. S. (1981). Maternal affectionate behavior and infant–mother attachment patterns. *Child Development, 52,* 1341–1343.

Trause, M. A., Voos, D., Rudd, C., Klaus, M., Kennell, J., & Boslett, M. (1981). Separation for childbirth: The effect on the sibling. *Child Psychiatry and Human Development, 12,* 32–39.

Trevarthen, C., & Hubley, P. (1978). Secondary intersubjectivity: Confidence, confiding and acts of meaning in the first year. In A. Lock (Ed.), *Action, gesture and symbol: The emergence of language* (pp. 183–229). London/New York: Academic.

Tronick, E., Als, H., & Adamson, L. (1979). Structure of early face-to-face communicative interactions. In M. Bullowa (Ed.), *Before speech.* Cambridge, Eng: Cambridge University Press.

Tronick, E. Z., & Gianino, A. (1986). Interactive mismatch and repair: Challenges to the coping infant. *Zero to three, bulletin of the national center for clinical infant programs* (Vol. 3).

Trout, M. D. (1983). Birth of a sick or handicapped infant: Impact on the family. *Child Welfare, 62,* 337–348.

Tuckman, J., Connon, H. E. (1962). Attempted suicide in adolescents. *American Journal of Psychiatry, 119,* 228–232.

U.S. Department of Education. (1985) *To assure the free appropriate public education of all handicapped children: Seventh annual report to Congress on the implementation of the Education of the Handicapped Act.* Washington, DC: United States Department of Education Office of Special Education and Rehabilitative Services.

U.S. Department of Health and Human Services, Public Health Service, National Center for Health Statistics (1984). National Center for Child Abuse and Neglect. Hyattsville, Maryland: Department of Health and Human Services Publications.

Vale, W., Spiess, J., Rivier, C., & Rivier, J. (1981). Charactrization of a 41-residue ovine hypothalamic peptide that stimulates secretion of corticotropin and [B]-endorphin. *Science, 213,* 1394–1397.

Vanderveer, A. H. (1949). The psychopathology of physical illness and hospital residence. *Quarterly Journal of Child Behavior, 1,* 55–77.

Van Praag, H. M. (1978). Amine hypotheses of affective disorders. In L. L. Iverson, S. D. Iverson, & S. H. Snyder (Eds.). *Handbook of psychopharmacology* (Vol. 13, pp. 187–297). New York: Plenum.

Van Praag, H. M., & de Haan, S. (1980). Depression vulnerability and 5-hydroxotryptophan prophylaxis. *Psychiatry Research, 3,* pp. 75–83.

Van Putte, A. W. (1979). Relationship of school setting to self concept in physically disabled children. *Journal of School Health, 49,* 576–578.

Van Tassel, E. (1984). Temperament characteristics of mildly developmentally delayed infants. *Developmental and Behavioral Pediatrics, 5,* 11–14.

Vaughan, G. F. (1957). Children in hospital. *Lancet, 1,* 1117–1120.

Vaughn, B., & Sroufe, L. (1979). The temporal relationship between infant heart rate acceleration and crying in an adversive situation. *Child Development, 50,* 565–567.

Vaughn, B. E., Kopp, C. B., & Krakow, J. B. (1984). The emergence and consolidation of self-control from eighteen to thirty months of age: Normative trends and individual differences. *Child Development, 55,* 990–1004.

Vermes, I., Kajtar, I., Szabo, E. (1979). Changes of maternal and fetal pituitary-adrenocortical functions during labor. *Hormone Research, 11,* 213–217.

Vernon, D. T. A., Schulman, J. L., & Foley, J. M. (1966). Changes in children's behavior after hospitalization: Some dimensions of response and their correlates. *American Journal of Diseases of Children, 111,* 581–593.

Vygotsky, L. (1962). *Thought and Language.* New York: Wiley.

Wallerstein, J. S. (1984). Children of divorce: Preliminary report of a ten-year follow-up of young children. *American Journal of Orthopsychiatry, 54,* 444–458.

Warr, P. (1982). Psychological aspects of employment and unemployment. *Psychological Medicine, 12,* 7–11.

Wasserman, G. A., & Allen, R. (1985). Maternal withdrawal from handicapped toddlers. *Journal of Child Psychology and Psychiatry, 3,* 281–287.

Wasserman, G. A., Allen, R., & Solomon, C. R. (1985a). At-risk toddlers and their mothers: The special case of physical handicap. *Child Development, 56,* 73–83.

Wasserman, G. A., Allen, R., & Solomon, C. R. (1985b). The behavioral development of physically handicapped children in the second year. *Developmental and Behavioral Psychiatry, 6,* 27–31.

Wasserman, G. A., Green, A. H., & Allen, K. (1983). Going beyond abuse: Maladaptive patterns of interaction in abusing mother–infant pairs. *Journal of the American Academy of Child Psychiatry, 22,* 245–252.

Waters, E. (1978). The reliability and stability of individual differences in infant–mother attachment. *Child Development, 49,* 483–494.

Waters, E., Wippman, J., & Sroufe, L. A. (1979). Attachment, positive affect, and competence in the peer group: Two studies in construct validation. *Child Development, 51,* 208–216.

Watson, J. S. (1966). The development of and generalization of "contingency awareness" in early infancy. *Merrill Palmer Quarterly, 12,* 123–125.

Watson, J. S. (1971). Cognitive-perceptual development in infancy: Setting for the Seventies. *Merrill Palmer Quarterly, 12,* 123–125.

Watson, J. S. (1972). Smiling, cooing and "the game." *Merrill Palmer Quarterly, 18,* 323–339.

Watson, J. S., & Ramey, C. T. (1969). Reactions to response-contingent stimulation in early infancy. *Merrill-Palmer Quarterly, 18,* 219–227.

Watson, J. S., & Ramey, C. T. (1972). Reactions to response contingent stimulation in early infancy. *Merrill-Palmer Quarterly, 18,* 219–227.

Weber, R. A., Levitt, M. J., & Clark, M. C. (1986). Individual variation in attachment security and Strange Situation behavior: The role of maternal and infant temperament. *Child Development, 57,* 56–65.

Wedell-Monnig, J., & Lumley, J. M. (1980). Child deafness and mother child interaction. *Child Development, 51,* 766–774.

Wehr, A., Jacobsen, F. M., Sack, D. A., Arendt, J., Tamarkin, L., & Rosenthal, N. E. (1986). Phototherapy of seasonal affective disorder. *Archives of General Psychiatry, 43,* 870–875.

Weinberg, W. A., Rutman, J., Sullivan, L., Penick, E. C., & Dietz, S. G. (1973). Depression in children referred to an educational diagnostic center: Diagnosis and treatment. *Journal of Pediatrics, 83,* 1065–1072.

Weinraub, M., & Wolf, B. M. (1983). Effects of stress and social support on mother-child interactions in single- and two-parent families. *Child Development, 54,* 1297–1311.

Weintraub, S., Winters, K. C., & Neale, J. M. (1986). Competence and vulnerability in children with an affectively disordered parent. In M. Rutter, C. E. Izard, & P. B. Read (Eds.). *Depression in young people.* New York: Guilford.

Weintraub, S., Neale, J. M., & Liebert, D. E. (1975). Teacher ratings of children vulnerable to psychopathology. *American Journal of Orthopsychiatry, 45,* 839–845.

Weir, C. (1979). Auditory frequency sensitivity of human newborns: Some data with improved acoustic and behavioral controls. *Perception & Psychophysics, 26,* 287–294.

Weiss, J. M., Glazer, H. I., Pohorecky, L. A., Bailey, W. H., & Schneider, L. H. (1979). Coping behavior and stress-induced behavioral depression: Studies of the role of brain catecholamines. In R. A. Depue (Ed.), *The psychobiology of the depressive disorders: Implications for the effects of stress* (pp. 125–160). New York: Academic.

Weiss, R. S. (1973). The contributions of an organization of single parents to the well-being of its members. *The Family Coordinator, 22,* 321–326.

Weiss, R. S. (1974). The provisions of social relations. In R. Zuben (Ed.), *Doing unto others.* Englewood Cliffs, NJ: Prentice-Hall.

Weissman, M. M., & Boyd, J. H. (1985). Affective disorders: Epidemiology. In H. I. Kaplan, A. M. Freedman, & B. J. Sadock (Eds.), *Comprehensive textbook of psychiatry/4th ed* (pp. 764–769). Baltimore: Williams & Wilkins.

Weissman, M. M., Gershon, E. S., Kidd, K. K., Prusoff, B. A., Leckman, J. F., Dibble, E., Hamovit, J., Thompson, W. D., Pauls, D. L., & Guroff, J. J. (1984a). Psychiatric disorders in the relatives of probands with affective disorders: The Yale University-National Institute of Mental Health collaborative study. *Archives of General Psychiatry, 41,* 13–21.

Weissman, M. M., & Klerman, G. L. (1977). Sex differences and the epidemiology of depression. *Archives of General Psychiatry, 34,* 93–111.

Weissman, M. M., Leckman, J. F., Merikangas, K. R., Gammon, G. D., & Prusoff, B.A. (1984b). Depression and anxiety disorders in parents and children: Results from the Yale family study. *Archives of General Psychiatry, 41,* 845–852.

Weissman, M. M., Merikangas, K. R., Wickramaratne, P., Kidd, K. K., Prusoff, B. A., Leckman, J. F., & Pauls, D. L. (1986). Understanding the clinical heterogeneity of major depression using family data. *Archives of General Psychiatry, 43,* 430–434.

Weissman, M. M., & Myers, J. K. (1978). Affective disorders in a US urban community: The use of research diagnostic criteria in an epidemiological survey. *Archives of General Psychiatry, 35,* 1304–1311.

Weissman, M. M., Paykel, E. S., & Klerman, G. L. (1972). The depressed woman as a mother. *Social psychiatry, 7,* 98–108.

Weissman, M., & Paykel, E. (1974). *The depressed woman: A study of social relationships.* Chicago, IL: University of Chicago Press.

Weissman, M. M., Prusoff, B. A., Gammon, G. D., Merikangas, K. R., Leckman, J. F., & Kidd, K. K. (1984c). Psychopathology in the children (ages 6-18) of depressed and normal parents. *Journal of American Academy of Child Psychiatry, 23,* 78–84.

Weissman, M. M., Wickramaratne, P., Merikangas, K. R., Leckman, J. F., Prusoff, B. A., Caruso, K. A., Kidd, K. K., & Gammon, G. D. (1984d). Onset of major depression in early adulthood: Increased familial loading and specificity. *Archives of General Psychiatry, 41,* 1136–1143.

Weisz, J. R. (1980). Developmental change in perceived control: Recognizing noncontingency in the laboratory and perceiving it in the world. *Developmental Psychology, 16,* 385–390.

Weisz, J. R., & Stipek, D. J. (1982). Competence, contingency, and the development of perceived control. *Human Development, 25,* 250–281.

Weller, E. B., Preskorn, S. H., Weller, R. A., & Croskell, M. (1983a). Childhood depression: Imipramine levels and response. *Psychopharmacology Bulletin, 19,* 59–69.

Weller, E. B., Weller, R. A., & Preskorn, S. H. (1983b). Depression in children. *Journal of the Kansas Medical Society, 84,* 117–119.

Welner, Z., Welner, A., McCrary, M. D., & Leonard, M. A. (1977). Psychopathology in children of inpatients with depression: A controlled study. *Journal of Nervous and Mental Disease, 164,* 408–413.

Werner, E. E., & Smith, R. S. (1979). An epidemiological perspective on some antecedents and consequences of childhood mental health problems and learning disabilities. *Journal of the American Academy of Child Psychiatry, 18,* 292–306.

West, L. J. (1975). Integrative psychotherapy of depressive illness. In F. F. Flach & S. C. Draghi (Eds.), *The nature and treatment of depression.* New York: Wiley.

White, R. W. (1959). Motivation reconsidered: The concept of competence. *Psychological Review, 66,* 297–333.

Whybrow, P. C., Akiskal, H. S., & McKinney, W. T. (1984). *Mood disorders: Toward a new psychobiology.* New York: Plenum.

Wiener, J. M. (1984). Psychopharmacology in childhood disorders. *Psychiatric Clinics of North America, 7,* 831–843.

Wiener, J. M., & Jaffe, S. (1977). History of drug therapy in childhood and adolescent psychiatric disorders. In J. M. Wiener (Ed.), *Psychopharmacology in childhood and adolescence* (pp. 9–40). New York: Basic Books.

Wikler, L., Wasow, M., & Hatfield, E. (1981). Chronic sorrow revisited: parent vs. professional depiction of the adjustment of parents of mentally retarded children. *American Journal of Orthopsychiatry, 51,* 63–70.

Williams, A. W., Ware, J. E., & Donald, C. A. (1981). A model of mental-health, life events, and social supports applicable to general populations. *Journal of Health and Social Behavior, 22,* 324–336.

Williamson, A. P., Montgomery, J. R., South, M. A., & Wilson, R. (1977). A special report: Four-year study of a boy with combined immune deficiency maintained in strict reverse isolation from birth. *Pediatric Research, 11,* 63–89.

Winnicott, D. W. (1956). Primary maternal preoccupation. In *Collected Papers* (pp. 300–305). New York: Basic Books.

Winnicott, D. W. (1960). The theory of the parent–infant relationship. In Winnicott, D. W. *The maturational process and the facilitating environment* (pp. 37–55). New York: International Universities Press.

Winokur, G., Cadoret, R., Dorzab, J., & Baker, M. (1971). Depressive disease: A genetic study. *Archives of General Psychiatry, 24,* 135–144.

Winokur, G., Clayton, P. L., & Reich, T. (1969). *Manic depressive illness.* St. Louis: Mosby.

Wolfe, D. A. (1985). Child-abusive parents: An empirical review and analysis. *Psychological Bulletin, 97,* 462–482.

Wolff, P. H. (1969). Observations on the early development of smiling. In B. M. Foss (Ed.), *Determinants of infant behavior* (Vol. 2., pp. 113–138). London: Methuen.

Wolkind, S. N., & De Salis, W. (1982). Infant temperament, maternal mental state and child behaviour problems. *Ciba Foundation Symposium, 89,* 221–239.

Wolock, I., & Horowitz, B. (1984). Child maltreatment as a social problem: The Neglect of neglect. *American Journal of Orthopsychiatry, 54,* 530–543.

Wortman, R. A. (1981). Depression, danger, dependency, denial: Work with poor, black, single parents. *American Journal of Orthopsychiatry, 51,* 662–671.

Wylie, R. C. (1979). *The self-concept: Theory and research on selected topics* (Vol. 2., rev. ed.). Lincoln: University of Nebraska Press.

Yarrow, L. J. (1964). Separation from parents during early childhood. *Review of child development research* (Vol. 1): National Institute of Mental Health.

Yarrow, L. J., & Goodwin, M. S. (1963). Effects of change in mother figure during infancy on personality development. *Family and child services* (progress report). Washington, D. C.

Young, L. (1964). *Wednesday's children: A study of child abuse and neglect.* New York: McGraw-Hill.

Zahn-Waxler, C., Cummings, E. M., Iannotti, R. J., & Radke-Yarrow, M. (1984a). Young offspring of depressed parents: A population at risk for affective problems. *New Directions for Child Development, 26,* 81–105.

Zahn-Waxler, C., Cummings, E. M., McKnew, D. H., Jr., & Radke-Yarrow, M. (1984b). Altruism, aggression, and social interactions in young children with a manic–depressive parent. *Child Development, 55,* 112–122.

Zalba, S. R. (1967). The Abused Child II: A typology for classification and treatment. *Social Work, 12,* (70–79).

Zaslow, M. J., Pederson, F. A., Cain, R. L., Suwalsky, J. T. D., Kramer, E. L. (1985). Depressed mood in new fathers: Associations with parent–infant interaction. *Genetic, Social, and General Psychology Monographs, 111,* 133–150.

Zill, N. (1977). *National survey of children: Summary of preliminary results.* Unpublished manuscript, Foundation of Child Development, New York.

Zis, A. P., Haskett, R. F., Albala, A. A., Carroll, B. J., & Lohr, N. E. (1985). Opioid regulation of hypothalamic-pituitary adrenal function in depression. *Archives of General Psychiatry, 42,* 383–386.

Zung, W. W. K. (1965). A Self-Rating Depression Scale. *Archives of General Psychiatry, 12,* 63–70.

Zussman, J. (1980). Situational determinants of parental behavior: Effects of competing cognitive activity. *Child Development, 53,* 172-800.

Author Index

Subject Index